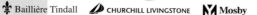

Differential Diagnosis in Abdominal Ultrasound

Commissioning Editor: Michael Houston
Project Development Manager: Sheila Black
Project Manager: Hilary Hewitt
Design Direction: Jayne Jones
Illustrator: Jenni Miller

Differential Diagnosis in Abdominal Ultrasound

Second Edition

R A L Bisset MB BS FRCR MHSM
Consultant Radiologist, North Manchester
General Hospital, Manchester, UK

A N Khan MB BS FRCP(Edin) MRCS DMRD FRCR MHSM
Consultant Radiologist, North Manchester General Hospital;
Lecturer in Diagnostic Radiology, Faculty of Medicine,
University of Manchester, Manchester, UK

with contributions from

Y S Al-Khattab MB BS FRCR
Consultant Radiologist, North Manchester General Hospital,
Manchester, UK

and

N B Thomas MB BS FRCR
Consultant Radiologist, North Manchester General Hospital,
Manchester; Professor of Radiology, Salford University,
Salford, UK

 W.B. SAUNDERS

London Edinburgh New York Philadelphia St Louis Sydney Toronto 2002

WB Saunders
An imprint of Harcourt Publishers Limited

© Harcourt Publishers Limited 2002

 is a registered trademark of Harcourt Publishers Limited

The right of R. A. L. Bisset and A. N. Khan to be identified as editors of this work
has been asserted by them in accordance with the Copyright, Designs and Patents
Act 1988

First edition 1990
Second edition 2002

ISBN 0 7020 2652 2

British Library Cataloguing in Publication Data
A catalogue record for this book is available from the British Library

Library of Congress Cataloging in Publication Data
A catalog record for this book is available from the Library of Congress

Note
Medical knowledge is constantly changing. As new information becomes available,
changes in treatment, procedures, equipment and the use of drugs become
necessary. The editors/authors/contributors and the publishers have, as far as it is
possible, taken care to ensure that the information given in this text is accurate
and up to date. However, readers are strongly advised to confirm that the
information, especially with regard to drug usage, complies with the latest
legislation and standards of practice.

Existing UK nomenclature is changing to the system of Recommended
International Non-proprietary Names (rINNs). Until the UK names are no
longer in use, these more familiar names are used in this book in preference to
rINNs, details of which may be obtained from the British National Formulary.

Printed in China by RDC Group Limited

The
publisher's
policy is to use
paper manufactured
from sustainable forests

Contents

Gamuts

Chapter 7 501

Preface to the first edition

In the spring of 1986 we undertook a retrospective review of 45 patients with apparent complex cystic hepatic mass lesions. Whilst conducting the review we became increasingly aware of the lack of specificity of many sonographic findings. When these features were considered in conjunction with the full clinical history, physical examination and results of other investigations, an accurate diagnosis was reached in a high percentage of cases. The lack of specificity makes the gamut approach to differential diagnosis very valuable. Since this time we have collected gamuts of differential diagnoses from the literature. Using these differential diagnoses in conjunction with all the other clinical information available, we have been able to make an accurate diagnosis or guide further investigation in the majority of cases examined. These differential diagnoses have been valuable in our clinical work and form the basis of this book.

R A L Bisset
A N Khan
1990

Preface to the second edition

It is now more than 10 years since the first edition of this book was published. In this time ultrasonography has become firmly established as a valuable means of diagnosis and in many areas it has become a natural extension of clinical examination. Over 22 000 general and obstetric sonographic examinations are now undertaken each year at North Manchester. Many more vascular and echocardiographic examinations are also undertaken in the cardio-respiratory unit. Ultrasonography is thus undertaken by a range of operators in varying clinical circumstances increasing the need for teaching, audit and quality control. The second edition of this book has been produced to provide a handbook sized source of information for those beginning a career in sonography and an aide-mémoire for the experienced operator, not least the authors themselves.

Rob Bisset
Ali Khan
March 2000

Dedication

We wish to thank our wives and children
　　Alison, Alexandra, Charlotte, Francesca and Cameron
　　Nazir, Sumaira and Suhail,
for their patience and understanding during our
work on this book.

This book is dedicated to the memory of John
Wolstencroft (1957–1989)

1

Introduction

Ultrasonography is a uniquely safe and non-invasive means of imaging internal anatomy. It is particularly suited to the demonstration of solid organs and fluid-filled structures because of their excellent sound transmission. Changes in internal anatomy such as organ size, shape, echogenicity, echopattern and internal architecture may be demonstrated. A wide range of processes may affect this relatively limited number of parameters, thus it is not surprising that many sonographic features are non-specific. The ultrasonographer must demonstrate as many normal and abnormal findings as possible and then interpret the abnormalities in the light of the patient's clinical history, physical findings and the results of other investigations. As a consequence the diagnostic accuracy is very operator dependent. The operator must have a skilled and thorough examination technique as well as an adequate knowledge of anatomy, pathology, medicine, surgery and allied subjects. Despite these difficulties the experienced ultrasonographer can frequently make a firm diagnosis or shorten the clinical differential diagnosis thus directing the clinician to further relevant investigations or treatment.

1.1 SONOGRAPHIC DIAGNOSIS

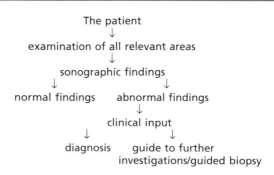

The patient
↓
examination of all relevant areas
↓
sonographic findings
↓   ↓
normal findings   abnormal findings
↓
clinical input
↓   ↓
diagnosis   guide to further
investigations/guided biopsy

1.1.1 INABILITY TO MAKE A SONOGRAPHIC DIAGNOSIS

The inability to make a sonographic diagnosis or making an error in diagnosis may occur for several reasons.

1. A disease may cause only microscopic changes in organ structure that are not visible at ultrasonography.
2. The scanner may be unable to resolve the pathological changes – it may be inadequate for the task on the grounds of age, construction or the use of an inappropriate transducer.
3. Incorrect gain settings or image processing may mask disease or make normal tissue appear abnormal. The sonographer should be fully aquainted with the workings of the scanner in order to achieve optimum image quality.
4. Inadequate patient preparation.
5. Unhelpful patient physique – obesity, scoliosis, etc.
6. Poor examination technique.
7. Failure to recognise visible sonographic findings.
8. Failure to correctly interpret the sonographic findings.

1.1.2 DIAGNOSTIC ACCURACY

Providing the scanner is capable of the required task the majority of variables affecting diagnostic accuracy are under the control of the ultrasonographer. Ultrasonography can therefore be a challenging and rewarding means of investigation from both the practical and intellectual points of view. The accuracy of ultrasonography is, in many areas, very high. It is inexpensive, non-invasive and mobile. The future of ultrasonography is thus assured. When scanning, the operator must attempt to answer all the clinical questions posed by the referring physician or surgeon. Frequently this is not possible but the skilled operator will go as far as the technique allows. It is important to answer not only the questions posed by the clinician but also the questions which have not been asked. It is a failure if, on answering a clinical question, the clinician immediately poses a further question related to the same area of examination that cannot be answered. For example, when reviewing the gallbladder, the pancreas and lower bile ducts should also be examined. When evaluating the upper abdomen in cases of acute upper abdominal pain it is always worth having a quick look at the pelvis. Even in the absence of any upper abnormality the presence of free fluid collecting in the pelvis will show that the patient's symptoms must be taken seriously however minor they may seem. The diligent sonographer can thus guide the clinician and should anticipate the needs of the clinician in each clinical situation.

1.2 PHYSICAL PRINCIPLES OF ULTRASOUND

Modern ultrasound scanners are generally user-friendly though some require a greater understanding of the basic physical principles of sonography than others in order to obtain the best possible images. Regardless of the nature of the scanner in use the operator should have a working knowledge of the physics of sonography in order to avoid artefacts and technical pitfalls. Ultrasonography relies on the echoes from an ultrasound beam to provide the information necessary to generate an ultrasound image of the body. Ultrasound is high-frequency sound above the frequency range that can be heard by the human ear (i.e. above 20 000 Hz). Generally the 2.5–12 MHz frequency range is used, the higher frequencies being used when scanning the breast, thyroid, eyes, muscles, ligaments, tendons and other superficial structures.

1.2.1 ULTRASOUND

Sound is energy in the form of waves of mechanical vibrations. Ultrasound waves can be characterised by their physical parameters such as frequency, wavelength, velocity, amplitude and intensity.

Frequency   The number of oscillations or cycles of the waveform per second. The units of frequency are hertz (Hz).
Wavelength   The length of one cycle or oscillation.
Velocity   The distance travelled by the ultrasound wave per unit time.

These parameters are related by the equation

$$\text{velocity} = \text{frequency} \times \text{wavelength}$$

Velocity   Ultrasound velocity is not constant but varies depending upon the nature of the medium through which it is travelling. Sound travels more rapidly through tissues which demonstrate a greater 'stiffness' (i.e. are more resistant to deformation by mechanical vibration) velocity being related to the density and elasticity of the tissue.

Medium	Velocity of sound (m/s)
air	330
fat	1450
water (20°C)	1480
brain	1540
liver	1550
muscle	1570

Ultrasound wavelength at a velocity of 1540 m/s

Frequency	Wavelength
2 MHz	0.77 mm
5 MHz	0.31 mm
10 MHz	0.15 mm

Power   The power of the ultrasound beam is the energy flow rate of the whole beam. The units of power are watts (W).

Intensity   The intensity of the ultrasound beam is the energy flow rate per unit area. Intensity is measured in units of watts per square centimetre (W/cm^2).

Amplitude   The amplitude of the ultrasound beam is the maximum variation in the ultrasound wave. Amplitude is used to describe the magnitude of a pulse. The ultrasound pulse is very brief being in the order of only 2–3 cycles in length, less than 1 µs. Power values averaged over a period of time will therefore appear quite low compared to peak intensity.

Echoes   Echoes occur when sound reaches an interface between tissues of different acoustic impedance. Acoustic impedance is a measure of the tissue's resistance to distortion by ultrasound. The acoustic impedance depends upon the tissue density and velocity of sound within the tissue. The intensity of the echo is proportional to the difference in acoustic impedance between the two tissues.

Tissue	Acoustic impedance ($g\,cm^{-2}s^{-1}$)
air	0.0004×10
fat	1.38×10
water (20°C)	1.48×10
liver	1.65×10
bone	7.80×10

Attenuation   As the ultrasound beam passes through the tissues the beam is attenuated and intensity falls. This is because of

● absorption of sound into the tissues and conversion to heat
● reflection of sound at tissue interfaces
● beam scattering and divergence.

The reduction in ultrasound beam intensity as sound waves pass through tissues is measured in decibels per centimetre (dB/cm). The attenuation per unit distance increases with increasing frequency. Higher frequency sound waves therefore cannot penetrate as far through tissues as lower frequencies. The depth of field available when imaging at higher frequencies is thus shorter than with lower frequencies. Also, since the intensity of the ultrasound beam falls as it passes through the body then the intensity of echoes arising deep within the body will be less than those arising from similar reflecting interfaces closer to the transducer. The 'half intensity depth' can be used to demonstrate ultrasound beam attenuation within tissues, it is the distance travelled by the ultrasound beam after which the beam intensity has fallen to half the original value:

Beam frequency	Water	Soft tissue
2 MHz	340 cm	1.5 cm
5 MHz	54 cm	0.5 cm
10 MHz	14 cm	0.3 cm

Ultrasound beam generation

Certain crystals and treated ceramics exhibit the piezo-electric effect which essentially means that they deform or change shape when an electric voltage or potential is applied across them. When the voltage is removed the crystal returns to its original shape. Varying the voltage across the crystal can therefore cause it to vibrate. Crystal vibration causes adjacent structures to vibrate resulting in a moving wave of mechanical vibration, this is SOUND. The ultrasound transducer which houses the crystal element(s) is carefully constructed using damping materials that absorb sound, and transmitting or coupling materials that facilitate the passage of sound in order to ensure that the ultrasound beam generated is directional. The frequency of the sound waves generated depends upon the size and configuration of the crystal and nature of the applied electrical potential. Ultrasound imaging uses very short pulses of sound only 2–3 cycles in length. The transducer element is then static. It may be caused to vibrate by returning sound waves or echoes. Just as a voltage can cause a piezo-electric crystal to deform and vibrate, sound waves reaching the transducer element and causing it to vibrate will generate a voltage across it. This voltage can be measured, thus the ultrasound transducer element can both generate the ultrasound beam and detect the sound echoes returning from within the body.

The ultrasound beam

The ultrasound beam is not uniform but changes configuration as it moves away from the transducer. Initially the beam converges after leaving the transducer. It is narrowest at the focal zone and then diverges. The near zone (between the transducer and the narrow focal zone) is longer with large-diameter transducers and higher sound frequencies. The ultrasound beam diameter is thus affected by

- ultrasound frequency
- distance from the transducer

- transducer diameter
- the use of mechanical or electronic focusing.

Beam focusing may be achieved by the use of

- a curved transducer element
- a lens
- electronic phased array transducers.

The ultrasound beam may be widened by the formation of 'sidelobes' around the main beam.

Ultrasound amplification

The scanner transducer emits a pulse of sound in a known direction and then awaits an echo in a manner analogous to radar. The longer the delay between the initial ultrasound pulse and the echo the deeper the reflecting surface. The greater the intensity of the echo the 'stronger' the reflector (i.e. the greater the difference in acoustic impedance between the tissues at the reflecting surface). The scanner amplification system must take the distance travelled by the ultrasound beam into account when analysing the echoes. Those which have travelled further will have been subject to greater attenuation and lost intensity. In order that echoes arising from tissue interfaces of equal reflectivity give rise to similar appearances on an ultrasound image, those that have travelled further are subject to greater amplification than those that arise closer to the transducer. This 'swept gain' or depth dependent amplification is essential in order that equally reflective interfaces at different depths within the body give rise to similar images.

Ultrasound resolution

The ultrasound pulse is very short both in terms of time and spatial length. The actual time the pulse lasts is called the temporal pulse length. The spatial pulse length of the ultrasound beam is the physical length of the ultrasound pulse.

Spatial pulse length = wave length × number of cycles in the pulse

A 3-cycle pulse of ultrasound with a frequency of 5 MHz (5 million cycles per second) within soft tissue (velocity of sound 1540 m/s) will last 0.6 μs in duration and will have a spatial pulse length of 3×0.031 mm $= 0.93$ mm. A very short and brief ultrasound pulse is needed to generate a high-resolution image. The resolution of the scanner is its ability to resolve adjacent structures as separate. The greater the resolution the smaller and closer the objects which can be differentiated. Resolution is not a constant

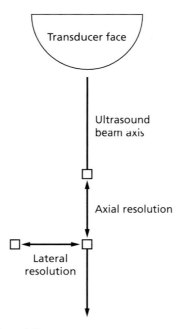

Figure 1.1 Ultrasound resolution.

phenomenon but depends upon the position of the objects in relation to the ultrasound beam and their distance from the transducer. It also differs in the axial and lateral planes (Figure 1.1).

Axial resolution
The axial resolution of the system is the resolution measured along the axis of the ultrasound beam, i.e. perpendicular to the probe face. It depends upon the brevity of the ultrasound pulse and the ultrasound wavelength. Increasing the ultrasound frequency reduces the wavelength and thus improves resolution. Unfortunately increasing the frequency increases beam attenuation and thus decreases beam penetration and the depth of view.

Lateral resolution
The lateral resolution of the system is a measure of the resolution of objects or echoes on a plane parallel to the transducer face, i.e. perpendicular to the axis of ultrasound beam. The lateral resolution depends upon the ultrasound beam width, the size of the transducer face relative to the ultrasound

wavelength and the distance from the transducer face. Lateral resolution decreases as the distance from the transducer face increases because of beam divergence. Beam divergence may give rise to artefacts since strong echoes arising outside the main ultrasound beam may be wrongly assumed to have arisen within the main beam.

Incorrect assumptions in image processing

The speed of sound is assumed to be 1540 m/s but it is in fact variable depending upon the nature of tissue through which it is passing. Sound is assumed to travel in a straight line but it may be refracted. All echoes detected by the scanner are assumed to have arisen on the main ultrasound beam axis but they may have arisen in adjacent tissues because of beam divergence.

Artefacts

An artefact may exist when any part of an image is not properly indicative of structures being imaged. This may be related to the information obtained on the screen not being real, being absent, at an improper location or improper brightness, size or shape. In order to achieve a high degree of diagnostic accuracy the ultrasonographer must be aware of the many artefacts that may be encountered during scanning. These occur because of the physical properties of the ultrasound beam, technical aspects of the scanner construction and assumptions made during image processing which are not always correct.

The origin of artefacts

Ultrasound waves are very high-frequency sound waves generated in the ultrasound probe or transducer by the piezo-electric effect. The ultrasound image is derived from echoes received when the ultrasound beam passes through the body. Each ultrasound pulse is very short and usually lasts less then 1 μs. The transducer then acts as a receiver detecting the echoes of the pulse of sound which it originally emitted. These echoes may arise in several ways.

Specular reflection

When an ultrasound beam encounters a tissue interface it may be reflected in a manner analogous to light hitting a mirror. This is termed specular reflection. The angle of incidence of the ultrasound beam is equal to the angle of reflection (Figure 1.2). The reflected beam is only returned to the ultrasound probe when the incidence beam is at 90 degrees to the tissue interface. The intensity of the reflected ultrasound echoes also depends on

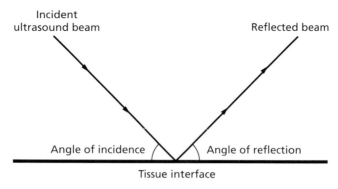

Figure 1.2 Specular reflection.

the angle of incidence. Thus when specular echoes are seen they are usually of high amplitude. For specular reflection to occur there must be an interface between tissues of different acoustic impedance. For soft tissues the acoustic impedance is largely dependent upon the amount of collagen and connective tissue stroma within the tissue. The greatest differences in acoustic impedance occur at air–tissue and tissue–bone interfaces. Reflection of sound is so great at these interfaces that the ultrasound beam is effectively blocked.

Backscatter echoes
Backscatter echoes occur when the size of the reflector is of the same order of magnitude as the ultrasound beam wavelength. The echoes are of low amplitude but return to the transducer with little regard for the angle of incidence of the ultrasound beam.

Rayleigh scattering
Rayleigh scattering is the process of ultrasound beam scattering which occurs when particles or tissue interfaces causing the scattering are very small in relation to the wavelength of the ultrasound beam (for example red blood cell diameter 6.3–7.9 μm × thickness 1.9 μm). The intensity of the scattered beam is dependent upon the fourth power of the ultrasound beam frequency and is thus greater at high frequencies. It is Rayleigh scattering that is used for Doppler flow studies. The Doppler theory is by no means new, it was first put forward by Christian Johann Doppler in 1842. The principle involves frequency and wavelength changes which occur when a waveform, in this case sound, is reflected by a moving target or tissue interface. As Figure 1.3 shows ultrasound waves reflected by a moving target will

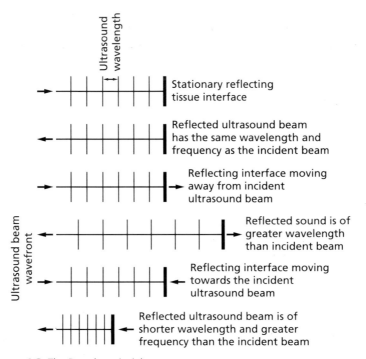

Figure 1.3 The Doppler principle.

show altered frequency and wavelength depending upon the direction of movement of the reflector relative to the incident beam and the difference in their velocities. The 'Doppler shift' in frequency may be used to measure the relative rate of blood flow through blood vessels. To ensure the optimum signal quality a high-frequency probe should be used and the sonographer should ensure that the axis of incident ultrasound beam is as close as possible to the axis of blood flow being analysed.

Reverberation

The transducer face, skin and coupling medium form acoustic interfaces. Sound passing from the transducer into the body and echoes returning to the probe from within the body may be reflected by these interfaces allowing the sound waves to be reflected back and forth. These 'reverberating' sound waves may act as new ultrasound pulses. The majority of echoes generated by the reverberating sound waves are too weak to be detected by the scanner. At times the echoes are strong enough to be detected and then artefactual reverberation echoes will be seen. These are seen as regular band echoes, usually in the near field at 90 degrees to the beam axis. They are usually multiple with regular spacing reflecting the distance between the reverberating tissue interfaces. They may occur with any strongly reflecting surface, for example the anterior wall of the fluid-filled bladder.

Artefacts seen in everyday scanning

Reverberation (see above).
Acoustic enhancement or shadowing.
Electronic noise.
Partial volume and beam width artefact.
Mirror image artefact.
Side lobe artefact.
Velocity artefact.
Refraction artefact.
Echogenic focal zone artefact.
Paralysis.
Comet tail artefact.

Acoustic enhancement

The 'swept gain' amplification system used in ultrasound scanners is designed to provide an image of even brightness when scanning homo-geneous tissue. To this background amplification the sonographer makes adjustments which take into account the nature of the tissues in the section under examination. Often different tissues will be present at the same depth in different areas of the ultrasound field. These tissues may attenuate the ultrasound beam differently and thus the intensity of the beam reaching the distal tissues may vary. This is most prominent when the beam passes through a fluid-filled structure such as the gallbladder. The fluid within the gallbladder causes very little attenuation of the ultrasound beam compared with adjacent tissues. The beam which has passed through the gallbladder is thus of greater intensity than the beam which has passed through an equal thickness of soft tissues which cause greater beam attenuation. The greater beam intensity distal to the fluid-filled structure will give rise to stronger echoes in the distal tissues and thus echoes arising distal to a fluid-filled structure may appear brighter or 'enhanced' compared to adjacent echoes at the same depth (Figure 1.4). Though acoustic enhancement is usually seen behind fluid-filled structures to a lesser extent it is seen distal to very uniform soft tissues.

Acoustic shadowing

Tissue interfaces which are very good ultrasound reflectors may completely obstruct the passage of the ultrasound beam. As the beam does not

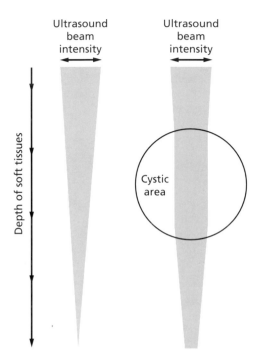

Figure 1.4 Distal acoustic enhancement. The ultrasound beam is attenuated as it passes through the body. When passing through fluid the ultrasound beam is subject to little if any attenuation. The beam is therefore stronger distal to a fluid-filled structure than distal to an equal thickness of solid tissue.

penetrate the tissues distal to this interface a shadow results. The reflecting interface is usually seen as a strongly echogenic band with an anechoic area running distally behind it. To cause shadowing the tissue interface concerned must be a similar size or larger than the width of the ultrasound beam. If a strong reflector is much smaller than the ultrasound beam width then the sound waves may pass around it and echoes may then be detected from the distal tissues (Figure 1.5). Gas, bones and calculi are the commonest cause of acoustic shadowing seen in everyday practice. It should be remembered however that small calculi may be seen as echogenic foci without shadowing and lack of shadowing does not exclude the diagnosis of a small calculus. As the ultrasound beam width is narrowest in the focal zone of the beam it is important that any areas of interest are kept within this zone. This will increase the chance of seeing shadowing distal to small calculi and also ensure that the area is viewed with the greatest possible scanner resolution.

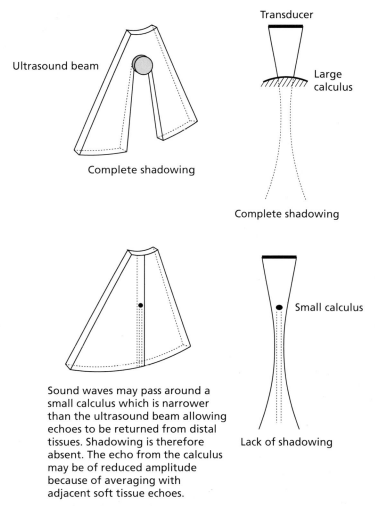

Figure 1.5 Acoustic shadowing.

Transducer

Ultrasound beam

Large calculus

Complete shadowing

Complete shadowing

Small calculus

Sound waves may pass around a small calculus which is narrower than the ultrasound beam allowing echoes to be returned from distal tissues. Shadowing is therefore absent. The echo from the calculus may be of reduced amplitude because of averaging with adjacent soft tissue echoes.

Lack of shadowing

Electronic noise

An ultrasound scanner, as with any other complex electronic apparatus, may suffer electronic interference from adjacent machinery. The artefacts produced by electronic noise are usually easily recognised, consisting of radiating lines and echogenic steaks forming patterns which are usually situated on the ultrasound beam axis. This may be a particular problem if the scanner is sited adjacent to an operating theatre where diathermy is in regular use, or next to a lift or other electric device.

Partial volume and beam width artefact

The ultrasound beam is of finite width. This may give rise to problems when both an object under examination and adjacent tissues lie within the same part of the ultrasound beam. Echoes arising from the object and adjacent tissues will be presented in the same part of the ultrasound image. This may cause problems, particularly when a cyst and soft tissues lie in the same part of the ultrasound beam. Echoes arising from within the soft tissues may give the appearance of debris within the cyst or the cyst may even appear solid and thus be missed (Figure 1.6). Small cysts narrower than the ultrasound beam usually cannot be differentiated from solid tissue. Similarly, very small echogenic foci within a fluid collection, for example microbubbles of gas within an abscess, may cause the fluid collection to appear solid owing to summation of echoes from that volume of tissue. In order to reduce the risk of misdiagnosis it is essential that all organs are examined in at least two planes preferably at right angles. In addition, changing the patient's position changes the position of abdominal organs in relation to each other. This can be a valuable method of diagnosis when sonographic appearances raise the possibility of the partial volume effect. Just as the partial volume effect may give rise to a misleading tissue echopattern the curved contour of adjacent organs may give rise to misleading appearances. The duodenal cap, for example, bulges into the gallbladder. If the gallbladder is only examined in single plane the resulting appearance (Figure 1.7) may be mistaken for a gallstone. To ensure that errors such as this do not occur, all areas should be examined in multiple planes with the patient lying in different positions.

Mirror image artefact

Mirror image artefacts arise when an image arises close to a curved and strongly reflecting tissue interface, for example the diaphragm. The ultrasound beam may then take two paths to reach an object in the field of view (Figure 1.8). The second path to the object via the curved reflecting surface is longer than the direct path and gives rise to a second image which lies distal to the curved reflector which caused the artefact. This problem occurs more frequently than usually realised and can result in incorrect diagnosis particularly of pelvic mass behind the bladder (if you look for mirror image artefacts they can be relatively easy to generate, particularly behind the neonatal bladder).

Side lobe artefact

The ultrasound beam is not uniform but narrows after leaving the transducer to become narrower in the focal zone. It then widens as it passes

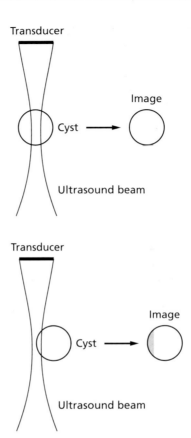

Figure 1.6 Partial volume or margin artefact. Scanning both solid tissue and the edge of the cyst simultaneously may give an artefactual appearance of debris within the cyst or the cyst may appear solid.

deeper into the body. Though the beam may be electronically or mechanically focused some sound waves diverge from the main beam. These diverging sound waves are known as the side lobes. They are less intense than the main beam but occasionally strong reflectors within the side lobes may give rise to echoes which may be detected by the transducer. The ultrasound scanner will assume that these echoes arose within the axis of the main beam and will project them as artefactual echoes on the final image. Narrower focused beams are less prone to side lobe artefacts or the partial volume effect.

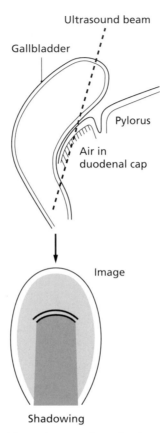

Figure 1.7 The ultrasound image is a two-dimensional representation of three-dimensional internal anatomy. Failure to examine the patient in multiple sections may lead to misdiagnosis. Each organ should be examined in at least two planes preferably at 90 degrees as performed with conventional radiography.

Velocity artefact

During image processing the ultrasound scanner assumes a constant velocity of sound within the tissues of 1540 m/s. This assumption is necessary to allow the calculation of distance from the time taken for an echo to return to the transducer. Unfortunately the speed of sound is variable and depends upon the nature of transmitting medium. The velocity of sound in fat, for example, is only 1460 m/s. The variation in the velocity of sound will give rise to distortion of the final image compared to the true internal

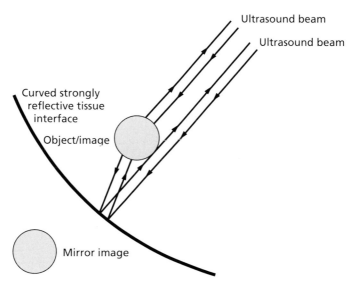

Figure 1.8 Mirror image artefact. The false image is seen beyond the curved specular reflector because of the second pathway taken by the ultrasound beam.

anatomy and may cause errors of 5 per cent or greater in the measurement of distance.

Refraction artefact

The ultrasound beam may be refracted in a manner similar to the refraction of light by a prism. The axis of the ultrasound beam is thus not always straight but may cut corners (Figure 1.9). This may lead to errors in the registration of the position of the origin of the ultrasound echoes on the image. Refraction of the ultrasound beam may also lead to beam splitting. This results in an area totally devoid of the ultrasound signal and thus an area of shadowing results on the final image (Figure 1.10). Refraction and refractive shadowing occur most frequently when the beam strikes the margins of a solid or cystic structure tangentially. This is seen particularly frequently at the gallbladder margin. The presence of refractive shadowing is highly dependent upon the angle of incidence of the ultrasonic beam and thus refractive shadowing is not constant if multiple sections are taken.

Echogenic focal zone artefact

As the ultrasound beam is narrowest in the focal zone the relative intensity of sound per unit area is greater here than elsewhere in the beam. Echoes

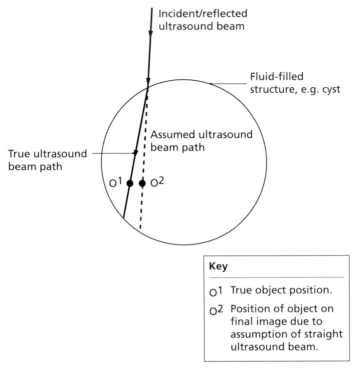

Figure 1.9 Cysts and fluid-filled structures may act as lenses refracting the ultrasound beam and leading to mis-registration of the position of the origin of echoes. This effect may occur to a lesser extent with solid structures.

arising from this area therefore may be of greater intensity than echoes arising from similar tissue interfaces elsewhere in the beam.

Paralysis

To generate the ultrasound signal an electrical potential of several hundred volts is applied to the transducer elements. The echo detected by the transducer is far weaker than the signal and it generates potentials from a few millionths of a volt to 1 volt. These signals are amplified and processed to produce the final image. The amplifier can be overloaded by the high potential used to generate the ultrasound signals and may be temporarily paralysed. This is seen as a block echo in the near field as paralysis occurs immediately after the ultrasound pulse. Paralysis is seen infrequently with modern scanners because of their advanced amplification design, but when

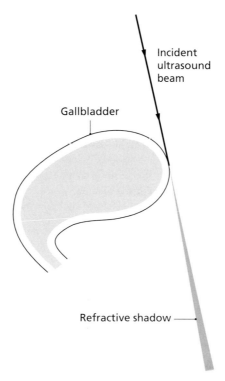

Incident
ultrasound
beam

Gallbladder

Refractive shadow

Figure 1.10 Refraction artefact – refraction shadow. A combination of reflection and refraction cause beam splitting giving rise to a 'refraction shadow' caused by an area devoid of ultrasound signal.

encountered it may be overcome by the use of a spacing substance to increase the distance between the transducer and the area of interest. The use of a spacer between the probe and skin surface is an underused technique to improve near field visualisation and avoid artefacts.

Comet tail artefact

The comet tail artefact is a form of intense reverberation which occurs between two adjacent surfaces, for example the sides of a surgical clip or a small stone. The resultant reverberation echoes are so close to each other that they tend to merge and give rise to a bright 'comet tail' echo extending distally into the ultrasound field behind the structure causing the reverberation.

Comment on technique

To ensure the greatest possible accuracy the ultrasonographer must

- be fully conversant with the operation of the ultrasound scanner in use, including the use of its controls and probes
- pay constant attention to gain and processing controls during the examination
- use a careful and thorough technique including changing the patient's position during the examination
- be fully aware of the physical artefacts and diagnostic pitfalls which may occur
- discuss the operation of the scanner with the medical physicist in charge of its maintenance; this is invaluable
- examine a phantom thoroughly; this can be rewarding and should form part of routine quality control.

Basic Doppler properties

The Doppler principal has already been discussed on p. 9. Here we briefly describe the various terms used in current Doppler technology.

Doppler shift

Doppler shift is a consequence of the Doppler phenomenon. Doppler ultrasound machines work on the principle that the sound wave reflected from a moving object has a different frequency than the sound wave that was sent out by the transducer. The difference between the incident and reflected frequency is called the Doppler frequency shift (DFS). Doppler shift can be calculated by the equation:

$$DFS = (2 \times IF \times BFV/SS) \times cosine\ O$$

where BFV is blood flow velocity, IF is the incident frequency, SS is the speed of sound and O is the angle between the ultrasound beam and the vascular flow. It is important to know that Doppler systems do not measure flow but determine blood velocity. There is only one variable on the right side of the Doppler equation – the BFV, all the other factors are known. The Doppler frequency is therefore directly proportional to BFV. Blood flow velocity can therefore be measured directly by Doppler instruments and expressed in units of either cm/s or m/s. For exact flow measurements to be made the instrument must know the Doppler angle. If the Doppler angle is high then there is the possibility of an erroneous flow measurement. The Doppler frequency shift is greatest if the sound and the moving object are in either the same or the opposite direction. In trigonometry the cosine of zero corresponds to an angle of 90 degrees. Hence, if the incident beam is at 90 degrees to the axis of blood flow no Doppler shift is observed. This fact is of particular importance in colour-flow Doppler. Velocity measurements become increasingly unreliable if the Doppler angle is reduced to below 30 degrees or increased beyond 60 degrees. Flow velocity should therefore be measured within 30–60 degree range.

Aliasing

When determining blood flow velocities, the overlap of forward components into the reverse frequency range, and vice versa, is called aliasing. In practical terms it represents the upper limit of Doppler shift that can be detected by pulsed instruments. If the Doppler shift frequency exceeds half the pulse repetition frequency (normally 5–30 KHz) the information provided by the system is faulty. If a high frequency shift is detected one should use a high pulse repetition rate, although this is compromised by increased depth of artefacts. Aliasing may be reduced or eliminated by increasing repetition frequency, increasing the Doppler angle, shifting the baseline, lowering operating frequency and the use of a continuous wave device.

Doppler instruments

Continuous wave Doppler

This easy to use and low cost system is the most basic diagnostic Doppler instrument. The system is fairly accurate in detecting blood flow and grading stenosis. These devices need separate emitting and receiving transducers, normally mounted on a single hand-held probe. Continuous wave Doppler (CWD) can detect very high velocities and thus there is no aliasing. One drawback of CWD is the lack of range or resolution. This limitation particularly applies when an artery and vein overlap. The CWD transducer picks up signal from both vessels simultaneously so that Doppler shift is superimposed. In these circumstances the clinical utility of CWD is severely compromised. The problem of poor resolution can be eliminated if the transducers are separated by a wide gap. However, this will make the probe unwieldy.

Pulsed Doppler

This system utilises one transducer which emits and receives. An ultrasound pulse of several wavelengths is transmitted into the body. Various tissues including red blood cells reflect the pulse which is received by the transducer. Since the sound velocity in tissue is known and presumed constant, with pulsed Doppler it is possible to process a particular range of received information and a 'Doppler shift' at one particular range can be obtained.

Duplex Doppler

Pulsed Doppler and continuous wave instruments are incorporated with real time B-mode system in the same probe to create 'duplex Doppler'. Although the two systems are mounted on the same system, the Doppler transducer may be separate from B-mode imaging or the same transducer may be used for both. There is usually a rapid electronic switching capability from one probe to the other, between B-mode and Doppler. Duplex Doppler with a separate mechanical sector imaging and a Doppler transducer is normally used for peripheral vascular work. A combination of phased array and Doppler transducer is used in cardiac work. Colour Doppler standard B-mode ultrasound imaging normally uses two pieces of information to construct an image, i.e. the time taken by the returning echo and the strength of the echo. There is other information in the returning echo such as 'Doppler frequency shift' which is normally not utilised. Colour duplex imaging records standard B-scan information and adds the magnitude and direction of Doppler shift. The reflected frequency of ultrasound may be greater or less than the incident ultrasound waves depending upon whether blood flow is towards (positive) or away (negative) from the deflecting transducer. With colour Doppler imaging positive and negative Doppler shift frequencies can be colour coded, depicting blood flow in different colours depending on whether blood flows towards the transducer (usually red) or away from the transducer (usually blue).

Power Doppler

Power Doppler is colour flow imaging that maps blood flow distribution rather than blood flow velocity. All flow is mapped with a single colour regardless of direction. The major advantages of power Doppler are its high sensitivity, lack of dependence on the Doppler angle and immunity to aliasing. The disadvantages of power Doppler are that velocity information is sacrificed with loss of grey scale information and degradation of temporal resolution.

Three dimensional ultrasound

Three dimensional (3D) ultrasound is an evolving technology, once used mainly as a research tool it is now beginning to be made available for clinical use. However its clinical usefulness remains to be proven and clinical trials are awaited. Baba and Okai define 3D ultrasound as imaging of the distribution of ultrasonic echo information in three-dimensional space. Three dimensional images can be reconstructed from any digital image, once each voxal can be located in a three-dimensional space. Various methods of data collection, reconstruction and image display have been used, but the optimum method is not yet known. Clinical utility at the moment is speculative but the following potential applications are in the pipeline.

1. Increased accuracy of volume measurements, for example bladder, stomach, prostate, endometrium, ovarian follicle and cancer tumour size. This is important particularly in evaluation of kidney tumours in a solitary kidney when kidney-sparing surgery is planned. Volumetric measurements of a transplanted kidney when combined with power Doppler imaging may prove useful in transplant kidney rejection, as it is known that when acute rejection occurs the kidney enlarges with uneven blood flow patterns.
2. Better replication of volume measurement; there is reduced inter-observer and intra-observer error as compared to conventional 2D ultrasound.
3. Better surgical planning; it may aid better staging of tumours.
4. Better understanding of 3D anatomy; this technique could be used in planning liver segment resection.

Ultrasound contrast agents

An ultrasound beam passing through the body may be absorbed, reflected or refracted. Ultrasound contrast agents can influence any of these para-meters. An ultrasound contrast agent may enhance the returning echo. The intensity of signal enhancement generated by an ultrasound contrast agent depends on its density and compressibility, on the contrast particle size and concentration, and on the frequency of the incident ultrasound beam. Water and saline are the simplest ultrasound contrast agents used to look at body cavities and the walls of hollow abdominal viscera when echofree liquid provides visualisation of luminal abnormalities. An impedance mismatch is maximal at the air–tissue interface. As a result many ultrasound contrast agents are based on stabilised gas bubbles. An early ultrasound contrast agent based on 'bubble technology' was freshly drawn up saline, when trapped air bubbles provided reflective surfaces. Toxicity of contrast agents is obviously an important factor in their development. Toxicity depends upon the biochemical structure, osmolarity, viscosity and particle size. The most promising agents are based on microbubbles or suspended reflective particles. There have been several recent advances in bubble technology. Bubble design varies; the bubbles can exist as free gas, or in an encapsu-lated or emulsion form. One drawback of microbubbles is the relatively short life of the bubbles. In order to increase their life span different stabilising agents have been used.

Gelatin, when used to stabilise microbubbles, makes a useful ultrasound contrast medium for cardiovascular work. Using high-energy ultrasound to create microbubbles can sonicate various agents. Conventional radiographic contrast can be sonicated in this way and used for intra-arterial injection during contrast echocardiography. Sonicated albumin microspheres have been used as an ultrasound contrast agent since the 1980s. There has been some concern over the possible antigenicity of the albumin component of the contrast agent. Despite this theoretical risk, in practice the contrast agent is well tolerated. Some of the microbubble echo enhancers that have evolved over the last 15 years are discussed below.

1. Echovist® (Schering), introduced more than a decade ago, is composed of galactose stabilised microbubbles. The disadvantage of this contrast is that it is not stable enough to cross the pulmonary barrier. Its contrast effect is therefore limited to the venous system and the right side of the heart. Echovist® has also found a use in hysterosalpingography.
2. Levovist® (Schering) is derived from Echovist® by the addition of palmitic acid and is a microbubble microparticle suspension in an aqueous carrier solution. The small amount of palmitic acid (0.1 per cent) stabilises the microbubbles and allows them to cross the pulmonary barrier and enter the arterial circulation where they stay for over 3 minutes. Since Levovist is hyperosmolar it may cause generalised flushing and transient non-specific local irritation of the vascular endothelium. Pain and tissue irritation may occur with extravasation at the injection site. In patients with cardiac decompensation special care should be taken because of the potential risk of osmotic overload. Levovist is contraindicated in galactosaemia, and in patients with a suspected or known right to left shunts. Its use in children under the age of 15 years is not recommended. Levovist® has been shown to increase the Doppler signal by 15 to 20 dB for up to 5 minutes. Like most other ultrasound contrast agents Levovist® can be used with B-mode as well as Doppler ultrasound.
3. Perfluoroctylbromide (PFOB) (Imagent® Alliance Pharmaceuticals) is a new echo enhancer composed of surfactants, sodium chloride, phosphate buffers and gaseous perfluorohexane. The contrast can be detected for several hours on ultrasound following intravascular injection. Perfluoroctylbromide remains echogenic in the liver and spleen for up to 2 hours since the agent is phagocytosed in the reticuloendothelial system. The dosage required is rather large and minor side effects such as allergic reactions and abnormalities of liver function tests may occur. These side effects may limit the clinical use of this contrast agent.

The clinical applications of ultrasound contrast agents are varied. The most obvious use is their application in cardiovascular disease. Many applications of dynamic ultrasound contrast enhancement in the abdomen have also evolved recently. Levovist® produces a significant increase in both colour Doppler and duplex Doppler signal from the main renal artery, allowing a more confident diagnosis of renal artery stenosis and renal artery occlusion. Contrast agents may also improve the visualisation and characterisation of tumours by increasing the visualisation of neo-vascularity.

Echo enhancers are being increasingly applied in the evaluation of tubal patency in sub-fertile patients. Another novel use to which ultrasound contrast agents can be put is in the assessment of vesicoureteric reflux in children. Many other agents are undergoing clinical trials and we are likely to see many more clinical applications.

Harmonic ultrasound imaging

Harmonic imaging is based on the principle that when the ultrasound beam strikes tissues, the tissues resonate at twice the frequency of the incident beam. The principle of harmonic imaging was a chance discovery during research on microbubbles. It became apparent that the shell of gas-filled microbubbles reflected ultrasound with greater efficiency as compared to the red blood cells. This phenomenon is explained by the fact that an incident ultrasound beam deforms the shell of the microbubble much like a bow stretches the string of a musical instrument. The microbubbles absorb the energy and then release it through vibrations with a range of frequencies higher than the incidental frequency. The most intense frequency is the 'second harmonic', so named because the frequency is twice the strength of the incident beam. Although the 'second harmonic' is very weak as compared to the original frequency it has tremendous advantages when captured. By selectively receiving a harmonic signal, noise created by the transducer surface can be eliminated resulting in a high-contrast image that renders extraordinary detail. Harmonics can be applied in conjunction with ultrasound contrast agents or used as 'native harmonic imaging' with grey scale ultrasound. A specific transducer design is required to produce harmonic imaging. One major advantage with harmonic imaging is that one can use a low-frequency probe in the obese but receive higher frequency images and therefore improve resolution.

1.3 FURTHER READING

Balen FG, Allen CM, Lees WR: Ultrasound contrast agents. Clin Radiol 49:77–82, 1994.
Carroll BA, Von Ramm OT: Fundamentals of current Doppler technology. Ultrasound Quarterly 6:275–298, 1988.
Cosgrove DO, Blomley MJK, Jayaram V, Nihoyannopoulos P: Echo-enhancing (contrast) agents. Ultrasound Quarterly 14:66–75, 1998.

Downey DB, Fenster A: Three dimensional ultrasound: a maturing technology. Ultrasound Quarterly *14*:25-40, 1998.

Schlief R, *et al*: In Advances in Echo Imaging using Contrast Enhancement. Eds Nanda NC and Schlief R Dordrecht Kluwer Academic Publishers, 1993.

Zwiebel WJ: Color Doppler imaging and Doppler spectrum analysis: principle, capabilities, and limitations. Semin Ultrasound CT MR *11*:84-96, 1990.

Zwiebel WJ, Fruechte D: Basics of abdominal and pelvic duplex: instrumentation, anatomy, and vascular Doppler signatures. Semin Ultrasound CT MR *13*:3-21, 1992.

2

Liver, biliary system, pancreas and spleen

2.1 LIVER

2.1.1 HEPATIC ANATOMY

The liver begins to form early in the fourth week of foetal life and by 9 weeks it fills most of the abdomen accounting for 10 per cent of foetal weight. At term the liver accounts for 5 per cent of foetal weight and in adult it accounts for approximately 2.5 per cent of body weight. It is the largest single organ in the body weighing 1.35–1.6 kg in adults. The liver lies in the right hypochondrium protected by the ribs. The upper border is approximately at the level of the nipple. The lower border extends down to the right 8th/9th costal cartilage. The greatest vertical (craniocaudal) length of the liver is up to 16 cm with a maximum normal anteroposterior diameter of around 11 cm. There is a great deal of variation in the size and shape of the liver depending upon individual build. The liver may have a relatively short vertical height or it may have a long slender extension inferiorly into the right iliac fossa (Riedel's lobe). This is more commonly seen in women than in men. It contains tissue from both anterior and posterior segments of the right lobe and receives blood supply from both the anterior and the posterior segmental portal vein branches. The liver extends from the right lateral abdominal wall across the midline well into the left hypochondrium. In infants and occasionally in adults the liver may extend to the left lateral abdominal wall overlying the spleen. This configuration may be mistaken for splenic laceration particularly if ascites is present giving rise to a trace of fluid between the liver edge and spleen. If a splenic laceration is suspected and a wedge of tissue is seen overlying the spleen then the medial edge of the wedge of tissue should be identified. If the tissue edge is part of the liver, portal tracts will become evident on scanning medially. The liver is also often slightly hypoechoic in comparison to the spleen. Misdiagnosis of splenic laceration is relatively common in young children in whom portal tracts may be too small to visualise near the liver edge. Anatomically the liver consists of a large right and a smaller left lobe separated by the interlobular fissure (Figure 2.1). By this classification the right lobe is 5 to 6 times larger than the left in terms of parenchymal mass. Two smaller lobes are also present. The caudate lobe lies posteriorly between the interlobular fissure and the inferior vena cava whilst the quadrate lobe lies between the interlobular fissure and the gallbladder anterior to the porta hepatitis. The caudate lobe may have a prominent papillary process which can mimic a pancreatic head mass. The functional (physiological or surgical) anatomy of the liver is more complex than the classical anatomical description and is based upon the hepatic vasculature. An imaginary line running from the gallbladder fossa through the middle hepatic vein and inferior vena cava divides the liver. This line reaches the superior surface of the liver to the right of the falciform ligament and divides the liver into two roughly equal halves. The quadrate lobe lies within the physiological left lobe and the caudate lobe lies between the right and left lobes. The line of division through the middle hepatic vein ('principal plane' or Cantlie's line) divides the portal venous, hepatic artery and bile duct branches. The recess of Rex, a relatively avascular plane with the left hepatic vein at its posterosuperior aspect divides the left lobe of the liver into

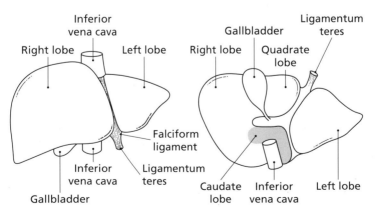

Figure 2.1 Line diagrams of the anterior surface (left) and inferior (right) surface of the liver showing the major anatomical landmarks.

medial and lateral segments. The right hepatic vein divides the right lobe into medial (anterior) and lateral (posterior) segments. A further imaginary line (horizontal) drawn through the left and right main portal vein branches may be used to divide the hepatic lobes into superior and inferior segments. The liver segmental anatomy (Figures 2.2a and b) as described by Couinaud (1957) and modified by Bismuth (1982) allows accurate localisation of hepatic masses relative to the hepatic vasculature. This is important as recent advances in liver surgery allow hemihepatectomy, segmental and subsegmental resections. The eight liver segments are numbered clockwise on the frontal view and counterclockwise from the inferior vena cava on a caudal to cranial view (Figures 2.2–2.5). Smith *et al.* (1993) have recently described a procedure for placement of liver mass lesions into Couinaud's liver segments by sonography. They image a plane that separates any two segments then rotate the probe 90 degrees. By keeping the separating boundary in the image they scan through the liver until the mass and boundary are seen in the same image.

Hepatic segments

The liver is divided into eight segments

1. caudate lobe
2. left lateral superior segment
3. left lateral inferior segment
4. a) left medial superior segment
   b) left medial inferior segment
5. right anterior inferior segment
6. right posterior inferior segment
7. right posterior superior segment
8. right anterior superior segment

Hepatic lobar agenesis

This is a rare congenital variant. Apparent absence of a hepatic lobe or apparent lobar hypoplasia is more commonly caused by prolonged biliary obstruction particularly cholangiocarcinoma or biliary stricture causing severe atrophy. Absence or occlusion of a hepatic or portal vein branch will also cause focal atrophy.

Hepatic ligaments and fissures

The liver has a fibrous capsule (Glisson's capsule) which extends into the hepatic parenchyma along the portal vein and bile duct branches. This

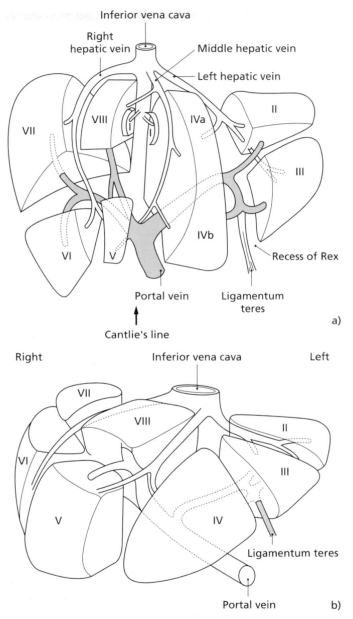

Figure 2.2 Schematic representation of the hepatic segments showing the relationship between segments and hepatic and portal veins. NB – as the diagram shows a 'flattened' 2D representation it should be remembered that segments VII and VI actually lie posteriorly behind and posterolateral to the right hepatic vein.

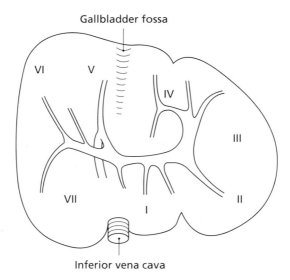

Figure 2.3 Liver viewed from below.

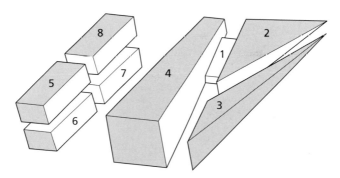

Figure 2.4 Schematic diagram of liver segments.

capsule is sensitive to pain and capsular stretching may cause pain during either liver biopsy or a sudden increase in liver size. The liver is also invested in a layer of peritoneum which is reflected onto the anterior abdominal wall and diaphragm as a series of ligaments or peritoneal folds. Extensions of the capsule into the substance of the liver give rise to the fissures. The fissures are echogenic because of the presence of fat and collagen and they may attenuate the ultrasound beam to the extent that tissues lying distally may appear hypoechoic. The falciform ligament extends from

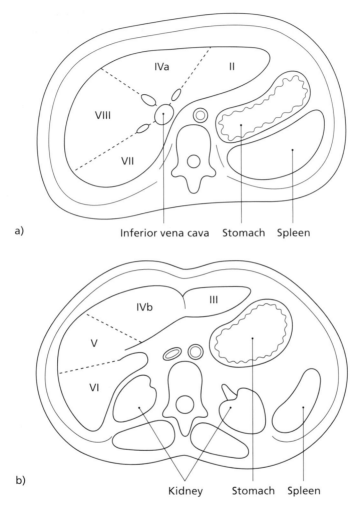

Figure 2.5 Hepatic segments – axial section, a) cranial aspect of the liver, b) caudal aspect of the liver.

the liver to the umbilicus, anterior abdominal wall and diaphragm. At the liver the falciform ligament is continuous with the ligamentum teres (the umbilical vein remnant) in the falciform fissure (the umbilical vein extends from the umbilicus to the left branch of the portal vein and from there via the ductus venosus to the left hepatic vein in the foetus). The falciform ligament contains fat and appears quite echogenic. The liver behind the falciform ligament usually appears hypoechoic because of sound attenuation by the ligament. The falciform fissure divides the medial and lateral aspects of the left lobe of liver. Reflections of the falciform ligament on the liver surface help to form the coronary ligaments at the 'bare area' of the liver. Compromise to normal portal venous drainage can result in reopening of the umbilical vein forming collaterals draining to the anterior abdominal wall around the umbilicus. Varices at the umbilicus (caput medusae) may be seen as a mass of serpiginous vessels radiating from the umbilicus. The ligamentum teres is seen as a linear echogenic band which runs from the antero-inferior surface of the liver to the left portal vein branch. The ligamentum venosus represents the ductus venosus lying between the caudate lobe and the lateral segment of the left lobe of the liver.

Ligaments are echogenic and may mimic

- lipoma
- sarcoma
- haemangioma
- paraganglioma
- cyst (by causing a hypoechoic area distally).

2.1.2 HEPATIC ULTRASONOGRAPHY

Elective hepatic ultrasound should be performed after an overnight fast at best or after 6 hours fasting as a compromise. This allows gallbladder distension, reduces portal vein calibre to its resting level (portal vein calibre and flow increase after eating) and also reduces the amount of gas in the upper gastrointestinal tract. Gas in the upper gastrointestinal tract is largely swallowed air. Swallowing is greatly reduced during sleep thus gas within the upper gastrointestinal tract is at a minimum on waking in the morning. As fasting is not always possible evaluation of the gallbladder after the patient has eaten may still yield useful information.

Abdominal ultrasound is generally undertaken with the patient supine but the ribs may obscure the liver. Inspiration may improve hepatic visualisation but can (particularly in patients with a 'barrel chest') cause the liver to move higher under the ribs, and in these patients 'pushing the abdomen out' may bring the liver down from under the ribs. The value of turning the patient from side to side should also be stressed and should form part of every examination to allow visualisation of the abdominal contents from several angles. A lateral decubitus position with the right side up may improve access to the liver and biliary system but will also increase gas within the pylorus, which may obscure the pancreatic head and the distal common bile duct. In addition to improving access to organs moving a patient during the examination allows organs to be evaluated from different angles and also alters the relationships of these organs. Examining the abdomen from different angles and different positions gives a more complete picture of the abdominal organs than simply examining the supine patient. The prone position used frequently in the early days of scanning should not be forgotten. The liver has a relatively homogeneous pattern of fine echoes, being slightly more echogenic than the kidney but less echogenic than the pancreas. The liver is usually isoechoic or slightly hypoechoic compared to the spleen. The caudate lobe may appear relatively hypoechoic because of sound attenuation by the falciform fissure. The liver has a branching pattern of vessels. The portal vein branches radiate from the porta hepatis. They have echogenic walls. The hepatic veins, which usually have no discernible walls, run posterosuperiorly to converge on the inferior vena cava. The bile ducts run with the portal veins but are not usually visible within the liver except close to the porta hepatis. Measured in the midclavicular line from the dome of the diaphragm the normal liver has a craniocaudal length of up to 16 cm. A length over 16 cm usually indicates significant hepatomegaly though the build of the patient and the configuration of the liver should also be considered. If the liver measures 16 cm or more it is abnormal in 75 per cent of patients. Longitudinal measurement alone is 87 per cent accurate in measuring hepatic size. As the liver enlarges it usually loses its sharp angular configuration becoming lobular in contour with a rounded inferior edge. Another sign of hepatomegaly is the extension of the inferior angle of the liver beyond the inferior aspect of the right kidney (except in Reidel's lobe). If the liver is 13 cm or less in the midhepatic plane (longitudinally) it is normal in size in 93 per cent of cases.

2.1.3 VARIATIONS IN LIVER SIZE

Causes of an enlarged caudate lobe

1. Primary cirrhosis of any kind; cirrhosis often has companion findings of right or left lobar atrophy, irregular lobular liver contour, ascites and varices (in cirrhosis and other causes of a shrunken liver there is often relative sparing of the caudate lobe which then looks large in relation to the remaining liver).
2. Hepatic venous occlusion. Venous drainage from the caudate lobe is maintained to the inferior vena cava by emissary veins thus the caudate is spared. An enlarged caudate lobe may narrow the intrahepatic portion of the inferior vena cava.

3. Focal mass lesions within the caudate lobe such as cysts, abscess or neoplasm may enlarge the caudate lobe. Fatty infiltration confined to the caudate lobe may mimic a tumour. Traumatic fractures of the caudate lobe may occur but are very rare.

Causes of liver atrophy with compensatory hypertrophy

Surgical resection.
Cirrhosis.
Hepatic vein obstruction and Budd–Chiari syndrome.
Portal vein obstruction.
Cholangiocarcinoma.
Intrahepatic biliary obstruction – intrahepatic cholelithiasis.
Liver metastasis – breast, colon, bile duct, squamous cell, tonsillar, renal, transitional cell.
Post-chemotherapy for hepatic tumours including selective chemoembolisation.
Lobar agenesis.

Causes of apparent hepatomegaly on clinical examination

True hepatomegaly.
Riedel's lobe.
Downward displacement – pulmonary over-inflation, pleural effusion, subphrenic collection.
Masses confused with the liver – renal mass, adrenal mass, para-aortic mass/lymph nodes, pancreatic mass/pseudocyst, ascites.

Causes of hepatomegaly in the neonate

Heart failure.
Infection – neonatal hepatitis.
Metastasis.
Primary neoplasia.
Metabolic defects.
Nutritional disorders.
Hepatoxins.
Biliary atresia.

2.1.4 DIFFUSE LIVER DISEASE THAT ALTERS HEPATIC ECHOGENICITY

The normal liver is slightly more echogenic than renal cortex and slightly less echogenic than the pancreas. In diffuse liver disease this relationship may change. Clinical assessment of liver echogenicity is a subjective comparison. This assessment is prone to error for three reasons

1. pathological processes may alter the echogenicity of the kidney or pancreas (both the liver and kidney are vascular organs and the kidney in particular can show non-specific changes in cortical echogenicity with acute illness)
2. there is considerable inter-observer variability
3. machine settings are variable (inherent or operator controlled).

Quantitative methods for measuring tissue echogenicity are available but at the moment this is a research tool and is cumbersome in the clinical setting. The liver may appear 'bright' (increased echogenicity) with steatosis (fatty change) with the formation of intracellular fat globules within the hepatocytes. Conversely the liver may appear hypoechoic in conditions that give rise to oedema and increased water content. When assessing diffuse liver disease one needs to examine the liver in at least two planes, usually transverse and longitudinal. In a 'bright' liver assess whether the echoes are fine or coarse and homogeneous or heterogeneous. One should also assess the degree of ultrasound beam attenuation and the echogenicity of the parenchyma relative to portal vein walls which may become invisible as hepatic parenchymal echogenicity increases. When ultrasound beam attenuation is increased the beam will fail to penetrate deeper tissues so it may not be possible to see the deeper aspects of the liver.

Hepatitis

Inflammation of the liver, or hepatitis, may take a large number of forms with a whole range of aetiologies. Clinically hepatitis is usually subdivided into acute and chronic forms.

Acute hepatitis – aetiology

- Infective hepatitis, for example viral, bacterial, parasitic or secondary to the toxic effects of infection elsewhere.
- Neonatal hepatitis, usually hepatitis A and B, rubella, cytomegalovirus, toxoplasmosis and spirochaetes.
- Toxic hepatitis, alcohol, chemicals, toxins, drugs and their metabolites.

Chronic hepatitis – aetiology

- Granulomatous, primary and secondary biliary cirrhosis, tuberculosis, histoplasmosis, sarcoid.

● Non-granulomatous, drug reactions, persistent active hepatitis (often viral).

Sonography

Ultrasound does not normally play a prominent role in the diagnosis of acute hepatitis as the liver may appear normal. However ultrasound is performed routinely in patients presenting with jaundice to rule out large-duct obstruction. Hepatomegaly is the most common manifestation of acute hepatitis. Some patients with acute hepatitis present with a decrease in liver echogenicity attributed to hydropic swelling of the hepatocytes and increased extracellular fluid. Marked contrast may be evident between the hypoechoic liver parenchyma and the echogenic portal tracts – the so called 'starry sky' appearance. The periportal fat and the fat around the falciform ligament may also appear relatively more echogenic than normal in relation to the liver parenchyma. The gallbladder is often incompletely distended even though the patient is fasting. In cases of acute hepatic insult the gallbladder wall is often oedematous and thickened (this is most commonly seen in acute alcoholic hepatitis after a heavy drinking binge and is a sign of the hepatic insult, not infective cholecystitis).

The gallbladder may not be visualised in neonatal hepatitis because of the lack of bile flow; lack of gallbladder visualisation is a non-specific sign which cannot be taken to indicate biliary atresia. Ascites may be present.

In acute alcoholic hepatitis the liver may appear 'bright'; this may be caused by coexistent fatty infiltration. Uncommonly acute hepatitis may give rise to areas of focal echogenicity which may be mistaken for masses, particularly in cytomegalovirus infection and alpha$_1$-antitrypsin deficiency. Purulent bacterial hepatitis is only diagnosed when abscesses form.

The liver may appear normal in chronic hepatitis. Cases of reduced parenchymal echogenicity have been recorded in chronic hepatitis but increased echogenicity occurs more frequently. In addition to generalised increased echogenicity areas of necrosis give rise to hypoechoic or anechoic foci and these features combined with regenerative nodules may give rise to a generally heterogeneous appearance. The portal vein walls may lose their normal echogenic appearance relative to hepatic parenchyma and may become ill defined because of inflammatory and fibrotic changes in the liver within the portal tracts. The general pattern of parenchymal changes may thus vary depending on the stage of disease process, particularly as a case of acute hepatitis may evolve into a more chronic form. The granulomas of tuberculosis, brucellosis and sarcoid may calcify. Always look closely at the hepatic margin as the first sign of established parenchymal disease may be loss of the smooth and sharp hepatic margins with the development of a slightly lobulated contour.

Opportunistic infection

Immune-compromised patients, particularly those with AIDS, are prone to systemic infections with *Candida albicans*, toxoplasmosis, cytomegalovirus and *Pneumocystis carinii*. In these infections tiny abscesses may diffusely involve the liver. Such abscesses may be of sufficient size to be seen on ultrasound. *C. albicans* infection may cause multiple tiny echogenic or target lesions although diffuse liver abscesses particularly of larger sizes tend to be hypoechoic. In AIDS patients with systemic *P. carinii* infections liver involvement may present as a generalised mottled appearance indistinguishable from neoplastic infiltration.

Causes of the 'starry sky' appearance of the liver

Acute hepatitis
Heart failure particularly in cardiac liver disease
Toxic shock syndrome
Opportunistic infections
Leukaemic infiltration
Diffuse lymphomatous infiltration
Diffuse neoplastic infiltration of the liver by primary or metastatic tumour

Diffuse disease may be due to confluence of areas of focal disease, infiltrating tumours or miliary metastatic deposits. The liver may appear 'moth eaten' with a patchy echopattern which may be of increased or decreased echogenicity or, commonly, the infiltrates are isoechoic. Hepatomegaly is usually present. Lymphoma and leukaemia are particularly prone to diffuse disease which usually appears hypoechoic though these changes do not always reflect the presence of metastases as reactive lymphocytic infiltration secondary to disease elsewhere may give rise to the same appearance. When the liver is extensively replaced by metastasis jaundice may occur because of inadequate liver function. Alternatively Hodgkin's disease may cause intrahepatic biliary obstruction at the canalicular level whilst lymphadenopathy may compress the extrahepatic biliary system. Even in the absence of jaundice liver function tests usually show some abnormality in the presence of liver metastatic disease.

Fatty liver

The accumulation of fat within the liver is a non-specific response to a wide variety of aetiologies. This diagnosis can be made histologically when the liver contains more than 7 per cent fat as lipid vacuoles appear in the cell cytoplasm. Fatty infiltration is usually related to a prolonged insult but may accumulate rapidly, for example parenteral nutrition, and in some instances it may also be rapidly reversible. Fatty liver is usually 'bright'. Increased echoes in the liver are due to increased collagen rather than fat although some workers believe fat itself is responsible. Ultrasound is not a very accurate means of diagnosing a fatty liver until the pathological changes are well established. A subjective assessment of liver echogenicity has a positive predictive value of 65 to 100 per cent and a negative predictive value of 67 to 94 per cent. The false positive rate is low but the sensitivity is only 60 per cent (90 per cent in severe cases). Liver brightness can be assessed by comparison with the right kidney which is normally less echogenic than the liver. Echogenicity can also be assessed by evaluating the appearance of the portal vessels.

- Grade I   slight (mild) diffuse increase in liver echogenicity but normally visualised intrahepatic vessels.
- Grade II   moderate increase in hepatic echogenicity with slight impairment of visualisation of the hepatic vessels.
- Grade III   marked increase in echogenicity with portal vein walls and the diaphragm hard to define. The deeper parts of liver may also be difficult to see.

Sonography

The liver is enlarged with increased strength and number of returning echoes resulting in a 'bright' liver. The overall parenchymal structure is rather fine. The increased echogenicity is not always uniform with regional differences. This is probably related to the fact that fatty infiltration can be patchy particularly with acute alcohol abuse, steroids, and malnutrition (for example cancer). The right lobe is most often affected. Band-like areas of fatty change may occur. Unlike a pathological mass, vessels passing through fatty areas show little or no displacement. Vascular structures including portal vein walls are less prominent than normal and there is increased attenuation of the ultrasound beam (diminished through transmission). The gallbladder wall may be ill defined. All these changes are non-specific and inconstant. In case of doubt fatty change in the liver can be confirmed most easily by computed tomography (CT) or magnetic resonance imaging (MRI). Paradoxical lack of ultrasound attenuation with gross fatty change in the liver has been described which serves to illustrate the role of scattering in attenuation of the ultrasound beam. The reported cases also demonstrate the importance of the use of a 5 MHz transducer where fatty change is diffuse and where reliance cannot be placed on increased attenuation alone.

Focal fatty infiltration and focal sparing of the liver

Fatty infiltration of the liver is often nonhomogeneous and may be focal, diffuse, nodular or multifocal. This may on occasion cause diagnostic problems. Focal fat may mimic echogenic liver masses. In this instance the 'fatty mass' may mimic lesions such as haemangioma, hepatocellular carcinoma, adenoma, focal nodular hyperplasia or a solitary metastatic deposit. Alternatively 'spared' normal areas of liver may mimic hypoechoic masses. Focal sparing is most often seen in the quadrate lobe beneath the capsule and in the perihilar region. Most ultrasound diagnostic problems arise with focal sparing. The features that suggest focal fatty infiltration or focal sparing are

1. geographic distribution of the fat or sparing
2. sharp angulated boundaries with normal tissue (tumours and abscesses tend to be more rounded)
3. absence of mass effect with no attempt at vessel displacement, distortion or encasement
4. there tends to be interdigitization of normal and fatty tissue, the distribution of the fat tends to be lobar or segmental.

In case of doubt radioisotope scanning or CT would confirm or refute the diagnosis. On isotope scanning with Tc-99m sulfur colloid no mass is seen. On CT the echogenic fatty areas on ultrasound corresponds to low attenuation areas on CT. Focal fat can also be confirmed by MRI.

Acute fatty liver of pregnancy

The liver size and liver histology remain normal in an uncomplicated pregnancy. In the second and third trimester there is some elevation of the serum liver enzymes but these are of placental origin. The serum bilirubin and aminotransferase levels stay within the normal range. Acute fatty infiltration of the liver in pregnancy typically becomes apparent after the 30th week of gestation. It is more common with twin pregnancy and pre-eclampsia. Patients present initially with non-specific constitutional symptoms followed in many instances by frank hepatic failure. The disorder is usually associated with a high mortality. However recently milder cases without frank hepatic failure with a good prognosis have been reported. The only known treatment is termination of pregnancy. On imaging the patient presents with a 'bright liver' on ultrasound associated with ascites. The liver echogenicity varies with the degree of fatty infiltration. Fatty change may be patchy.

Congenital generalised lipodystrophy

This is a rare hereditary disorder associated with muscular hypertrophy, lack of adipose tissues and hepatomegaly. There is fatty infiltration of the liver, hypertriglyceridaemia and insulin resistant diabetes mellitus. Ultrasound show a hyperechoic liver.

Causes of fatty infiltration of the liver

Toxic – alcohol, steroids, chemotherapy, tetracycline, chlorinated hydrocarbons, halothane.

Nutritional – obesity, starvation, intravenous feeding.

Metabolic – diabetes mellitus, glycogen storage disease, galactosaemia, lipid storage disease, lipodystrophy, porphyria tarda.

Infections – viral hepatitis, chronic systemic infections.

Cryptogenic – acute fatty infiltration of pregnancy, ulcerative colitis.

Genetic – Asians from the Indian subcontinent particularly women, cystic fibrosis.

In clinical practice obesity, diabetes melitus, alcohol, chemotherapy and steroids are the most commonly encountered causes of fatty liver.

Causes of diffusely increased liver echogenicity – 'bright liver'

Normal variant.

Fatty infiltration.

Cirrhosis.

Diffuse infiltration – glycogen storage disease, Gaucher's disease.

Miliary granulomata – tuberculosis.

Extensive malignant infiltration.

Infectious mononucleosis.

Portal tract fibrosis.

Acute alcoholic hepatitis.

Severe viral or other hepatitis.

Cardiac failure and venous congestion.

Hyperalimentation.

Malnutrition.

Brucellosis.

Wilson's disease.

Fructose intolerance.

Reye's syndrome.

Tyrosinaemia.

Steroid therapy particularly in conjunction with cytotoxic drugs.

Radiotherapy (the majority of patients show no detectable change).

Massive hepatic necrosis

This represents fulminant hepatitis with an extremely poor prognosis resulting in death 2 to 3 weeks from the onset. About 50 to 65 per cent result from viral hepatitis. Acute fatty infiltration, ischaemia, drugs, hypothermia,

Wilson's disease and Reye's syndrome are other causes of massive hepatic necrosis. The only effective treatment is liver transplantation though haemoperfusion through an artificial liver allows systemic support until the liver recovers in a manner analogous to dialysis support in renal failure. The ultrasound features depend upon the cause but usually show an oedematous liver with a 'starry sky' appearance associated with ascites.

Hepatic fibrosis

Hepatic fibrosis, like fatty infiltration of the liver, is a non-specific response to various toxins, metabolic disorders, hepatitis and a variety of other causes. Histologically there is diffuse scarring in the liver that is preceded by necrosis of hepatocytes and other cellular elements. Unlike fatty change hepatic fibrosis is irreversible. Ultimately hepatic fibrosis leads to cirrhosis. Hepatic fibrosis in infants is a progressive condition that may be associated with autosomal recessive polycystic kidney disease. Most children with hepatic fibrosis eventually develop portal hypertension and splenomegaly. These children are at increased risk of hepatocellular carcinoma.

Sonography
Initially most livers with hepatic fibrosis appear normal on ultrasound. The liver may of course be 'bright' as fatty infiltration and hepatic fibrosis can co-exist. Hepatic fibrosis in isolation may cause only slight increase in hepatic echogenicity with increased periportal echogenicity. Hepatic fibrosis may progress to cirrhosis, when such a change occurs ultrasound may demonstrate the characteristic features of cirrhosis.

Causes of hepatic fibrosis
Alcohol abuse.
Hepatitis, usually viral.
Toxins.
Drugs.
Metabolic disorders.
Immune deficiency.
Intestinal bypass.
Hepatic venous obstruction, for example Budd–Chiari syndrome.
Cryptogenic.
Autosomal recessive polycystic kidney disease.

Prominent periportal echoes

Acute cholecystitis.
Chronic cholecystitis.

Cholangitis.
Recurrent pyogenic cholangitis (oriental cholangiohepatitis).
Infectious mononucleosis.
Lymphoma.
Hepatocellular carcinoma.
Periportal fibrosis.
Cholangiocarcinoma, particularly Klatskin tumours.
Cystic fibrosis.
Schistosomiasis.
Pneumobilia – enterobiliary fistula, sphincterotomy.
Liver transplantation, normal finding.
Hepatoportal sclerosis.
Langerhans histiocytosis.

Hepatoportal sclerosis

Hepatoportal sclerosis is characterised by thickening of the portal tracts with extending fibrous septa. The portal vein radicals have patchy or generalised wall thickening. Portal vein thrombosis is not uncommon. In idiopathic portal hypertension portal pressure is increased in the absence of both histologic lesions of the liver and obstruction of the portal vein. It is suggested that idiopathic portal hypertension and hepatoportal sclerosis are the early and late stages of the same disease. In some patients hepatoportal sclerosis is attributed to a precise cause such as arsenic, copper sulphate, vinyl chloride monomer, and azathioprine or hypervitaminosis A. Ultrasound shows well-demarcated bands of increased echogenicity surrounding the portal tracts. The gallbladder wall may also show marked thickening.

Increased periportal echoes in neonates

Acute hepatitis.
Cytomegalovirus infection.
Biliary atresia.
Idiopathic neonatal jaundice.
Alpha$_1$-antitrypsin deficiency.
Nesideroblastosis.
Langerhans histiocytosis.

Cirrhosis

Cirrhosis is a chronic liver disease with parenchymal destruction, fibrosis and nodular regeneration. A variety of toxins, viral infections, metabolic disorders and autoimmune disease may cause cirrhosis. Essentially the causes of cirrhosis are the same as hepatic fibrosis. Histology of a cirrhotic liver reveals a combination of hepatocyte necrosis and fibrotic scarring with nodules of regenerating liver tissue. These changes distort hepatic architecture further reducing the efficiency of the surviving liver. Pathologically cirrhosis may be divided into micro- and macronodular forms depending upon the size of regenerating nodules, though in the late stages of cirrhosis the two forms merge as microscopic nodules enlarge. The two commonest causes of liver cirrhosis are alcoholic damage and viral hepatitis. Cirrhosis may be complicated by portal hypertension, hepatocellular carcinoma and frank hepatocellular failure. Childhood cirrhosis is usually secondary to cystic fibrosis, chronic hepatitis, biliary atresia, Budd–Chiari syndrome, drugs and metabolic disorders (Wilson's disease, glycogen storage disease, tyrosinaemia, galactosaemia, and $alpha_1$-antitrypsin deficiency).

Sonography

In the early stages of liver damage the liver may be enlarged but then it returns to normal size or shrinks. The caudate lobe is often relatively spared and may appear enlarged (caudate lobe is usually half the width of the right lobe measuring from the lateral edge of the caudate lobe to the free edge of each lobe). In effect the right lobe of liver shrinks more than the caudate lobe. The normal ratio of the caudate lobe to the right lobe is less than 0.6. This ratio is 84 per cent sensitive for the diagnosis of cirrhosis and nearly 100 per cent specific. This ratio is most sensitive in cases of cirrhosis due to hepatitis B and least sensitive in alcoholic cirrhosis. There is no single ultrasound appearance that suggests cirrhosis. In mild cases the liver may appear normal but most advanced cases will show ultrasound changes particularly of increased echogenicity with a lobular contour. The parenchyma appears 'bright' or abnormally echogenic with a fine echotexture or coarse with a heterogenous texture. This appearance may be partly related to associated fatty infiltration of the liver. The liver margin may appear nodular in outline and loss of the normal sharp contour is one of the earliest sonographic findings. There often is good through transmission of the ultrasound beam. Duplex and colour Doppler show increased flow in the dilated hepatic artery which may have a tortuous 'corkscrew' appearance in patients with cirrhosis and portal hypertension. The degree of ultrasound abnormality correlates poorly with the degree of liver dysfunction as the latter depends not only upon liver cell necrosis but also upon disordered hepatic architecture and efficiency of regenerative nodules. Regenerating nodules may give the liver surface an uneven appearance. This may also be seen in cystic fibrosis and malignancy. Increased hepatic echogenicity reduces the apparent echogenicity of the portal vein walls and may make adjacent renal parenchyma relatively hypoechoic. In all cases of suspected hepatic abnormality the portal vein (normal diameter less than 1.5 cm) and the splenic vein (the normal diameter of 1 cm should show alteration in calibre with respiration) should be examined for signs of portal hypertension and the splenic size should be noted. Frank ascites may be present and varices may be detected on grey scale imaging at various anatomical sites, confirmed with duplex and colour Doppler. There is an increased incidence of gallstones in patients with portal hypertension. The incidence of gallstones is even higher in patients with biliary cirrhosis with or without portal hypertension (35 per cent). Increased hepatic echogenicity is seen more frequently in micronodular than macronodular cirrhosis though the latter is associated with a greater incidence of hepatocellular carcinoma, which may complicate up to 5 per cent of cases. Ultrasound changes are least marked in primary biliary cirrhosis. Regenerating nodules are rarely seen sonographically and when identified may be indistinguishable from hepatocellular carcinoma. Ultrasound is over 80 per cent accurate at showing parenchymal abnormality in biopsy proven cases of cirrhosis. However cirrhosis and fatty liver cannot be reliably differentiated sonographically.

Causes of cirrhosis

Hepatitis – alcoholic, viral, autoimmune.

Biliary disorders – chronic biliary obstruction, primary biliary cirrhosis, sclerosing cholangitis, biliary disease of childhood, ulcerative colitis.

Metabolic disorders – haemochromatosis, Wilson disease, glycogen storage disease, alpha$_1$-antitrypsin deficiency, abetalipoproteinemia, galactosaemia, tyrosinaemia, hereditary fructose intolerance, intestinal bypass.

Parasitic causes – schistosomiasis.

Drug-induced causes.

Cardiovascular disorders – passive cardiac congestion, Budd–Chiari syndrome, veno-occlusive disease, Osler–Rendu–Weber syndrome.

Miscellaneous – sarcoid, cryptogenic, familial, hereditary tetany, juvenile polycystic kidney disease.

Glycogen storage disease

Six categories of glycogen storage disease are described, the classification depends upon the clinical presentation and biochemical abnormalities. It is a disorder of carbohydrate metabolism and is inherited in an autosomal recessive manner. Type 1 Von Gierke disease is the most prevalent and is due to lack of glucose-6-phosphatase, which prevents glycogenolysis. Sonography reveals hepatomegaly and a bright liver because of fatty change and glycogen deposition. Focal lesions within the liver may represent hepatic adenoma (40 per cent), focal nodular hyperplasia or hepatocellular carcinoma. Cirrhosis may ensue with longer survival.

Wilson's disease

Also termed hepatolenticular degeneration, this is an autosomal recessive disorder caused by excessive copper retention. Copper deposition causes a multisystem disease involving the liver, kidneys, eyes, brain and joints. There are no specific ultrasound appearances of liver involvement and the features of cirrhosis and portal hypertension are indistinguishable from cirrhosis of other aetiology. Wilson's disease may be complicated by hepatocellular carcinoma.

Haemochromatosis

This is a genetically determined abnormality of iron metabolism. Haemochromatosis may also occur secondary to alcoholic cirrhosis or multiple blood transfusions, thalassaemia or chronic excessive oral iron ingestion. Clinically patients present with cirrhosis, skin pigmentation, diabetes (bronze diabetes), arthropathy, later ascites and cardiac failure. There are no specific sonographic features of liver involvement. Sonography may reveal signs of cirrhosis and portal hypertension. CT is more specific (60 per cent sensitivity for iron). There may be a diffuse or focal increase in liver attenuation (100 to 140 HU (Hounsfield Units)). On MRI there is signal loss in the liver on the T1 weighted images equal to or less than background noise. With secondary haemochromatosis the signal loss in the liver on T1 weighted imaging is greater than background noise. The intensity in the spleen is usually normal. Hepatocellular carcinoma may complicate haemochromatosis.

Schistosomiasis

Schistosomiasis is a common parasitic infestation worldwide and is a major cause of portal hypertension. *Schistosoma mansoni* is the most common of several schistosomes that may infect humans. The cercariae enter the portal venous system through the gut and then lodge in the portal veins and liver where they mature into adult worms. The adult worms may live 10 to 15 years. The ova shed by these adult worms migrate into the portal radicals where they cause granulomatous periphlebitis leading to fibrosis, cirrhosis and portal hypertension. It is one of a few liver conditions, which cause a fairly characteristic ultrasound appearance. Sonography reveals a highly echogenic periportal band because of periportal fibrosis. Transverse scans through the portal vein branches demonstrate a 'bull's-eye' appearance. This is caused by the central echolucent portal vein branch being surrounded by periportal fibrosis. There is often hepatosplenomegaly, hyper-echoic gallbladder fossa and a thickened gallbladder wall. The characteristic sonographic features of portal hypertension invariably occur in late cases. Infection with *Schistoma japonicum* results in the formation of characteristic calcified septated appearances of the periportal and pericapsular regions of the liver on CT and ultrasound, referred to as tortoise-shell appearance.

Liver radiation

The liver may show changes caused by external radiation within weeks of exposure. There are geometric echogenic areas related to fatty change corresponding to radiotherapy ports. CT shows low-density areas corresponding to the areas exposed.

2.1.5 FOCAL LIVER LESIONS THAT ALTER HEPATIC ECHOGENICITY

Sonography is fairly sensitive at detecting focal liver lesions. The accuracy of sonographic detection depends on a variety of factors besides the technical problems of liver accessibility, the build of the patient and the presence of co-existing diffuse liver disease such as fatty infiltration, cirrhosis or liver oedema. Factors directly related to the focal lesion that determine the clarity of detection are the size, location and echogenicity of the lesion. Focal lesions may be hypoechoic, hyperechoic, isoechoic, anechoic or complex. A small anechoic or hyperechoic lesion may be easily detected whereas an isoechoic lesion can only be visualised by its mass effect on surrounding structures. A lesion near the dome of the diaphragm may be easily missed, particularly if it lies anteriorly or very close to the lateral border of the liver. The differential diagnosis of a focal liver lesion is fairly extensive (see below). In order to narrow the differential diagnosis one needs to look at other features such as the number of lesions, the internal architecture such as the presence of septae, debris, calcification (including the pattern of calcification) and the relationship to known anatomic structures, for example the gallbladder, bile ducts, etc. The use of colour flow and pulsed Doppler adds another useful facet. Doppler ultrasound detects the presence and pattern of blood flow within or surrounding the mass lesion, adding further characterisation.

Differential diagnosis of focal liver lesions

Pseudo-lesions – normal or hypertrophied caudate lobe, ligamentum venosus and surrounding fat, 'daisy-chain' lymph nodes in hepatoduodenal ligament, echogenic fat in the hepatoduodenal ligament, regenerative nodules in a damaged liver.

Congenital anomalies (these may not present until adolescence or adulthood) – congenital cyst, liver polycystic disease, Caroli's disease (focal biliary dilatation may mimic multiple focal lesions), choledochal cyst (juxta-position is not truly intrahepatic), mesenchymal hepatic hamartoma,* haemangioma,* hepatic teratoma,* portal vein aneurysm,* hepatic adenoma,* hereditary haemorrhagic telangiectasis.

Metabolic disorders – focal fatty infiltration, focal fatty spring.

Haematological disorders – myeloma deposits, extramedullary haematopoiesis, hypereosinophilic syndrome, leukaemia deposits.

Vascular disorders – aneurysm of portal vein, cavernous malformation of portal vein, hepatic artery aneurysm, hepatic artery pseudoaneurysm, infarct.

Trauma – haematoma, biloma, hepatic tear or laceration.

Infections – bacterial, parasitic (amoebiasis, *Echinococcus granulosus*, *Echinococcus multilocularis*), viral (herpes simplex virus), opportunistic (*Candida*,† *Pneumocystis carinii*,† cytomegalovirus, toxoplasmosis†).

Angiomyolipoma.

Biliary cystadenoma.

Cystic lymphangioma.

Dysontogenic cysts.

Peribiliary cysts.

Epithelioid haemangioendothelioma.

Malignant primary tumours – hepatocellular carcinoma, fibrolamellar carcinoma, cholangiocarcinoma, lymphoma, biliary cystadenocarcinoma, hepatoblastoma, angiosarcoma, malignant mesenchymoma, undifferentiated sarcoma, malignant metastatic.

Miscellaneous masses – inflammatory pseudo-tumours, focal nodular hyperplasia.

Multiple benign masses – cysts (congenital or acquired), haemangioma, abscesses, Caroli disease, regenerative nodules, adenomas, focal nodular hyperplasia, Langerhans' cell histiocytosis, peliosis hepatis, peribiliary cysts, bile duct varices, infarcts.

Multiple malignant tumours – metastasis, lymphoma, multicentric hepatocellular carcinoma, incidental haemangiomas and cysts with a primary or metastatic neoplasm.

Hepatic calcification

Right upper quadrant abdominal calcification may occur in all age groups. The commonest cause is gallstones but above the level of the gallbladder calcification is usually in the liver or rarely in the lung in the posterior

---

* These anomalies have been detected antenatally.
† Opportunistic infections may occur in the immune compromised, e.g. AIDS and chemotherapy patients, but can also occur rarely in immune competent patients.

sulcus. Ultrasound is quite sensitive at detecting liver calcification. The accuracy of detection of calcium deposits depends upon their size, exact location, configuration and density. Calcification within the liver may or may not shadow, depending upon the size and density of the deposits and the frequency and type of transducer used. There are many causes of hepatic calcification which can broadly be divided into two groups

1. those found in the neonate
2. those found in the older child and adults.

Sonographic features are not specific but assessment of the pattern of distribution and nature of the calcification and the presence of a mass or cyst may help to narrow the differential diagnosis. The anatomical location is also important, for example portal vein distribution, subcapsular, multifocal parenchymal, intraduct biliary. The differential diagnosis of hepatic calcification includes pneumobilia, gas within an abscess, gas within the portal vein or gas in an infarcted tumour (this follows chemoembolisation).

Causes of liver calcification in children and adults

Infections – tuberculosis (48%), coccidioidomycosis, histoplasmosis, *Schistosoma japonicum*, brucellosis, syphilitic hepatitis, toxoplasmosis, cat-scratch disease, herpes simplex virus, systemic *Pneumocystis carinii* infection, gumma, *Armillifer armillatus* (porocephalosis), old pyogenic abscess, old amoebic abscess, chronic granulomatous disease of childhood, *Echinococcus granulosus* cyst (33%), *Echinococcus multilocularis*, *Dracunculus medinensis* (rare, mostly in the abdominal/thoracic wall), paragonimiasis.

Vascular causes – hepatic artery aneurysm, portal vein thrombosis or phlebolith (following umbilical vein infusion), intrahepatic haematoma, subcapsular haematoma, ischaemic liver injury, hepatic artery thrombosis (following infusion), calcified thrombus within the intrahepatic inferior vena cava.

Biliary causes – intrahepatic calculi, porcelain gallbladder, Caroli disease, biliary atresia without jaundice following surgery (probably calculi).

Benign tumours – acquired cyst, congenital cyst, cavernous haemangioma, capsule of regenerative nodules, liver adenomatosis, infantile haemangioendothelioma.

Malignant primary tumours – hepatocellular carcinoma, hepatoblastoma (10–20%), fibrolamellar carcinoma, cholangiocarcinoma, epithelial haemangioendothelioma.

Malignant metastatic tumours – mucinous (colon, breast, stomach and psammomatous cystadenocarcinoma of the ovary), thyroid carcinoma, melanoma, pleural mesothelioma, carcinoid, leiomyosarcoma, insulinoma, osteosarcoma, neuroblastoma, teratoma, chondrosarcoma, phaeochromocytoma.

Miscellaneous causes – haemochromatosis, sarcoidosis, amyloid, patients on ambulatory peritoneal dialysis, capsular calcification (meconium peritonitis, pseudomyxoma peritonei, lipoid and barium granuloma, it has also been reported in cirrhosis and pyogenic infections).

Causes of neonatal liver calcification

Infections and transplacental infections – cytomegalovirus infection, herpes simplex virus, toxoplasmosis, maternal varicella infection, neonatal fulminant syphilitic hepatitis.

Primary and metastatic tumours – haemangioma, hamartoma, hepatocellular carcinoma, hepatoblastoma.

Vascular anomalies – calcified thrombus (portal vein, ductus venosus following umbilical vein catheterisation), haematoma, ischaemic liver necrosis *in utero*.

Abscess.

Biliary calcification.

Miscellaneous causes – idiopathic, meconium peritonitis.

Hyperechoic liver masses

Ultrasound pseudo-lesions – ligamentum ductus venosus, fat around the hepatoduodenal ligament.

Metabolic causes – focal fatty infiltration, haemochromatosis.

Trauma – haematoma, laceration, infarct.

Infections – abscess, erythromycin hepatitis (multiple poorly defined hyperechoic foci), hepatitis (particularly cytomegalovirus and alpha$_1$-antitrypsin deficiency), *Echinococcus granulosus, Echinococcus multilocularis.*

Neoplasia – haemangioma, adenoma, focal nodular hyperplasia, lipoma, angiomyolipoma, adenolipoma, myelolipoma, hepatocellular carcinoma, hepatoblastoma, angiosarcoma, epithelial haemangioendothelioma, leiomyosarcoma, malignant fibrous histiocytoma, undifferentiated (embryonal) sarcoma.

Metastasis (echogenic) – hepatocellular carcinoma, carcinoid, cholangiocarcinoma, renal cell carcinoma, islet cell tumours, colon (may be hyper- or hypoechoic but often bright, cauliflower-like lesions), Kaposi's sarcoma.

Metastasis (calcified) – mucinous adenocarcinoma, ovarian cystadenocarcinoma, breast carcinoma treated, carcinoid, osteogenic sarcoma, ovarian teratocarcinoma, chondrosarcoma, medullary carcinoma of the thyroid, neuroblastoma, pancreatic islet cell tumour, leiomyosarcoma.

Miscellaneous conditions – myeloma deposits, cryosurgery defects, hypereosinophilic syndrome, fibrosis.

Anechoic and hypoechoic intrahepatic masses

Ultrasonic pseudo-lesions – normal caudate lobe.

Congenital causes – congenital cyst (with or without cholesterol crystals or haemorrhage), infected cyst, Caroli disease.

Metabolic causes – focal fatty sparing.

Infections – abscess, hydatid cyst, focal hepatitis.

Trauma – focal hepatic necrosis (irregular margins, may have internal echoes and abnormal adjacent parenchyma), haematoma (anechoic during acute haemorrhage and during clot liquefaction), biloma.

Vascular causes – infarct, aneurysm.

Neoplastia – adenoma, focal nodular hyperplasia, haemangioma, hepatocellular carcinoma, lymphoma, sarcoma, epithelial haemangioendothelioma, metastasis (melanoma, pancreas, lung and cervix, parenchyma around the anechoic area may be abnormal), myeloma.

Miscellaneous causes – inflammatory pseudo-mass, extra-medullary haematopoiesis, hypereosinophilic syndrome.

Complex hepatic masses

Congenital masses – haemorrhagic or infected cyst.

Trauma-induced masses – haematoma, infarction (which may also be post embolic).

Infective masses – abscess (pyogenic or amoebic), *Echinococcus granulosus*, *Echinococcus multilocularis*.

Neoplastic masses – Virtually any primary or metastatic, benign or malignant tumour may have a complex appearance particularly if complicated by haemorrhage.

Target or bull's-eye liver lesions

Focal nodular hyperplasia (colour Doppler may be helpful in differentiating this from other liver mass lesions by showing blood flow in the hypoechoic rim. However hepatocellular carcinoma can have a similar blood flow).

Atypical haemangioma.

Adenoma.

Hepatocellular carcinoma.

Virtually any metastasis but especially bronchogenic carcinoma, breast, carcinoid, colon.

Lymphoma.

Leukaemia.

Myeloma.

Kaposi's sarcoma.

Infections – septic emboli, systemic candidiasis,* toxoplasmosis,* cytomegalovirus,* systemic *Pneumocystis carinii.**

* These infections usually occur in immune compromised patients such as AIDS patients. In candidiasis a 'wheel-within-a-wheel' appearance may be seen early in the course of the liver abscesses. These appearances represent a peripheral hypoechoic ring with an inner echogenic wheel and a central hypoechoic nidus. The central nidus is said to represent necrosis in which fungal elements are concentrated. The exact mechanism in the causation of target lesions by infections is not clear. The central echogenic area may be related to fibrosis or early calcification, while the outer hypoechoic ring may represent oedema.

The presence of a halo suggests a more aggressive lesion which is related to a combination of normal compressed perifocal liver tissue and proliferating concentrated neoplastic cells.

Target or bull's-eye liver lesions in children

Tumours – hepatocellular carcinoma, metastasis from bowel, liver adenoma in glycogen storage disease.
Infections – pyogenic liver abscess, amoebic abscess.

Hepatic pseudo-lesions and pseudo-mass lesions

Focal fatty infiltration
This is seen as a focal area of increased echogenicity with angulated margins and interdigitation with normal liver tissue.

Focal fatty sparing
This is seen as irregular areas of reduced echogenicity particularly at the porta hepatis owing to focal sparing in fatty infiltration. These areas of normal liver tissue may be irregular, ovoid or spherical in shape.

Hypoechoic caudate lobe
This is a normal variant caused by acoustic shadowing by fibrous tissue in the ligamentum venosus.

Papillary process of the caudate lobe
The distal margin of the caudate lobe is often prolonged into a narrow process. On axial CT the connection of this process with the caudate lobe may be missed and this normal process may be erroneously diagnosed as an enlarged lymph node. A similar appearance may be caused on axial ultrasound scans.

Hypoechoic quadrate lobe
This is usually a sign of diffuse fatty infiltration with relative sparing of the quadrate lobe.

Falciform ligament
The appearance of a pseudo-lesion is caused by fat around the falciform ligament appearing as an echogenic mass at the junction of the right and left lobes. This is the commonest pseudo-lesion in the liver; it is confusing

on axial scans but the cause is quite apparent on longitudinal or oblique scans.

'Daisy chain' nodes

Demonstration of normal lymph nodes in the hepatoduodenal ligament (daisy chain nodes) is possible in 77 per cent of normal subjects. These may be isoechoic to the liver, hyperechoic or, rarely, hypoechoic. They are seen frequently in young individuals and should not be misinterpreted as pathological masses. They usually form a 'C' shape around the distal hepatic artery.

Echogenic fat in the hepatoduodenal ligament

This may be a normal finding but is usually secondary to pericholecystic inflammation, for example cholecystitis pancreatitis or a perforated peptic ulcer.

Perihepatic fat

Normal variation in the amount of intra-abdominal fat and its distribution in relation to the liver borders may cause indentation of the hepatic margin simulating disease. This is seen most frequently between the liver and the right kidney and between the left lobe and chest wall.

Air in the biliary tree

Air may be introduced into the biliary tree spontaneously by a fistulous communication between the bowel and biliary tree, or following an endoscopic retrograde cholangiopancreatography biliary stenting or sphincterotomy. Air in the bile ducts usually has a linear branching pattern which may mimic calcification or even metastasis.

Diaphragmatic slips

The diaphragm may appear to interdigitate with the liver, particularly with a broad ultrasound beam. The slips are seen as echogenic lines at the liver margin. Changing the plane of scanning will usually show the diaphragmatic origin of the insertions impressing the liver margin.

Liver–splenic interface

The lateral aspect of the left lobe of the liver may lie adjacent to or just above the medial aspect of the spleen and may be mistaken for a hypoechoic mass such as an abscess or haematoma. The left lobe of the liver overlies the medial aspect of the spleen more often than suggested by anatomy texts, particularly in children. Fluid within the abdomen may be mistaken for splenic laceration if seen in the left upper quadrant. This mistake is avoided if, on seeing tissue adjacent to the spleen you always show the margins of each structure. As you scan medially portal branches will become evident in the liver.

Hepatic cysts

Liver cysts are common although less common than renal cysts. Liver cysts may be subdivided into developmental, traumatic, infective and neoplastic types. While most cysts have a lining, traumatic cysts, which are really pseudocysts, have no lining. With most solitary hepatic non-parasitic cysts no cause is apparent. When the cysts are multiple they are often associated with cystic disease in other organs (60 per cent of polycystic liver disease has renal cysts, while 25 to 33 per cent of patients with autosomal dominant renal polycystic disease have hepatic cysts). Infantile renal polycystic disease is associated with hepatic fibrosis and not macroscopic cystic liver disease. Congenital cysts are said to be malformed bile ducts with an average size of 3 cm that are usually lined with a columnar epithelium. Solitary simple hepatic cysts occur in up to 22 per cent of patients on ultrasound examination and are found in 50 per cent of postmortems. Most hepatic cysts occur in the 50 to 80 year age group with a female to male ratio of 4 : 1. They may grow in size to 20 cm and contain serous fluid. The cysts are epithelial lined and have a fibrous capsule with an outer vascular layer.

The majority of hepatic cysts are asymptomatic. Cysts may become symptomatic from their mass effect (55 per cent), hepatomegaly (40 per cent), abdominal pain (30 per cent) or jaundice (9 per cent). Solitary cysts in children are rare and are usually congenital. Acquired cysts are either inflammatory, neoplastic or traumatic, while multiple cysts are often associated with polycystic disease. They are seen as spherical or oval anechoic masses. They have sharp well-defined borders and give rise to distal acoustic enhancement, which may make the posterior border appear prominent. In simple benign cysts the wall is not visible at sonography. Small cysts may not be detectable as reverberation echoes or the partial volume effect may make them appear solid. Sonography is quite accurate at differentiating solid from cystic masses and is more accurate than CT in showing internal cyst morphology. Sonography shows the presence or absence of internal echoes, septa, debris and wall irregularity. If the cyst wall is prominent or irregular an alternative diagnosis such as an abscess, tumour necrosis, hydatid cyst or a lymphoma deposit should be considered. Rarely simple cysts may show septae, which are usually secondary to trauma and internal haemorrhage. Beware of anechoic solid lesions, for example metastasis which will show little or no posterior enhancement.

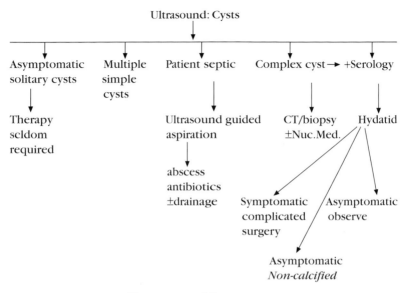

Management of liver cysts

Smooth-walled well-defined liver cysts

These represent fairly well-defined cysts with no intraluminal wall irregularity, good through sound transmission and no formed elements within the cyst:

Normal/anatomical variants – normal intrahepatic gallbladder, normal portal or hepatic vein in cross section.

Congenital or developmental solitary cyst – polycystic liver disease, choledochal cyst, Caroli's disease (careful examination will usually show these to be multiple ectatic bile ducts and not cysts).

Acquired cysts – infective, abscess, *Echinococcus granulosus* cyst, vascular, hepatic artery aneurysm, portal vein aneurysm, arteriovenous malformations (these can be congenital but may not present until middle age, or they can be acquired by trauma), infarct, post-traumatic or liquified haematoma (acute haematoma is briefly cystic but rapidly becomes echogenic then later liquefies), biloma (this may follow accidental injury or liver biopsy).

Multiseptate cystic hepatic lesions

Neoplastic lesions – metastases (for example ovarian cystadenocarcinoma, pancreatic cystadenocarcinoma, mucinous adenocarcinoma (stomach, colon), squamous cell carcinoma, leiomyosarcoma and melanoma, they may be from a primarily cystic tumour or necrosis within a large metastasis, this is the commonest cause in the authors' clinical practice), biliary cystadenoma, biliary cystadenocarcinoma, hepatic hamartoma, mesenchymoma, teratoma, cavernous haemangioma, cystic hepatoblastoma.

Inflammatory lesions Hydatid cysts, pyogenic abscess, amoebic abscesses – these are the commonest causes in many tropical and subtropical countries.

Benign cysts (particularly after internal haemorrhage or infection) – congenital, hepatic polycystic disease, foregut, traumatic, cavitating infarct, haematoma, biliary.

Miscellaneous lesions – infantile peliosis hepatitis.

Caroli's disease

Caroli's disease is a rare developmental disorder with segmental non-obstructed bile duct dilatation associated with infantile polycystic disease. The disease usually presents itself in childhood with recurrent cholangitis and lithiasis in dilated bile ducts. Sonographically it may mimic polycystic disease because multiple liver cysts are seen. In Caroli's disease the cystic dilated ducts may be seen to communicate, calculi cast shadows with biliary wall protrusions causing partial or complete bile duct bridging. Scintigraphy with Tc-99m HIDA may be a useful adjunct to imaging, to differentiate between polycystic disease and Caroli's disease.

Hepatic trauma

Injury to the abdominal viscera may be caused by blunt abdominal trauma or penetrating wounds. The solid organs and retroperitoneal segments of the bowel are more prone to injury than bowel suspended on a mesentery as the latter is more mobile. Liver injury occurs more easily in children than in adults as the ribs are more flexible allowing force to be transmitted to the liver. Also the liver is not fully developed, having a weaker connective tissue framework than in adults. Blunt hepatic trauma is the second most common abdominal injury leading to death with a 10 to 20 per cent mortality rate. Hepatic injury is associated with splenic injury in 45 per cent of patients. Up to 10 per cent of patients who have received blunt abdominal trauma have liver injuries. Steering column injury may cause trauma to a whole liver lobe. Deceleration injuries produce shearing forces that may tear hepatic lobes from each other often involving the inferior vena cava and hepatic veins. Interventional radiology procedures such as percutaneous biopsy, cholangiography or biliary drainage (transjugular intrahepatic portosystemic shunt) procedure and percutaneous alcohol injection can cause capsular tears, haematoma, bile leaks, bilomas, arteriobiliary or venobiliary fistulas and haemoperitoneum. In the neonate hepatic injury may be unsuspected. In neonatal deaths 9.6 per cent of post mortems show evidence of liver trauma especially subcapsular haematoma.

Hepatic haematoma

Haematoma of the liver may occur as a result of blunt trauma (for example road traffic accident), penetrating injury, biopsy, rupture of aneurysm, pseudoaneurysm, adenoma, hepatocellular carcinoma, B cell lymphoma, coagulopathies, systemic lupus erythematosis, polyarteritis nodosa, amyloid, patients who have received long-term haemodialysis, metastatic chorio-carcinoma, cavernous haemangioma, sickle cell disease, interventional radiology procedures, peliosis, and organic phosphate toxicity. Spontaneous rupture and haemorrhage has also been reported in pre-eclampsia and eclampsia in the third trimester. Three categories of hepatic haematomas occur

1. rupture into the liver and its capsule
2. separation of the capsule by a subcapsular haematoma
3. central hepatic rupture.

Parenchymal laceration and intrahepatic/subcapsular haematoma may be life threatening. With stab and gunshot wounds the haematoma forms along the track. Subcapsular haematoma may also follow lithotripsy. Trauma may cause acute or delayed haemorrhage with parenchymal laceration. An expanding haematoma may lead to delayed liver rupture and resolving haematomas may give rise to hepatic cysts. In addition laceration of the biliary system may lead to the formation of biliary fistulas or bile collections. Sonography of hepatic haematomas shows a poorly defined hypo-echoic mass. During active bleeding, blood is anechoic although there is less distal acoustic enhancement behind a newly formed haematoma than posterior to a bile collection. As blood clots the haematoma changes, becoming echogenic with a heterogeneous echopattern. Later the clot breaks down and liquefies forming anechoic areas giving a complex cystic appearance. Fluid/debris and fluid/fluid levels have been reported within resolving haematomas. Chronic persistence of a fluid collection after trauma suggests other complications such as cyst or biloma formation. Subcapsular haematomas usually appear multilocular regardless of the cause and may displace or compress normal liver tissue. Liver laceration is seen as irregular clefts; the appearance of the clefts may vary from anechoic to echogenic depending upon the age and extent of the blood or haematoma. Over 80 per cent of hepatic haematomas and lacerations are managed conservatively.

Hepatic infarction

Hepatic infarction is uncommon because of the dual blood supply. Infarction can of course be deliberately created by chemoembolisation of primary or metastatic liver tumours as an alternative treatment to surgery. Spontaneous liver infarction has been reported in diseases associated with embolic phenomenon, i.e. atrial fibrillation, rheumatic heart disease, bacterial endocarditis and left atrial myxoma. There is also an association with the trauma, the contraceptive pill, eclampsia, sepsis, sickle cell crises, anaesthesia and polyarteritis nodosa. An important complication of orthoptic liver transplantation is hepatic artery thrombosis which may occur in up to 10 per cent of transplants. Infarction shows as a wedge or segment, a sharply demarcated hypoechoic area. Rarely an infarct may cavitate or get infected in which case its echopattern may change to a more complex or multicystic mass. In a transplanted liver the hypoechoic infarcts may liquefy and show as intrahepatic fluid collections. Gas formation within infarcts may make the infarct hyperechoic. A conventional radiograph or CT may show the air with advantage. Computed tomography is particularly good at showing vascular changes in the liver with segmental areas of poor enhancement post-contrast.

Hepatic foregut cysts

Hepatic foregut cysts of embryonic origin are rare within the liver. They are histologically similar to bronchial and oesophageal cysts and are lined by ciliated epithelium. These cysts have been associated with portal hypertension secondary to extrinsic compression. In common with other foregut cysts these masses are typically well defined, being anechoic or hypoechoic with good through transmission.

Cystic masses at the porta hepatis in children and adults

Enlarged gallbladder.
Hepatic cyst.
Choledochal cyst.
Biloma.
Pancreatic pseudocyst.
Hepatic artery aneurysm.
Hepatic artery stenosis with post-stenotic dilatation.
Portal vein aneurysm.
Portal vein stenosis with post-stenotic dilatation.
Peribiliary cysts – hepatic hilar cysts, mucinous bile duct hamartoma.

Bile duct varices.

Hepatic foregut cysts.

Duodenal duplication cysts.

Subcapsular hepatic haematoma.

Cystic liver and bile duct tumours – biliary cystadenoma, biliary cystadenocarcinoma, mesenchymal hamartoma, malignant mesenchymoma, lymphangioma, undifferentiated sarcoma.

Loculated fluid collections.

Right adrenal cyst.

Upper pole right renal cyst.

Post-stenotic dilatation inferior vena cava stenosis.

Dysontogenic cysts – dysontogenic cysts represent a form of hamartomatosis which frequently occurs with cysts of the pancreas and kidney, the liver contains multiple epithelialised cysts of varying sizes.

Peliosis hepatis

Peliosis hepatis is characterised by multiple blood-filled spaces in the liver parenchyma. These spaces vary in size from a few millimetres to several centimetres. Only the larger spaces are resolved with ultrasound. These spaces are usually lined with endothelium and may communicate with sinusoids. Peliosis hepatitis manifests itself with hepatomegaly, signs of cirrhosis, portal hypertension, hepatic failure or shock because of hepatic rupture. Peliosis is associated with cancers elsewhere, tuberculosis, AIDS and AIDS-related complex, and certain drugs such as corticosteroids, anabolic steroids and azathioprine.

Hereditary haemorrhagic telangiectasia

Hereditary haemorrhagic telangiectasia or Osler–Weber–Rendu syndrome is an autosomal dominant disease with an estimated incidence of 1–2:100000. The cardinal features of the disease are telangiectasis, arteriovenous malformations and aneurysms. Over 60 per cent of patients are symptomatic by the age of 16 years. Presentation is with skin telangiectasis, epistaxis, haematemesis, haematuria, high output cardiac failure, symptoms related to pulmonary arteriovenous maformations and portal hypertension. Sonography may reveal enlargement of the main hepatic artery as well as the intrahepatic arteries. Increased echogenicity from fatty infiltration and cirrhosis may occur. Cystic spaces within the liver parenchyma representing arteriovenous malformation may be evident. Dilated hepatic arteries and portal vein branches may be confused with dilated bile ducts. Application of duplex Doppler and colour flow Doppler reveals the true nature of these tubular structures. Signs of portal hypertension may be apparent both on grey scale as well as Doppler ultrasound.

Bile duct varices
See p. 115.

Peribiliary cysts
These are synonymous with hepatic hilar cysts and mucinous hamartoma of bile ducts (see pp. 66–67). Benign hepatic tumours are more common than malignant tumours in neonates and infants, however in adults and older children malignant tumours and metastases are more common. In young children infantile haemangioendothelioma and mesenchymal hamartoma are the two most common benign tumours. Absolute diagnosis is not usually possible as appearance of tumours, tumour infection, haematoma, etc. overlap. If in doubt perform a biopsy (if permitted by the hepatic surgeon who may not want any interfence with the liver prior to consideration of surgery).

Infantile haemangioendothelioma

Haemangioendothelioma is the commonest hepatic neoplasm in the neonate. The majority of these (often multiple) tumours present with hepatomegaly and liver masses in children less than 6 months old, with a male to female ratio of 1:1.4 to 1.2. They are vascular tumours, which may be associated with skin haemangiomas in 24 per cent cases. With highly vascular tumours infants may present with high output cardiac failure or Kasabach–Merritt syndrome, a haemorrhagic diathesis caused by platelet sequestration by the tumour and disseminated intravascular coagulopathy. Haemolysis may also occur. The tumour is classified into three subtypes

1. the tumour shows orderly neo-vascularity of small blood vessels
2. the tumour shows a more aggressive proliferation of blood vessels
3. the appearances are those of a cavernous haemangioma with dilated endothelial lined vascular spaces.

Infantile haemangioendothelioma appears to be unrelated to the adult form of cavernous haemangioma. The haemangioendothelioma of later childhood may become sarcomatous without significant alteration in its radiological appearance. The sonographic appearance of infantile haemangioendothelioma depends upon the degree of its vascularity. The size of these tumours varies from a few millimetres to several centimetres but with an average size of 3 cm. The liver is usually diffusely involved, but occasionally unifocal or multifocal disease is present. Hypoechoic, hyperechoic and complex patterns all have been described. Vascular spaces within the tumour are particularly large and may be seen as anechoic or hypoechoic areas. Calcification, which is usually speckled, may be seen in up to 16 per cent of cases if carefully looked for. There is high flow within the enlarged upper abdominal aorta, coeliac axis and the hepatic veins demonstrable on colour flow and duplex Doppler. The tumour is also vascular with high flow on Doppler analysis.

Mesenchymal hamartoma

This is the second most common tumour in young children. These tumours represent an interface between haemangioma and a pure mesenchymal tumour. Like hamartomas elsewhere, these tumours contain elements of mesenchymal cells and in the liver present as a huge abdominal mass. The mean age at presentation is 16 months with a male to female ratio of 2:1. Sizes recorded vary from 1 to 22 cm. A tumour weighting 7 kg has been recorded. Approximately 75 per cent of children are symptomatic presenting with increasing abdominal distension. Physical examination in these children reveals an abdominal mass or hepatomegaly. In the rare instance with predominant angiomatous elements, a high output cardiac failure as with a haemangioendothelioma may occur. Malignant mesenchymomas occur, but are fortunately rare, affecting older children more than the benign form. Solitary case reports of hepatic mesenchymal hamartomas in older children and young adults have appeared in medical literature but this is extremely rare. Recurrence following complete resection or malignant transformation has not been reported. A presumptive diagnosis can be made preoperatively by normal laboratory values and combination of ultrasound and CT. Sonographically the appearances are those of a well-defined tumour with some echogenic foci, but cystic spaces with septations are more prominent. These tumours may mimic hydatid cysts, although the latter are rare in the age group affected by hepatic hamartoma. These tumours may enlarge suddenly because of fluid accumulation from necrosis or degeneration. Approximately 20 per cent are pedunculated. With predominantly angiomatous tumours, increased flow within the supplying arteries is to be expected and associated significant colour flow within the tumour can occur. Spontaneous regression of mesenchymal hamartoma during observations using ultrasound has been described. These masses are intrahepatic; other large masses in this age group are usually extrahepatic, for example mesenteric lymphangioma, duplication cysts, cystic leiomyomas and enteric cysts.

Liver haemangioma

Liver haemangioma is the most frequently encountered benign liver tumour, occurring in 1 to 10 per cent of the population. They occur in all age groups but are particularly common in adults and in females, with a female to male ratio of 5 : 1. One autopsy series put the frequency at 7.3 per cent. In females the incidence rises with multiparity. In 10 to 20 per cent of cases the tumours are multiple. They may undergo degeneration fibrosis and calcification. Haemorrhage into the tumour is rare but massive haemorrhage and rupture has been described. Giant cavernous haemangioma of the liver is associated with the risk of rupture and severe haemorrhage because of pressure during pregnancy and delivery. Association with focal nodular hyperplasia and Rendu–Osler–Weber syndrome has been implicated. Oestrogens may affect haemangioma growth and as a result haemangiomas can enlarge during pregnancy. These benign tumours are said not to grow over time except uncommonly in pregnancy. However recent reports show that these tumours can grow significantly over time both in males and postmenopausal women with no exogenous or endogenous oestrogen supply, although such growth is unusual. Involution has been described with corticosteroid therapy. In children cavernous haemangioma of the liver may rarely present with cardiac failure or failure to thrive. Kasabach–Merritt syndrome (see p. 60) has been recorded but is rare. Most haemangiomas are less than 3 cm (32 per cent) in diameter and are incidental findings in adults. They do not cause symptoms or biochemical abnormalities unless large. When larger than 4 cm they are classed as giant haemangiomas. The majority of these tumours are subcapsular (70 per cent) with 25 per cent found in the left lobe. Most are round (75 per cent) while 14 per cent are oval and 11 per cent are lobulated. Pedunculated tumours occur rarely. Rare instances of spontaneous rupture have been described. Microscopy shows multiple vascular spaces lined by a single layer of endothelium separated by fibrous septa.

Capillary haemangiomas

These tumours contain numerous small vessels and are seen as echogenic foci with well-defined margins. They are very commonly encountered in middle-aged women. Size is variable but they tend to be small often being situated superficially. They often show posterior acoustic enhancement but this is less prominent than with cysts and may only be seen on close examination.

Cavernous haemangiomas

Cavernous haemangiomas are less commonly seen in clinical practice than the frequently encountered echogenic capillary haemangiomas. Sonographically large sinusoidal vessels give a lobulated hypo- or anechoic appearance, though internal echoes may occur and distal acoustic enhancement is not always seen. When haemorrhage occurs within these tumours the ultrasound appearances become complex. Fluid–fluid levels have been recorded and echogenic and complex lesions cannot be reliably differentiated from metastases. Giant cavernous haemangioma is a great mimic and on imaging alone it may sometimes be impossible to differentiate it from a metastatic deposit, primary hepatocellular carcinoma, an adenoma, abscess and even a complicated hydatid cyst. A 'target' or a multicystic appearance has rarely been described. In a fatty liver haemangiomas are often hypoechoic. Colour Doppler studies may show a 'spot' pattern of internal flow in 10 to 50 per cent of tumours. Haemangiomas usually show little change in appearance over prolonged periods. Spontaneous regression has been recorded. Other imaging may be required to confirm the diagnosis of cavernous haemangioma. On angiography the hepatic artery is usually normal in size. There are large, irregular, well-defined sinusoidal spaces which retain contrast. The filling is from the periphery to the centre. Contrast CT has been shown to be reliable in differentiating haemangiomas from other tumours, however hypervascular metastases may be difficult to differentiate. Furthermore, on a diagnostic CT small lesions may not be easy to characterise. When haemangiomas occur in a fatty liver they may appear hyperdense on unenhanced CT, thus hindering their characterisation by contrast enhancement. In up to 46 per cent of haemangiomas atypical enhancement patterns occur which are indistinguishable from malignant liver tumours, though this may simply reflect the lack of a full series of pre-contrast, post-contrast and delayed post-contrast sections. Magnetic resonance imaging can be quite distinctive with a high signal lesion on T_2 weighted sequences and an enhancement pattern identical to that seen on early and delayed post-contrast CT sections. As with CT, peripheral enhancement with a centripetal 'fill-in' may be demonstrated with delayed imaging following the administration of intravenous gadolinium DTPA. Nevertheless limitations apply, similar to those for CT, when faced with hypervascular malignant tumours. Blood pool scintigraphy has been shown to be very sensitive (90 per cent) and specific (100 per cent) for large lesions but accuracy is reduced with smaller lesions. The sensitivity may be further improved with single photon emission tomography. The technique is not reliable for deep lesions and lesions less than 2 cm in diameter. If the diagnosis is still in doubt with non-invasive imaging laparoscopic ultrasonography is the technique of choice at the authors' institution.

Liver adenomas

These are uncommon tumours usually occurring in adults but also affecting children particularly in association with other abnormalities such as exogenous hormones, glycogen storage disease or Fanconi's anaemia. Eight per cent of patients with type Ia glycogen storage disease (von Gierke's disease) develop hepatic adenomas which are often multiple. Young females on the contraceptive pill are at risk, although adenomas have also been described in men on androgens and anabolic steroids. Association with pregnancy and diabetes mellitus has also been described. True hepatic adenomas consist of sheets of normal or atypical hepatocytes, other cells are either few or absent. Fibrous septa are unusual. These tumours are very vascular with thin-walled endothelial-lined vessels dispersed throughout the lesion. They are often smooth and lobulated tumours and large at the time of presentation (8 to 15 cm). They quite often present with a right upper quadrant pain or signs of acute haemorrhage within the tumour. An acute haemoperitoneum may occur. Pregnancy may increase tumour growth and may rarely lead to a rupture. Spontaneous regression has been described. As the risk of malignant transformation and major haemorrhage or rupture is small, surgical resection is often undertaken. Recurrence after surgical resection has been described. Histological diagnosis on fine needle biopsy can be difficult as the biopsy may only consist of normal hepatocytes, the clue being the loss of normal hepatic architecture.

Sonographic features are variable particularly if haemorrhage and necrosis have complicated the adenoma. The most frequent appearance is of an echogenic mass which is well defined and relatively uniform in appearance, though hypoechoic and anechoic areas may be seen. A hypoechoic rim (target lesion) may also be seen. Appearances may be particularly unusual in adenomas associated with an underlying liver abnormality such as glycogen storage disease. In these cases the adenomas may appear poorly defined, hypoechoic and inhomogeneous on a background of a 'bright' liver. Adenomas in glycogen storage disease may show marked sound transmission compared to adjacent liver. Isoechoic tumours may occur which may be difficult to identify. Colour and duplex Doppler may show intratumoural venous flow and peritumoural arterial and venous flow. There are no specific ultrasound features that differentiate hepatic adenoma from focal nodular hyperplasia. Percutaneous biopsy is risky as haemorrhage may follow. Radionuclide studies can be helpful in differentiating adenoma from focal nodular hyperplasia. A Tc-99m sulphur colloid scan showing uptake in the lesion is supportive of focal nodular hyperplasia. In 75 per cent of adenomas a sulphur colloid scan shows a photon-deficient mass.

Biliary cystadenoma

Biliary cystadenomas are uncommon benign cystic tumours which most frequently occur in middle-aged women with a female to male ratio of 4 : 1 and a peak incidence in the fifth decade. Although benign they have shown a malignant potential therefore the treatment of choice is surgical resection. Patients most commonly present with abdominal swelling, palpable mass and jaundice. The tumours originate in the bile ducts and may arise either from the extrahepatic ducts (15 per cent) or more commonly from the intra-hepatic bile ducts (85 per cent). Pathologically they present as a multi-loculate cystic tumour with proteinaceous contents and a fairly well-defined wall. Histologically there is a lining of a single layer of cuboidal or tall colum-nar biliary type epithelium with papillary projections. Macroscopic nodules and papillary projections from the septations or cyst wall are said to be more common in cystadenocarcinoma but rare in cystadenoma. Sono-graphically these masses are seen as ovoid mainly cystic tumours with irregular borders, which appear multiloculated with internal septations. Fluid–fluid levels or low level echoes may be seen within the cysts. The presence of thick septa, mural or septal nodules and the presence of dis-crete soft-tissue masses increase the likelihood of malignant change. The presence of thick amorphous calcification is also a pointer to cystadeno-carcinoma. There are no specific colour or duplex Doppler features reported for cystadenoma although angiography does show a small cluster of abnormal vessels distributed peripherally in a mainly avascular mass. The differential diagnosis is from a liver abscess, hydatid cyst, necrotic metastasis, cystic mesenchymal hamartoma and intrahepatic haematoma. Echinococcal cysts may appear similar to cystadenomas, but the internal locules in hydatid cysts tend to be of a smaller and more uniform size. Serological tests may be useful in differentiating the two entities.

Focal nodular hyperplasia

Hyperplastic nodules of liver parenchyma occurring in focal nodular hyper-plasia contain all the normal cellular elements of liver tissue but lack normal hepatic architecture and are thus poorly functioning. This benign tumour may occur in all age groups but is rare in children; the peak incidence is in the third to fifth decades of life with a male to female ratio of 1.2 : 4. It is the second most common benign tumour constituting approximately 8 per cent of primary liver tumours in autopsy series. They are usually less than 5 cm in diameter with an average size of 3 cm. The tumours are usually soli-tary but may be multiple in 7 to 20 per cent of patients. The tumour is usually well circumscribed but non-encapsulated. It frequently contains a central stellate scar and radiating fibrous septae which divide the tumour into lobules. Histologically the lesion is composed of abnormally arranged normal hepatocytes, numerous bile ducts and vascularised fibrous septa and Kupffer cells. Calcification is occasionally seen. There is no malignant poten-tial and therefore treatment is conservative. The majority of patients are asymptomatic and the liver function tests are usually normal, however a small minority (10 per cent) may have vague abdominal pain because of the mass effect. Association with hepatic haemangioma has been described in patients on the contraceptive pill. Other conditions described in association with focal nodular hyperplasia are vascular anomalies and neuro-endocrine tumours, these conditions include congenital heart disease, glioblastoma, astrocytoma, phaeochromocytoma and multiple endocrine syndromes. Sonographically approximately half the tumours appear hypo-echoic, nearly half appear echogenic while the remainder have a mixed heterogeneous appearance. Most of the lesions appear well defined. The central scar is usually not visible but when seen it is not specific for focal nodular hyperplasia because it may be seen in other liver masses both benign and malignant. The majority of tumours are vascular on angio-graphy. Colour flow and power Doppler show an increased blood flow radiating from a centrally feeding artery. These appearances are similar to the conventional angiography pattern of blood flow. Power Doppler is said to be more sensitive in detecting feeding arteries within hypervascular lesions. Resistive index values (resistive indices in the present context) in the feeding arteries (mean = 0.51) appear to be significantly different from those in the main hepatic artery and its intrahepatic branches (mean = 0.68). The mean resistive index difference is usually 0.19, indicative of sig-nificant arteriovenous shunting within the tumour. Because of the increased vascularity percutaneous biopsy carries an increased risk of haemorrhage. Both the echopattern of focal nodular hyperplasia and the results of the ultrasound-guided needle biopsy are non-specific. As focal nodular hyper-plasia contains Kupffer cells, 58 to 70 per cent will show normal uptake on sulphur colloid scintigraphy. Also 40 to 70 per cent of patients will show normal or increased uptake on Tc HIDA while the rest show a photon defi-cient mass. On MRI focal nodular hyperplasia tends to be isointense on both T_1- (60 per cent) and T_2- (34 per cent) weighted images while the central scar appears hyperintense on T_2-weighted images. This triad is seen in only 9 per cent of cases but when present the diagnosis of focal nodular hyper-plasia is almost certain.

Bile duct hamartoma (von Meyenberg complexes)

Multiple bile duct hamartomas (MBDH) are rare congenital defects which may cause single or multiple non-specific hepatic lesions that may be con-fused with metastasis, small abscesses or dilated ducts. The basic lesion in MBDH is a greyish nodule 0.5 to 1.5 cm but it can be a larger cyst. These nodules represent dilated tortuous bile ducts embedded in fibrocollagenous stroma. These features are characteristic of this disease and support the close association between liver cysts and biliary hamartomas. It has been postulated that a polycystic liver may result from cystic dilatation of bile duct hamartomas.

Rare association with carcinoid, cholangiocarcinoma and with long-term treatment with danazol has been described. The sonographic features are variable, visibility on ultrasound correlating with larger lesion size. The lesions may be hypoechoic, hyperechoic, cystic or more complex. Colour flow and duplex Doppler findings have not been described. Angiography shows no neo-vascularity or arteriovenous shunting but grape-like clusters of rings of vessels have been shown. In patients with a known primary malignancy it may not be possible to rule out liver metastasis on imaging because of the non-specific features. Biopsy may be the only way to achieve a definitive diagnosis. The diagnosis is usually made by wedge or core-needle biopsy; fine-needle aspiration is usually non-diagnostic.

Benign lipomatous liver tumours

Lipomas are rare primary benign tumours derived from mesenchymal elements. Non-capsulated they usually merge with hepatic parenchyma. There is no gender predilection and the tumours are distributed over a broad age range. On sonography they are invariably hyperechoic, small, round or oval and well defined usually occurring in a non-cirrhotic liver. Because of the reduced acoustic transit in fat these tumours may shadow. There is no malignant potential. On CT the appearances are those of a hypodense mass. Other liver fatty tumours include angiomyolipomas, adenolipomas and myelolipomas depending upon the mix of adenomatous, angiomatous and/or myomatous tissue. Like lipomas these tumours are echogenic and well defined, however angiomyolipomas can be heterogeneous depending upon the tissue mix. Liver lipomas and angiomyolipomas may be associated with tuberous sclerosis. Angiomyolipomas of the liver may be very vascular depending upon its angiomatous tissue mix. It is therefore expected that some of these tumours will show increased flow detectable on colour and power Doppler. The differential diagnosis includes haemangioma, echogenic metastasis or focal fatty infiltration. Sound attenuation, if present behind the mass, excludes a haemangioma. An ultrasound-guided fine needle aspirate is recommended to obtain a tissue diagnosis of angiomyolipoma. Foci of fat have been described in adenomas but non-fatty masses usually predominate. Hepatocellular carcinoma may undergo fatty change just as normal liver.

Regenerative macronodules

The liver possesses a remarkable power of regeneration following injury although liver regeneration may be disorganised resulting in the presence of nodules. Diffusely distributed regenerative nodules 2 to 3 mm in size are the usual feature of cirrhosis of the liver. In macronodular cirrhosis the nodules are large, usually 2 to 16 cm, but despite their size the nodules are often hard to delineate as their echopatterns are similar to normal liver tissue. The presence of the nodules may be deduced by distortion of hepatic architecture. When seen macronodules are well-defined, rounded, intrahepatic lesions. They are isoechoic or slightly hyperechoic compared to the liver parenchyma. When macronodules are seen they present an important diagnostic problem as they occur in the same group of patients prone to the development of a hepatocellular carcinoma. Therefore, when a focal lesion is seen in a cirrhotic liver it is presumed to be a hepatocellular carcinoma until proven otherwise. It has been said that ultrasonically discernible focal masses in a cirrhotic liver should be considered neoplastic and treated aggressively to prevent their progression to frank malignancy even if not malignant at presentation. Macronodules may show normal or decreased activity on 99m sulphur colloid scan depending upon their Kupffer cell content while hepatocellular carcinomas cause photon deficient areas provided they are large enough to be resolved. Doppler usually shows no evidence of neo-vascularity or hyperperfusion.

Nodular regenerative hyperplasia

Nodular regenerative hyperplasia (NRH) is a distinct pathological entity that should not be confused with regenerative nodules of a cirrhotic liver, focal nodular hyperplasia or a hepatic adenoma. Nodular regenerative hyperplasia is often associated with a variety of vasculitidies such as rheumatoid arthritis, Felty's syndrome, systemic lupus erythematosus, polyarteritis nodosa and other conditions which include systemic infections, tuberculosis, malignancies such as adenocarcinoma of the pancreas and colon and myelo- or lymphoproliferative disorders. It has also been associated with azathioprine treatment. Nearly one half of the patients have portal hypertension and recently an association with pulmonary hypertension has also been described. Nodular regeneration around the porta hepatis can compress the portal vein thus causing portal hypertension. Nodular regenerative hyperplasia is found in 0.6 per cent of autopsies and is thus presumably under diagnosed during life. Unlike focal nodular hyperplasia nodular regenerative hyperplasia may bleed and large nodules may rupture and cause haemoperitoneum. Histologically nodular regenerative hyperplasia can be distinguished from micronodular cirrhosis by the absence of fibrous bands between nodules. The nodules are of varying sizes, composed of morphologically normal hepatocytes arranged in abnormal cell plates. Diagnosis is important to prevent confusion with hepatic adenoma, hepatocellular carcinoma and regenerative nodules of cirrhosis, as management is very different. The prognosis of nodular regenerative hyperplasia and associated portal hypertension is much better than portal hypertension with cirrhosis. Nodular regenerative hyperplasia should be considered when patients present with 'idiopathic portal hypertension'. Sonography of the nodules reveals variable echogenicity with or without features of portal hypertension. Computed tomography often shows hypodense nodules with no significant contrast enhancement.

Angiography reveals vascular nodules which may fill from the periphery resembling haemangiomas. These nodules may take up Tc-99m sulphur colloid. There are features in common with focal nodular hyperplasia, hepatocellular carcinoma and metastases. Multiple needle biopsies under ultrasound or laparoscopic guidance biopsy is usually helpful.

Liver adenomatous hypertrophy

Edmondson first described liver adenomatous hypertrophy as a liver parenchymal nodule of regenerative nature following post-necrotic cirrhosis. Most are associated with viral hepatitis. Recent improvements in imaging resolution have made possible the detection of small nodules in cirrhotic livers. These nodules may represent adenomatous hypertrophy, regenerative nodules or hepatocellular carcinoma. It is obviously important that these mass lesions are distinguished as their management is different. It is particularly important that discrimination is made between adenomatous hypertrophy and hepatocellular carcinoma. The original description of adenomatous hypertrophy was that it is regenerative, of limited growth and benign in nature. However, recent histological studies have shown that adenomatous hypertrophy can grow gradually and finally progress to hepatocellular carcinoma. But in spite of malignant potential adenomatous hypertrophy is usually managed conservatively as most patients with adenomatous hypertrophy have viral cirrhosis and treatment is avoided to prevent further liver damage. Histological examination of adenomatous hypertrophy reveals a liver parenchymal nodule containing portal and biliary elements. Kupffer cells are rarely present. Unlike most hepatocellular carcinomas adenomatous hypertrophy appears hypovascular on angiography. On sonography adenomatous hypertrophy appears as ill-defined, inhomogeneous, echogenic masses. Colour flow and power Doppler show continuous flow but without pulsatility. This is in contradistinction to hepatocellular carcinomas which show both continuous and pulsatile flow in over 75 per cent of patients with a tumour size over 2.5 cm. Power Doppler appears to be more sensitive in showing blood flow within small tumours.

Solid non-neoplastic liver masses

Extramedullary haematopoiesis is the response to a need for increased blood cell production because of either inadequate production in the bone marrow or shortened red cell life span. Conditions that may provoke extramedullary haematopoiesis include thalassaemia, myeloproliferative disease, aplastic anaemia, marrow replacement syndromes, disseminated carcinomatosis, multiple myeloma, Albers-Schönberg's disease and myeloid metaplasia. The sites of extramedullary haematopoiesis are usually the sites of foetal erythropoiesis. These include the liver, spleen, lymph nodes, adrenal glands, mediastinum, lung, heart and thymus. Often large, ill-defined masses that are sonographically hypoechoic are seen in the liver. The medical history will often suggest the patient's underlying medical diagnosis. If doubt exists a needle biopsy may be performed under ultrasound guidance.

Hypereosinophilic syndrome

Hypereosinophilic syndrome is a spectrum of disorders characterised by marked eosinophil leucocytosis without identifiable cause. There is usually no organ dysfunction. Clinical manifestations include pulmonary symptoms, features of cardiac dysfunction, immune disorders, weight loss and fever. Sonography reveals pleural effusions, hepatosplenomegaly, a coarse echo-pattern or multiple focal nodules 1 to 3 cm in size, which may be hypo-, hyper-, or isoechoic. The nodules may be well defined or may have irregular ill-defined borders. The nodules are hypodense on CT.

Langerhans' cell histiocytosis

This term refers to proliferation of a unique histiocyte the Langerhans' cell. This global name replaces histiocytosis X, eosinophilic granuloma, Hand–Schüllar–Christian disease and Letterer–Siwe disease. Multiple systems are involved thus symptomatology depends on the site and extent of involvement. Common sites of involvement include the bone marrow, lung, skin, liver, spleen and lymph nodes. Hepatic involvement is associated with high mortality. Sonography reveals hepatomegaly with hyperechoic irregular nodular lesions. Periportal fibrosis because of sclerosing cholangitis may result in increased periportal echogenicity. Hypoechoic nodules may be seen in the spleen and the pancreas may be the site of cystic lesions. The liver lesions are hypodense on CT, hyperintense on T_1-weighted magnetic resonance images and hypointense on T_2-weighted images.

Inflammatory pseudo-tumours

These rare masses usually occur in children and young adults. The majority have been reported in the lungs but a number of cases have now been seen at extrapulmonary sites. Histologically they feature proliferation of mononuclear inflammatory cells, eosinophils, lymphocytes, mesenchymal cells and myelofibroblasts. Clinical presentation is with abdominal pain, fever, weight loss, anaemia and hepatomegaly. Sonography may show hepatomegaly associated with a well-defined hypoechoic or heterogenous mass usually involving the right lobe. No Doppler frequency shifts or colour flow Doppler changes have been described in pseudo-tumours.

Hepatic metastases

Metastasis is the commonest neoplasm in an adult liver, the liver being the second most common site for metastatic cancer spread after lymph nodes. In Europe and the United States a focal liver lesion is much more likely to represent a metastatic deposit than a primary malignancy. The liver may be the site of metastatic deposit from virtually any primary malignant neoplasm but the most common primary sites are the colon (30 per cent), stomach (22 per cent), pancreas (21 per cent), breast (14 per cent) and lung (13 per cent). In children the commonest liver metastases are from a neuroblastoma, Wilms' tumour and leukaemia. The majority of liver metastases are multiple involving both lobes in 77 per cent of patients, only 10 per cent being solitary. Multiple tumours often show a range of sizes suggesting that tumour seeding has occurred in episodes. Growing metastases compress adjacent liver parenchyma causing atrophy and forming a connective tissue rim. Large metastases often outgrow their blood supply causing hypoxia and necrosis at the centre of the lesion. Approximately half the patients with liver metastases have clinical signs of hepatomegaly or ascites; liver function tests tend to be insensitive and non-specific. Fortunately the sensitivity of ultrasound approaches that of bolus CT at 90 per cent while intraoperative sonography and laparoscopic ultrasound are the most sensitive tests available for detecting liver focal lesions. The sensitivity of intraoperative ultrasound is even better than CT arterial portography. The pathological anatomy of metastases resembles the primary tumour, often showing the same degree of vascularity. Most metastases are hypovascular but some primaries characteristically have hypervascular metastases. These include metastases from carcinoid, leiomyosarcoma, neuroendocrine tumours, renal carcinoma, thyroid carcinoma, choriocarcinoma, pancreas, ovary, breast and colon. Blood flow is said to increase relative to the normal parenchyma in all metastases, even the hypovascular tumours. The larger metastases tend to displace the surrounding vessels and may compress or occlude the portal vein branches but neo-vascularity, vascular encasement and arteriovenous shunting is rare. The sonographic appearances of metastases are quite variable reflecting the large spectrum of tumour types. Generally metastases cause hepatomegaly though this may not be evident until the disease is advanced. Intrahepatic masses may alter hepatic shape and the liver surface may appear nodular or lobular. This latter sign is non-specific and also occurs in cystic fibrosis and liver infiltration. In general the ultrasound appearance of liver metastases is non-specific and a biopsy may be required for tissue diagnosis. However, the presence of multiple hepatic nodules of different sizes within the liver is nearly always caused by metastases. Also, biopsy should not be undertaken percutaneously if there is a chance of curative hepatic resection. There has been an attempt to use colour and duplex Doppler arterial flow patterns around liver masses in an effort to improve the specificity of ultrasound examination. Unfortunately Doppler cannot always differentiate between other masses (for example haemangioma) and metastases since the latter are mostly hypovascular. However there has been some success in differentiating hepatocellular carcinoma from metastases since Doppler shifts greater than 5 kHz are said to be specific for hepatocellular carcinoma. Moreover a 'basket type' pattern has been described for hepatomas on colour flow Doppler. Doppler shift of up to 4 kHz has been described in vascular metastases. On colour flow Doppler a hypovascular mass with venous or arterial flow meandering around the mass, a 'detour sign', is occasionally seen around metastases reflecting their mass effect in displacing such vessels. While colour Doppler is of limited value in adding specificity to ultrasound diagnosis it can be invaluable to localise areas of vascularity in order to optimise the site for biopsy.

Hepatic metastases: echopatterns

These changes may be focal or diffuse. There is relatively poor correlation between sonographic appearance and tumour histology, although 'cauliflower' masses are often from the colon and a search of the abdomen may find a bowel mass. The echopattern is dependent on tumour vascularity, cellular composition, the degree of tissue invasion and the presence or absence of necrosis, fibrosis and fatty change. Metastases complicated by haemorrhage, necrosis or infection may result in dramatic changes in their configuration and echopattern.

Isoechoic metastases

Isoechoic and infiltrating metastases are difficult to identify. They may sometimes only be identified because of their mass effect as shown by irregularity of the liver surface, displacement or compression of intrahepatic blood vessels or segmental bile duct obstruction. There may be other tell-tale signs of malignancy, for example hepatic hilar lymphadenopathy, ascites, peritoneal metastases, or the primary site may be recognised such as a mass in the pancreas. A sonolucent ring sign may also be useful. A small hypoechoic mass in the liver adjacent to the gallbladder may demonstrate a hump or an edge sign, or a 'gallbladder compression sign'. A hump or edge sign may indicate the presence of a superficial mass placed near the outer surface.

The gallbladder compression sign is because of the compressive effect of a mass causing protrusion into the gallbladder as a result of an adjacent mass. These signs latterly described are non-specific signs of space-occupying lesions within the liver and may be caused by benign as well as malignant lesions. The gallbladder compression sign has also been described as a normal variant although this is exceptionally rare.

Echogenic metastases

Echogenic metastases contain multiple tortuous vessels and tend to be hypervascular, the echogenicity is most probably related to the number of blood–tissue interfaces rather than the blood-vessel walls themselves. The most common primary tumours that cause echogenic metastases are from the gastrointestinal tract, renal cell carcinoma, carcinoid, choriocarcinoma, pancreatic islet cell tumours, chloromas (leukaemic) and AIDS-related Kaposi's sarcoma. In children metastases from neuroblastoma, hepatoblastoma, leukaemia, hepatoma and Wilms' tumour may be densely echogenic.

Tumours responding to therapy may show increased echogenicity but more often show a reduction in size.

Hypoechoic metastases

These metastases tend to be hypovascular comprising uniform tissue and cellularity. Virtually any primary tumour can cause this pattern of metastases but particularly lymphoma, melanoma or carcinoma of the pancreas, lung and cervix.

Cystic metastases

Cystic metastases can cause diagnostic difficulties as they may mimic other pathology such as abscesses, haemorrhagic infarcts, haematomas, simple cysts and hydatid cysts. However there are tell-tale signs that may suggest the true nature of these lesions. These lesions display a degree of complexity in the form of mural nodules, thickened walls and septae and fluid-debris levels. These features are not present in simple hepatic cysts. A detailed clinical history may help exclude haematomas, hydatid cysts and abscesses from consideration. Two groups of patients tend to get cystic metastases

1. those patients who have a primary neoplasm that has a cystic component such as mucinous cystadenocarcinoma of the colon, stomach, pancreas or ovary
2. patients with metastases undergoing central necrosis, when low level echoes and walls irregularity is seen – squamous cell carcinoma, leiomyosarcoma, melanoma and testicular carcinoma have a propensity to undergo extensive central necrosis.

Target bull's-eye metastases

In this pattern of metastases there is a hypoechoic ring or halo that surrounds a hyperechoic or isoechoic mass. The halo is most probably related to a combination of compressed normal hepatic parenchyma around the mass and a zone of cancer cell proliferation. The presence of a halo usually suggests a more aggressive behaviour. Bronchogenic carcinoma characteristically cause 'target-type' metastases, however this pattern is non-specific and can be found with metastases from the breast and colon as well as primary malignant (hepatocellular carcinoma) and benign (adenoma in glycogen storage disease) liver neoplasms. A similar appearance has been described with liver abscesses.

Calcified metastases

These metastases appear densely echogenic and if calcification is sufficient will give rise to distal acoustic shadowing. The calcification and echogenicity results from intratumoural mucin, necrosis or phosphatase activity. This pattern of metastases can occur from many primary sites (see gamut, p. 77) but is particularly common with carcinoma of the colon of the mucin-secreting type, pseudomucinous cystadenocarcinoma of the stomach and, rarely, adenocarcinoma of the breast or melanoma. In children neuroblastoma is the commonest metastasis, it is usually hypoechoic but may show calcification and can be echogenic.

Diffuse or infiltrative metastases

Diffuse hepatic malignancy is seen less frequently than focal disease. Diffuse disease may be due to confluence of areas of focal disease, infiltrating tumours or miliary metastatic deposits. The liver may appear 'moth eaten' or diffusely heterogenous or, uncommonly, the infiltrates are isoechoic. Diffuse metastases are very difficult to detect at sonography particularly on the background of fatty infiltration which may occur as result of cirrhosis or chemotherapy. Lymphoma and leukaemia are particularly prone to diffuse disease which may appear hypoechoic, although these changes do not always reflect the presence of metastases as reactive lymphocytic infiltration secondary to disease elsewhere may give rise to the same appearance. A diffuse pattern is also commonly seen with carcinoma of the breast, lung and melanoma. When the liver is extensively replaced by metastases jaundice may occur because of inadequate liver function, this may be because of a lack of normal liver tissue or distortion of the hepatic architecture particularly bile ducts and vessels. Alternatively Hodgkin's disease may cause intrahepatic biliary obstruction at the canalicular level whilst the lymphadenopathy may compress the extrahepatic biliary system. Even in the absence of jaundice the liver function tests shows some abnormality in the presence of diffuse intrahepatic malignancy.

Leukaemia

Non-specific reactive hepatomegaly is not unusual in both lymphatic and myeloid leukaemia. Chloromas are rare solid extramedullary tumours histologically composed of granulocyte precursor cells. They usually have a mass effect. They have been reported in intracranial, intrathoracic and intra-abdominal sites. Chloromas mostly occur in children. Hepatic chloromas are extremely rare. In the few reported cases they have been described as hypoechoic or hyperechoic masses. The hyperechoic mass may mimic haemangiomas. Chloromas may rarely show central necrosis, which presents as echogenic centres (like candida abscess).

Lymphoma

Lymphoma usually causes diffuse infiltrates of the liver and spleen; focal involvement is less common. Hepatomegaly may be reactive as only 50 per cent of patients with known lymphoma and hepatomegaly have histological evidence of hepatic lymphoma. Steatosis is found in up to 70 per cent of livers following chemotherapy for lymphoma. The diffusely infiltrating type of liver lymphoma is difficult to image with ultrasound as it may cause subtle architectural distortion or no ultrasound abnormality at all. Primary lymphoma of the liver is an unusual entity, but its incidence appears to be rising. This may reflect its appearance in the rising numbers of immuno-compromised patients such as patients with AIDS or organ transplantation. Primary lymphoma (confined to solitary organs) is much more common with non-Hodgkin's lymphoma. Focal hepatic lymphoma is usually hypo-echoic but 'target' and hyperechoic patterns have been described in non-Hodgkin's but not Hodgkin's lymphoma. Burkitt's lymphoma can also cause hypoechoic liver masses. These masses are usually large at diagnosis. On CT the lymphoma deposits are hypovascular and thus become more obvious post-contrast.

AIDS-related liver tumours

Non-Hodgkin's lymphoma and Kaposi's sarcoma are common complications of HIV infection. Kaposi's sarcoma may be the consequence of gamma-herpesvirus infection while non-Hodgkin's lymphoma appears to be related to herpes virus. Epstein–Barr virus is also implicated in the development of non-Hodgkin's lymphoma. The incidence of Kaposi's sarcoma in AIDS patients is 0.5 to 0.9 per cent between the ages of 1 to 19 years but increases with age and is higher in males. Black children and adolescents who reported homosexual intercourse with other males have a threefold increase in the incidence of Kaposi's sarcoma. Non-Hodgkin's lymphoma is more common than Kaposi's sarcoma in children. Primary non-Hodgkin's lymphoma and Kaposi's sarcoma affecting the liver are uncommon. However in autopsy series in patients with Kaposi's sarcoma and AIDS 34 per cent of patients have liver involvement, although the incidence diagnosed at imaging is much lower. Non-Hodgkin's lymphoma usually presents with multiple hypoechoic masses within the liver and is no different to that presenting as a primary hepatic lymphoma in non-AIDS patients. It should however be remembered that liver abnormalities are frequent in AIDS patients and include changes that may follow with

1. coincidentally acquired hepatotropic viruses
2. complications related to therapy
3. changes associated with a chronic debilitating disease or
4. complications related to immune compromise, for example infections, neoplasms or iatrogenic complications.

Kaposi's sarcoma in the liver manifests itself as 5 to 12 mm hyperechoic nodules, although hypoechoic masses have been reported. Three-quarters of patients with AIDS-related Kaposi's sarcoma have abdominal lymphadenopathy, which cannot be differentiated from non-Hodgkin's lymphoma, inflammation or infection on imaging. A biopsy is usually required for this purpose.

Hepatic myeloma

Extramedullary myeloma deposits are extremely rare, a few cases of liver involvement have been reported. Ultrasonography shows hepatomegaly with single or multiple hypoechoic solid masses but 'target' lesions and hyperechoic masses have also been reported. A fine-needle aspirate may demonstrate numerous mononuclear cells characteristic of myeloma. Doppler studies on liver lesions have not been described but colour Doppler on a breast myeloma deposit showed evidence of neo-vascularisation mimicking breast cancer.

Echogenic liver metastases

It should be noted that some metastases can show both echogenic and hypoechoic metastases.

Mucinous adenocarcinoma of the colon.
Pancreatic carcinoma (usually hypoechoic but may become echogenic as calcification occurs).
Gastric carcinoma (usually hypoechoic).
Hepatocellular carcinoma.

Neuroblastoma.
Cholangiocarcinoma.
Treated breast carcinoma.
Renal cell carcinoma.
Carcinoid.
Choriocarcinoma.
Pancreatic islet cell tumours.
Wilms' tumour (usual spread is to the lung).
Kaposi's sarcoma.
Myeloma deposit.
Hepatic chloroma.

Calcified liver metastases

Mucinous adenocarcinoma stomach, pancreas, colon and rectum.
Ovarian serous cystadenocarcinoma.
Neuroblastoma.
Leiomyosarcoma (usually of the stomach).
Carcinoid.
Endocrine pancreatic carcinoma.
Medullary carcinoma of the thyroid.
Melanoma.
Osteogenic sarcoma.
Treated breast cancer.
Bronchogenic carcinoma.
Pleural mesothelioma.
Renal cell carcinoma.
Testicular carcinoma.
Lymphoma.
Chondrosarcoma.
Ovarian teratocarcinoma.

NB Calcification tends to be amorphous unlike solid calcification in granuloma.

Hypoechoic liver metastases

Lymphoma (especially AIDS related).
Hepatocellular carcinoma.
Pancreatic carcinoma.
Lung (particularly adenocarcinoma).
Cervix.
Melanoma.
Nasopharangeal carcinoma.

Kaposi's sarcoma (rare, most are hyperechoic).
Myeloma deposits.

Cystic liver metastases

Mucinous cystadenocarcinoma colon.
Cystadenocarcinoma ovary.
Cystadenocarcinoma pancreas.
Melanoma.
Leiomyosarcoma (may be difficult to separate left lobe cystic mass from gastric leiomyosarcoma on ultrasound).
Squamous cell carcinoma.
Testicular carcinoma.
Carcinoid.
Granulosa cell ovarian tumour.

Heterogeneous echogenicity liver metastases

Breast.
Colon and rectum.
Hepatocellular carcinoma (especially when complicated by haemorrhage).
Stomach (especially anaplastic).
Carcinoid.
Cervical cancer.
Melanoma.
Bronchogenic carcinoma.

Malignant hepatic tumours

Malignant hepatic neoplasms can be classified into primary and metastatic neoplasms. Metastatic neoplasia accounts for the majority of liver tumours occurring twenty times more frequently than primary hepatocellular carcinoma. Primary malignant tumours may arise from several cell types of either epithelial or mesenchymal origin. Hepatoblastoma (57 per cent) and hepatocellular carcinoma (43 per cent) are the most common primary malignant liver tumours in children. Others include rhabdomyosarcoma, teratocarcinoma, angiosarcoma and mesenchymal sarcoma arising from the bile ducts and supportive elements within the liver.

Hepatoblastoma

Hepatoblastoma is the most common primary hepatic malignancy in childhood. The majority of cases present at less than 3 years of age usually as an enlarging abdominal mass. However, it can occur in young adults and sporadic cases have been reported in patients in their early fifties. Men are more often affected then women. Hepatoblastoma is an aggressive neoplasm with markedly elevated alpha fetoprotein in up to 90 per cent of cases, metastases occur in the lungs early in the disease. There is an association with other conditions such as hemi-hypertrophy, macroglossia and sexual precocity. Two cell types are described

1. epithelial – containing foetal or embryonal malignant hepatocytes
2. mixed – containing more differentiated epithelial cells with foci of mesenchymal differentiation.

Prognosis is dependent upon histology with foetal type carrying the best prognosis and mixed variant with primitive embryonal cell fairing badly. Coarse calcification is present in 50 per cent of hepatoblastomas. As with other primary tumours imaging is non-specific. The right lobe is the commonest site for these tumours which may be seen as homogeneous, but are more commonly heterogeneous echogenic masses with areas of cystic necrosis, haemorrhage and calcification. The tumours are often 10 cm or more at presentation. The appearances are non-specific but invasion of vessels may give an indication of the mass's malignant nature. Biopsy is usually required for tissue diagnosis and may be performed at surgery. Colour and power Doppler usually show hyper-vascularity and Doppler frequency shifts are common because of neo-vascularity. Sonography may overestimate inferior vena caval involvement and therefore contrast venography may be required for further assessment. The differential diagnosis is haemangioendothelioma, metastatic neuroblastoma and hepatocellular carcinoma.

Hepatocellular carcinoma

Hepatocellular carcinoma is the most common hepatic primary tumour and the second commonest liver tumour in children. In the United Kingdom and the United States it is uncommon although its incidence appears to be rising. It is particularly common in southeastern Asia, Japan, sub-Saharan Africa, Greece and Italy. In adult cases in the United Kingdom up to 90 per cent of patients give a history of underlying cirrhosis or other liver disorders although recently we have seen an increasing number in females in their late forties and early fifties with hepatocellular carcinoma with no known predisposing factors. The most common predisposing factors in the United States are alcoholic cirrhosis, haemochromatosis and steroid use. The most common predisposing factor in Asia, Africa, Greece and Italy is chronic hepatitis B virus infection, while in Asia and Africa aflatoxine B1 is an additional risk factor. Other predisposing factors worldwide include hepatitis C, cirrhosis secondary to primary haemochromatosis, primary biliary cirrhosis, Wilson's disease, Gaucher's disease, glycogen storage disease type I, tyrosinosis, thorium dioxide (Thoratrast) exposure, biliary atresia, exposure to anabolic steroids, benign inferior vena caval obstruction and alpha$_1$-antitrypsin deficiency. The contraceptive pill has also been implicated. The highest incidence has been reported in Japan, where hepatocellular carcinoma is said to occur in 4.8 per cent of the population. The risk of developing hepatocellular carcinoma appears to be high in haemochromatosis macronodular cirrhosis and lower in alcoholic micronodular cirrhosis. In at risk subjects a focal hepatic lesion should be regarded as hepatocellular carcinoma until proven otherwise.

Patients may present with non-specific symptoms or may be found incidentally, while others may present with right upper quadrant pain, hepatomegaly or sudden deterioration in hepatic function in an already compromised liver. Paraneoplastic syndromes are rare but appear more commonly with hepatocellular carcinomas than with other malignancies; these include hypoglycaemia, hypercalcaemia, polycythaemia, hypercholesterolaemia and carcinoid syndrome, while in children sexual precocity may occur. Alpha fetoprotein is elevated in over a quarter of the patients, however 46 per cent of patients with hepatocellular carcinoma in the 3 to 5 cm range have a normal level alpha fetoprotein. Since most patients with hepatocellular carcinoma have underlying cirrhosis it is important to classify the degree of cirrhosis as it has a bearing on treatment and ultimate prognosis. The degree of cirrhosis is classified according to Child criteria based on a number of clinical and biochemical parameters which include serum bilirubin and albumin levels, the presence of ascites, the presence of portosystemic encephalopathy and the nutritional status of the patient. The patient is put into one of three categories, A, B or C, with A carrying the best prognosis and C the worst. Hepatocellular carcinoma progression may result in intrahepatic metastases and complete or partial portal vein thrombosis. Extrahepatic metastases to lungs, bones, lymph nodes and the adrenal gland is a late occurrence. Pathologically a hepatocellular carcinoma may appear single massive, nodular, multifocal or diffuse (infiltrating). There is a variant of an encapsulated tumour which responds well to surgery and has a better prognosis. Recently the Liver Cancer Group of Japan has proposed a further subdivision of the nodular type into four subgroups depending upon the macroscopic appearance: single nodular, single nodular with proliferation into the surrounding parenchyma, multinodular fused and multinodular. This classification is useful in anatomical classification and forecasting prognosis. Calcification has been reported in up to a quarter of the patients. The tumour may occasionally invade the bile ducts mimicking a cholangiocarcinoma. Invasion of vascular structures is frequent, particularly of the portal vein. In approximately 4 per cent of patients the inferior vena cava and right atrium may be invaded via the hepatic veins. Sonographic appearances are variable and depend upon the size, histological type of the tumour, growth rate and the presence of calcification, haemorrhage, necrosis and as to whether the tumour is vascular or avascular. The underlying cirrhosis, for example haemochromatosis and fatty change, also determines the ultrasonic features. The incidence of each appearance varies in each series and there are no characteristic appearances. Sonographically hepatocellular carcinoma may be identical to extensive metastatic disease. Regenerative nodules, haemangiomas, focal fatty sparing and adenomatous liver hypertrophy may all mimic hepatocellular carcinomas.

Ultrasonography is quite a sensitive means of demonstrating hepatic malignancy but multifocal hepatocellular carcinoma can be quite subtle and angiography will usually show far more lesions than suspected at sonography, CT or magnetic resonance scanning. As a result a normal ultrasound scan cannot entirely exclude hepatocellular carcinoma. Small hepatocellular carcinomas under 3 cm usually have a solid composition without necrosis and may present as a hypoechoic mass with or without a degree of posterior enhancement. Larger tumours show a more heterogeneous echopattern as a result of necrosis and fibrosis. The presence of pseudoglandular proliferation, fat within the tumour and sinusoidal dilatation gives rise to a more echogenic tumour. The diffuse infiltrative type of hepatocellular carcinoma may be difficult to detect particularly when it is superimposed upon underlying parenchymal liver disease. The clues to the diagnosis may be subtle and the only giveaway may be intrahepatic venous thrombosis, mass effect as shown by irregularity of liver surface, displacement or compression of intrahepatic blood vessels or segmental bile duct obstruction. Small hypoechoic hepatocellular carcinomas may be shown by a 'gallbladder compression sign', a hump sign or an edge sign (see page 168). Duplex and colour Doppler sonography are a valuable aid to the diagnosis of hepatocellular carcinoma. Generally speaking the main blood supply of hepatocellular carcinoma comes almost exclusively from the hepatic artery and hepatic angiography shows varying degrees of neo-vascularity. Important criteria described for diagnosing hepatocellular carcinoma on Doppler sonography include arterial pulsatile flow, afferent tumour vessels and continuous efferent vessels.

Recent advances in imaging have made it possible to detect small masses within cirrhotic livers. These lesions should be considered to be hepatocellular carcinoma until proven otherwise but there are a significant number of other lesions such as haemangioma, focal fatty sparing, regenerative nodules and adenomatous liver hypertrophy that are relatively common in cirrhotic livers. Adenomatous hypertrophy contains multiple portal venous channels and produces the same volume of portal flow as does the rest of the parenchyma of the cirrhotic liver. Differentiation between adenomatous hypertrophy and hepatocellular carcinoma is not always possible but rests with differences in hepatic arterial flow compared to portal venous flow. Colour flow sonography may reveal a 'basket pattern' composed of small peripheral vessels surrounding and penetrating nodules seen on grey scale images. There is arterial pulsating flow in 75 per cent of hepatocellular carcinomas smaller than 25 mm but not in adenomatous hypertrophy. Another study has described continuous arterial flow in 68 per cent of hepatocellular carcinomas smaller than 3 cm but not in adenomatous hypertrophy. Thus small hepatocellular carcinomas have a dominant arterial blood flow as compared to adenomatous hypertrophy even if angiography does not reveal tumour blush. Colour signals have been described in 34 per cent of hepatocellular carcinomas less than 2 cm. Both pulsatile and continuous flow in nodules are seen significantly more often with power Doppler which is 3 to 5 times more sensitive than colour flow sonography in detecting tumour blood flow. The Doppler peak velocity signals are normally more than 250 cm/s. Doppler shifts more than 5 kHz are said to be specific for hepatocellular carcinoma, on the other hand vascular metastases may cause Doppler shifts up to 4 kHz. The hepatic tumour index may be useful in differentiating large hepatocellular carcinomas from metastases. The hepatic tumour index is defined as the ratio of the peak systolic velocity in the tumour to the peak systolic velocity in the hepatic artery. On Doppler ultrasound the hepatic arterial branch supplying a hepatocellular carcinoma has a lower impedance than the branch not supplying the tumour. When this index was 1.0 or greater the sensitivity for distinguishing hepatocellular carcinoma from metastases is 76 per cent with a specificity of 92 per cent and accuracy of 82 per cent; and 76 per cent sensitivity, 100 per cent specificity and 82 per cent accuracy in distinguishing hepatocellular carcinomas from haemangiomas. Ultrasound, CT, MRI and angiography are complimentary in imaging hepatocellular carcinoma providing different information about tumour morphology. The sensitivity of CT and ultrasound is similar in the detection of hepatocellular carcinoma but CT shows spread of the tumour better than ultrasound and is therefore better at staging. Ultrasound also tends to underestimate hepatic involvement in 38 per cent of cases. In the diagnosis of hepatocellular carcinoma lipiodol CT has been shown to be the most sensitive imaging modality (90 to 97 per cent) for all size lesions. However the specificity of lipiodol CT is lower at 76.9 per cent since lipiodol uptake may occur in metastases, haemangioma or adenomatous hyperplastic nodules. But despite the limitations of lipiodol CT it is the most sensitive modality available which can detect lesions smaller than 1 cm preoperatively. Laparoscopic ultrasonography is gaining favour in the authors' institution as the most reliable means of assessing hepatic pathology when CT, MRI and abdominal sonography are inconclusive, it has the advantage of allowing biopsy under direct vision if appropriate, and cautery can be applied to the biopsy point to prevent seeding.

Screening for hepatocellular carcinoma

Sonography alpha fetoprotein levels have been proposed as screening methods for hepatocellular carcinoma in the at-risk population. Sonography appears to be more sensitive than alpha fetoprotein in diagnosing hepato-cellular carcinoma. Tumours detected by alpha fetoprotein are usually large. It has been shown that a steady rise in alpha fetoprotein is much more likely to be associated with hepatocellular carcinoma than normal or fluctuating alpha fetoprotein levels. In alpha fetoprotein detected hepatocellular car-cinoma only 29 per cent of cases are judged to be resectable. It has been shown that a combination of alpha fetoprotein and ultrasound-based screen-ing does not significantly improve survival rates in hepatocellular carcinoma patients. However it should be remembered that most hepatocellular car-cinomas are a complication of cirrhosis, and the degree of cirrhosis itself may determine survival rates. There is however little doubt that ultrasound can detect early tumours as small as 1 cm, but only in 35 per cent of patients. At the present stage of knowledge and on the basis of cost benefit ultra-sound screening for hepatocellular carcinoma cannot be justified. One study has estimated the screening cost at $25 000 per case of hepatocellu-lar carcinoma detected and $750 000 if the patient undergoes surgery!

Fibrolamellar hepatocellular carcinoma

Fibrolamellar hepatocellular carcinoma is a distinct variant of primary hepa-tocellular carcinoma which represents 2 per cent of all the primary hepa-tocellular carcinoma while it makes up 25 to 50 per cent of hepatocellular carcinoma in the age group 5 to 35 years (mean 23 years). There is no gender predilection. Unlike the classic hepatocellular carcinoma there is usually no underlying cirrhosis or elevation of alpha fetoprotein. They are 4 to 20 cm well-circumscribed slow-growing desmoplastic tumours that calcify and may develop a central scar. The prognosis is much better than that for the classic hepatocellular carcinoma with a 48 per cent resectabil-ity rate and 63 per cent of patients survive at 5 years. Sonographic appear-ances are variable but the tumour is usually well defined and may be of hyperechoic, isoechoic or hypoechoic appearance. The central scar and punctate calcification (rare in hepatocellular carcinoma) may be identified on ultrasound. The central scar is a non-specific occurrence that may be seen in other tumours such as hepatocellular carcinoma, focal nodular hyperplasia, adenoma and haemangioma. The angiographic and computed tomographic features are usually those of a very vascular tumour.

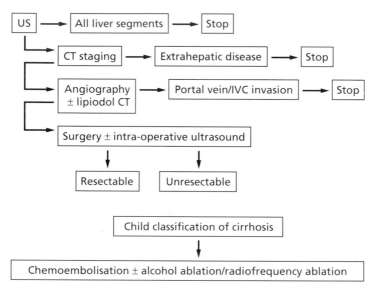

Figure 2.6 Management of hepatocellular carcinoma.

Cholangiocarcinoma

Cholangiocarcinoma is the second most common primary liver malignancy. The intrahepatic type accounts for 8 to 13 per cent of all cholangiocarcinomas. The majority of cholangiocarcinomas involve the extrahepatic biliary tree or the porta hepatis (Klatskin tumour). Several conditions predispose to the development of a cholangiocarcinoma including ulcerative colitis, sclerosing cholangitis, choledochal cyst, Caroli's disease, clonorchis sinensis infection, cholecystolithiasis, hepatolithiasis, biliary papillomatoses, Thorotrast exposure, autosomal dominant polycystic disease, congenital hepatic fibrosis, familial adenomatous polyposis, alpha$_1$-antitrypsin deficiency and haemochromatosis. Clinical presentation is with abdominal pain, palpable mass, weight loss and jaundice. The average age at presentation is 50 to 70 years with a slight male predominance. Macroscopically the tumours may be massive, nodular or diffuse type, the latter mimicking sclerosing cholangitis. The Thorotrast-related tumours are mostly cited in the mid-peripheral portion of the liver while the non-Thorotrast-related cholangiocarcinomas are located in the hilar region. Histologically the tumour consists of an adenocarcinoma arising from the biliary epithelium with a desmoplastic reaction; mucin and calcification may be present. The tumour infiltrates locally along the duct or into the adjacent liver parenchyma. The tumour may spread directly to adjacent structures such as the stomach. Metastatic spread to regional lymph nodes (usually at the porta) may occur in up to 15 per cent of patients. Intrahepatic metastases are rare. Unlike extrahepatic or hilar cholangiocarcinoma the intrahepatic variety presents late as it causes focal segmental biliary obstruction and atrophy. The patient may have a history of chronic abdominal pain but in the absence of external signs the diagnosis is often delayed. At presentation the tumour is usually at least 3 cm in diameter but the tumour mass is usually quite difficult to define having a similar echopattern and CT density as normal hepatic parenchyma. The diagnosis is suggested by the presence of dilated bile ducts radiating peripherally from the point of obstruction. With modern surgical techniques an increasing number of tumours are resectable but the 5-year survival is only 30 per cent. Cholecystolithiasis is present in up to half the patients but the cause for the relationship is not known. Sonographically the majority of tumours are ill-defined, homogeneous or heterogeneous, generally isoechoic masses. The diagnosis is suggested by the mass effect and the presence of biliary dilatation. Follow-up scans show progressive biliary dilatation and if the ducts are large enough intraluminal thickening, focal irregularity or polypoid intraluminal masses may be observed on rare occasions. The degree of focal atrophy can be quite severe when lesions have been present for some time and the atrophic lobe or segment can be quite small and echogenic, often being mistaken for a mass. Rarely, predominantly cystic intrahepatic cholangiocarcinomas have been reported. These tumours usually have some solid elements and intramural irregularity. The tumours are usually avascular or hypovascular. Invasion of the portal or hepatic veins occurs relatively late. Angiography shows a minor tumour blush in up to half the tumours with stretched or encased arteries. The diagnosis of cholangiocarcinoma when it occurs on the background of sclerosing cholangitis may be difficult even with the application of modern imaging and brush biopsy techniques. Certain tumour markers, particularly a combination of carcinoembryonic antigen (CEA) and carbohydrate antigen 19-9 (coeliac axis 19–9), are said to identify most occult tumours and therefore improve patient selection when orthotopic liver transplantation is planned. An ultrasound-guided fine needle aspirate is considered safe and may be useful in obtaining tissue diagnoses of intrahepatic mass lesions. These lesions are normally too peripheral to be sampled by brush cytology although bile cytology may be useful. An unusual entity of a combined hepatocellular and cholangiocarcinoma may occur with imaging features of both hepatocellular carcinoma and a cholangiocarcinoma. The sonographic features include round or ovoid hypoechoic masses with a central hyperechoic area (target appearance) reported in all patients in one series. These tumours are hypovascular with a central hypervascular portion on angiography. Lipiodol CT shows partial retention of the iodised oil within the tumour corresponding to the hepatocellular carcinoma component. Intra-operative ultrasound is useful in detecting occult liver tumours and planning resection.

Biliary cystadenocarcinoma

Biliary cystadenomas and cystadenocarcinomas, which usually present as large multiloculated tumours, most probably represent part of the same spectrum of disease since malignant transformation in a cystadenoma has been described and local recurrence after surgical excision of adenoma has been reported. Both tumours most probably originate in ectopic nests of primitive biliary tissue. These tumours usually arise from intrahepatic bile ducts (85 per cent). The tumours are 3.5 to 25 cm in diameter at presentation, are well encapsulated and composed of multiloculated cysts lined by biliary-type epithelium. The tumours are usually mucinous resembling mucinous pancreatic and ovarian tumours. There is a male to female ratio of 1:5, with most tumours occurring in fifth decade. Most patients present with right quadrant mass, pain and signs of biliary obstruction. The sonographic features are those of a large solitary complex mass that contains locules, septae, papillary projections and fluid–fluid levels. Differentiation from cystic metastases and other cystic neoplasms is not possible on imaging, and aspiration biopsy or surgery is required to obtain a tissue diagnosis. Rarely a microcystic variety may be encountered which may appear solid because of multiple tissue interfaces. A unilocular cystic lesion has been described which may need differentiation from an abscess or hydatid cyst.

Angiosarcoma

Hepatic angiosarcomas represent 1 to 3 per cent of all the primary liver cancers. A quarter of the patients have a history of exposure to chemical carcinogens, the most frequent being Thorotrast and vinyl chloride. Others include arsenicals, radium, steroids and possibly copper. There is also an association with haemochromatosis and von Recklinghausen disease. At autopsy 40 per cent of patients with angiosarcoma have hepatic fibrosis or cirrhosis, although the exact relationship with chronic liver disease and angiosarcoma remains obscure. Among the Thorotrast-related malignancies 43 per cent are cholangiocarcinomas, 38 per cent are angiosarcomas and 15.7 per cent are hepatocellular carcinoma. The peak incidence occurs in the seventh decade with a male to female ratio of 4:1. Patients present with abdominal pain, rapid weight loss, general debility and jaundice. Catastrophic intraperitoneal bleeding is a feature in a quarter of the patients. Consumptive coagulopathy or disseminated intravascular coagulation may occur because of local consumption of blood elements within the tumour.

The alpha fetoprotein is not elevated. Macroscopically the tumours display multifocal or multinodular lesions.

Tumour size is usually over 5 cm, but large grossly haemorrhagic tumours with areas of necrosis are seen in 30 per cent of cases. They are aggressive tumours with early metastatic spread to the lungs, spleen, regional lymph nodes, peritoneum, marrow and thyroid. Portal vein invasion and haemorrhagic ascites are common. Histologically the tumour is made up of malignant endothelial cells that from the vascular channels and sinusoids associated with surrounding atrophy. Imaging studies are non-specific unless there is a history of Thorotrast exposure when a conventional radiograph of the abdomen or CT shows increased density of the liver, spleen and upper abdominal lymph nodes. The increase in density may be diffuse or punctate. When this appearance occurs in combination with liver lesions the differential diagnoses include cholangiocarcinoma, angiosarcoma and hepatocellular carcinoma. Childhood hepatic angiosarcoma occurs in the age range of 1 to 7 years with slight female predominance. The usual presenting features are an abdominal mass with or without associated symptoms. The histological picture is that of large hepatocellular whorls of spindled sarcoma cells intermingled with blood vessels, bile ducts and collagen. The prognosis in both childhood and adult angiosarcoma is poor; the mean survival time in a child is 10 months and in adults 6 months. Sonography reveals large solid, single or multiple nodules of mixed or hyperechoic nature, the degree of heterogeneity depends on the degree of internal haemorrhage and necrosis. Angiography reveals a vascular blush around the periphery and puddling within the tumour in the late arterial phase. There is no arterial encasement. No colour flow Doppler studies have been described. Percutaneous biopsy should be avoided as catastrophic haemorrhage may occur.

Epithelial haemangioendothelioma

Metastatic spread is usually to the spleen, mesentery, regional lymph nodes, lungs and bone. The survival times vary from 5 to 10 years after diagnosis. Macroscopically epithelial haemangioendothelioma consists of multifocal nodules varying in size from a few millimetres to several centimetres distributed throughout the liver which may eventually coalesce and replace most of the liver parenchyma. The nodules at the periphery have a particular propensity to coalesce. Histologically there are dendritic spindle-shaped and epithelioid round cells in a matrix of myxoid and fibrous stroma. The neoplastic cells invade the sinusoids and other vascular structures. These tumours are also vasoformative and synthesise factor VIII-related antigen. Histologically these tumours may be mistaken for veno-occlusive disease. Sonographically epithelial haemangioendothelioma presents as multiple mainly hypoechoic nodules, most placed peripherally so that may become confluent. There may be capsular retraction associated with peripheral nodular lesions. However isoechoic, hyperechoic and target lesions have been described. Calcification is found in 15 per cent of cases. Extensive hepatic involvement is associated with hypertrophy of the uninvolved liver and splenomegaly. Duplex and colour Doppler may reveal invasion or occlusion of portal and hepatic veins. Coalescent peripheral hepatic masses with capsular retraction are highly suggestive of epithelial haemangioendothelioma. Angiography reveals a tumour of mixed hyper- and hypovascularity with invasion of hepatic and portal veins.

Undifferentiated (embryonal) hepatic sarcoma

Undifferentiated embryonal sarcoma is the most common malignant mesenchymal liver tumour in children and the fourth most frequent liver tumour of childhood. It usually occurs in older children, 90 per cent occurring in the 6 to 15 year age range although 5 per cent occur in infants less than 2 months old. Sporadic cases have been reported up to the age of 30 years. There is no gender predilection. Clinical presentation is with a right upper quadrant mass, fever, leucocytosis, mild anaemia and abnormal liver function tests. The prognosis is poor and most children die within 12 months. The tumours are usually 7 to 20 cm, well defined and mostly within the right lobe (75 per cent). Histologically primitive undifferentiated spindle sarcoma cells are arranged in whorls or sheets with foci of haematopoiesis. Sonographically these tumours are seen as large heterogeneous masses with multicystic areas due to necrosis and haemorrhage, separated by small echogenic solid areas. The cysts are rather large (usually up to 4 cm), but these cysts can be tiny giving a hyperechoic solid appearance.

Other sarcomas

Each of the hepatic mesenchymal elements has the potential for malignant proliferation. For example, a leiomyosarcoma may originate from the liver capsule. Leiomyosarcoma and malignant fibrous histiocytoma are extremely rare and usually affect middle-aged adults. The ultrasound appearances are variable. These tumours are usually large at presentation and are slow growing. The sonographic pattern may be hyperechoic or hypoechoic, diagnosis is usually not possible without a biopsy. Rhabdomyosarcoma, which usually affects children, gives rise to a solitary, relatively well-defined heterogeneous mass of reduced echogenicity. In certain cases cystic spaces with septations may be apparent. Sarcomatous change has been described in epithelial tumours such as hepatocellular carcinoma and cholangiocarcinoma.

2.1.6 LIVER TRANSPLANTS

Sonography of liver transplants

Ultrasound is widely used in the preoperative and postoperative assessment of liver transplantation. The role of ultrasound in the preoperative patient is to establish the presence of malignancy, the extent of diffuse liver disease and the patency of the inferior vena cava, hepatic and portal veins. Mass lesions within the liver are frequently seen on the background of diffuse disease. Analysis can be difficult as biopsy risks spreading malignancy prior to surgery. If histological confirmation is necessary biopsy can be undertaken at laparoscopic sonography, as laparoscopy allows cautery to the biopsy site reducing the risk of seeding to the peritoneum. The biopsy needle can be introduced into the abdomen via a sheath thus preventing seeding to the abdominal wall.

Normal appearance after liver transplantation

The surgical procedure of liver transplantation involves anastamosis of the hepatic artery, portal vein, the bile duct and the inferior vena cava. When a variant of donor hepatic artery is encountered a single donor hepatic artery is anastamosed to the recipient hepatic artery or aorta. There is often discrepancy of size when the donor portal vein is anastamosed to the recipient which results in portal vein irregularity. The appearance of the inferior vena cava depends upon the surgical technique used. If the hepatic inferior vena cava is removed *en bloc*, then the inferior vena cava anastamosis will be suprahepatic and infrahepatic. These anastamotic sites often calcify. A 'piggyback' procedure may be used when the recipient inferior vena cava is left *in situ*. In this instance, the suprahepatic donor inferior vena cava is anastamosed to a common lumen fashioned by the union of surgically joined hepatic veins of the recipient whilst the intrahepatic inferior vena cava of the donor is oversewn. A Roux-en-Y choledochojejunostomy is fashioned or the donor bile duct can be anastamosed directly to the recipient bile duct. A stent is routinely left *in situ* when the choledochojejunostomy is fashioned. This echogenic tubular structure is visible on ultrasound. There is often air in the biliary tree. The gallbladder is normally excised. The transplanted liver often has a diffuse heterogeneous echopattern associated with increased periportal echogenicity. Focal liver lesions such as a haemangioma may be an incidental finding in the donor liver. A right pleural effusion is common after such major surgery and may also be associated with a paralysed right hemidiaphragm as phrenic nerve injury occurs in up to a third of the patients. Similarly ascites is a common finding, this may loculate and may cause subhepatic or subphrenic collections. If the right pleural effusion enlarges after 3 days a subphrenic collection should be considered. Doppler ultrasound remains the mainstay of postoperative liver transplant but may be difficult to interpret. No detectable flow or a reversal of diastolic flow in the hepatic artery is usually of no diagnostic significance. It has been suggested that intense flow in the hepatic artery in the immediate postoperative period may in fact be an ominous sign. The portal waveform in the transplant liver may mimic hepatic artery flow because of its pulsatility. A helical flow form is recorded in 43 per cent of liver transplants and should not be confused with hepatofugal or bidirectional flow. The hepatic vein waveforms can be monophasic/non-pulsatile. However, if there is change in the flow pattern from a normal triphasic pattern to a non-pulsatile wave form a number of possibilities should be considered including rejection, hepatitis, cholangitis and venous-flow obstruction.

Graft rejection

Sonography is not sufficiently sensitive or specific in the diagnosis of rejection and hence ultrasound-guided liver biopsies are frequently performed to diagnose rejection.

Vascular complications

The major vascular complications following liver transplantation can be diagnosed by conventional duplex scanning. However colour Doppler imaging allows a more rapid visualisation of blood vessels and facilitates a more precise placement of Doppler sample volume. The three most common vascular complications of liver transplantation are hepatic artery thrombosis (6 to 10 per cent), portal vein thrombosis (1 to 7 per cent) and the development of hepatic artery aneurysm. Conventional pulsed Doppler can demonstrate hepatic artery patency in 92 per cent of patients. False positive diagnosis of arterial thrombosis has been reported due to sluggish flow caused by live oedema. Colour Doppler is helpful in reducing sampling error. Portal vein thrombosis (PVT) may be asymptomatic but may present with signs of acute portal hypertension-ascites or bleeding varices. Duplex Doppler can provide evidence of portal vein thrombosis. On real time imaging a spectrum of changes may be noted with portal vein thrombosis besides signs of portal hypertension. The portal vein thrombus may be directly visible with variable echogenicity from hyperechoic to echopoor. Colour flow Doppler is also quite sensitive (89 per cent) in detecting portal vein thrombosis with an accuracy of 92 per cent. Colour Doppler imaging also is useful in identifying hepatic artery dilatation that usually accompanies portal vein thrombosis. Stenosis of the portal vein at the anastamotic site may create a confusing picture because of the post-stenotic jet phenomenon with colour flow and pulsed Doppler. The helical flow detected in this situation can be misdiagnosed as hepatofugal flow.

A hepatic artery pseudoaneurysm is a life-threatening condition, early diagnosis is therefore essential. The aneurysm appears as a focal area of vessel dilatation, which will show a flash of colour with colour flow Doppler. Stenosis of the inferior vena cava occurs in up to 2.6 per cent of patients. The stenosis may be supra- or infrahepatic. This results in a localised acceleration of flow velocity at the stricture. Suprahepatic stenosis can cause graft dysfunction which can be difficult to identify because of difficulty in obtaining a suitable Doppler angle. Indirect signs of inferior vena cava stenosis are therefore sought, such as flat monotonous Doppler tracings in the inferior vena cava and hepatic veins reflecting dampened transmission of cardiac pulsation. Contrast cavography may be necessary to substantiate inferior vena cava stenosis. Inferior vena cava thrombosis is uncommon but when it occurs it carries a poor prognosis.

Biliary complications

Biliary complications occur in 38 per cent of liver transplants, these include stricture, obstruction, bile leaks and cholangitis. Since the sole blood supply to the biliary tract is from the hepatic artery, hepatic artery occlusion/stenosis should be considered when biliary complications develop. Sonography has a low sensitivity for biliary obstruction in the transplant patient. Nevertheless ultrasound is the initial examination performed in graft dysfunction, it may detect bile duct dilatation, mucocoele of the cystic duct and bile leaks. The detection of sludge in the bile ducts of transplant patients is important as it is frequently related to cholangitis (13 per cent) and hepatic artery occlusion (30 per cent). In biliary obstruction ultrasound may reveal grossly dilated intrahepatic bile ducts, lack of normal intrahepatic duct tapering, bile duct strictures and increased periductal echogenicity. With an intrahepatic bile duct diameter of 2 mm or more in a transplant liver, biliary obstruction should be considered.

Malignant disease

Cancer develops in 5 per cent of hepatic transplant patients; half of these cases are non-Hodgkin's lymphoma. These cancers are related to the antirejection drugs. With non-Hodgkin's lymphoma ultrasound findings include a hypoechoic mass or masses within the liver associated with lymphadenopathy. Patients who have undergone liver transplantation for a hepatocellular carcinoma have a 40 per cent risk of tumour recurrence within 3 years. A neoplasm in the donor liver may pass undetected on preoperative imaging but immune suppression may allow rapid growth within weeks of transplantation.

2.1.7 HYPOECHOIC PERIPORTAL ENCASEMENT

Transplanted liver
Malignant lymphadenopathy
Che(diak-Higashi) Syndrome
Cholangitis*
Obstructive jaundice*
Congestive cardiac failure*
Blunt abdominal trauma*
Periportal encasement refers to hypoechoic bands surrounding the portal vein and its intrahepatic radicals related to lymphatic oedema that has been shown in a few cases that have been biopsied.

2.1.8 CHEDIAK-HIGASHI SYNDROME

This is a rare autosomal recessive disorder. The cardinal features of the syndrome include partial oculocutaneous albinism, photophobia, recurrent fever and immune deficiency. Most affected children die before the age of 10 years from recurrent pyogenic infections. About 85 per cent develop a lymphoma-like disease associated with hepatosplenomegaly, lymphadenopathy and bleeding diathesis.

2.1.9 SEGMENTAL LIVER TRANSPLANTATION IN CHILDREN

The lack of timely availability of small donor organs is a major cause of death in children who are in need of liver transplantation. This lack of availability of small livers has led to the ingenious technique of segmental liver transplantation, which involves reducing an adult liver allograft. Left lobe liver transplantation is the most common form in which the donor organ may be cadaveric or harvested from a live donor. There are several unique features and potential complications of segmental liver transplantation. The cut surface of the line of separation of the right and left lobes is obtained by blunt dissection with ligation of blood vessels and ducts. The raw cut surface is sealed by application of fibrin glue. The cut surface appears heterogeneous or echogenic on ultrasound. Fluid collection along the cut surface is frequently encountered, which may represent sterile seroma, abscess or

---

* Periportal lymphoedema has been demonstrated on MRI and CT, it is therefore more than likely that ultrasound may show periportal hypoechoic bands.

biloma. The echogenicity of the fluid varies with the nature of the fluid collection, where indicated aspirated fluid under ultrasound guidance may be analysed. The biliary drainage of the left lobe transplant is fashioned by a Roux-en-Y choledochojejunostomy. A multi-fenestrated radiopaque stent secured by soluble sutures is placed across the anastamosis. The stent is usually passed into the gut approximately 1 month after placement. The stent is readily identified with ultrasound. The 'portahepatis' of the left lobe transplant lies on the lateral cut surface. The left and main portal veins are anastamosed end-to-end into the recipient portal vein. The hepatic arterial anastamosis is made end-to-side between the donor coeliac axis and recipient inferior abdominal aorta. This lateral placement of the new 'portahepatis' results in a very long circuitous route of the blood supply of the transplanted organ, which may lead to vascular compromise as a result of compression from the comparatively large donor organ in a child and mesenteric or intestinal oedema. Thus, if Doppler ultrasound shows compromised flow within the portal vein or hepatic artery immediately after surgery, this may be related to extrinsic compression. In such instances ways of reducing the intra-abdominal pressures should be explored.

2.1.10 INTRAOPERATIVE AND LAPAROSCOPIC ULTRASOUND

Intraoperative ultrasound of the liver has the highest sensitivity for the detection of focal liver abnormalities with a 96 per cent accuracy versus 84 per cent for transabdominal ultrasound. It is more accurate than any other known imaging modality at the present stage and is used in the authors' unit for cases not adequately diagnosed and staged by ultrasound, CT and MRI. Intraoperative ultrasound is an important diagnostic tool in patients undergoing hepatic resection for colorectal metastases allowing careful evaluation of the normal liver segments to exclude occult metastases in the segments that will be left *in situ*. The high accuracy is almost entirely accounted for by the contact scanning with complete organ coverage free from artefact with the use of a high frequency transducer and colour flow Doppler. Intraoperative ultrasound detects 25 to 35 per cent additional lesions as compared to preoperative ultrasound. Most significantly 40 per cent of these lesions detected by intraoperative ultrasound are neither visible or palpable and would presumably be missed. Intraoperative ultrasound has also been shown to be a sensitive means of detecting hepatocellular carcinoma particularly if sonographic contrast agents are used to improve Doppler images. Operative sonography is also used routinely during cryotherapy – the intraoperative freezing of metastases. The tip of the cryotherapy probe is placed within the centre of the metastasis which is then frozen with liquid nitrogen. As the metastasis freezes it becomes echogenic being seen as an echogenic sphere forming around the tip of the probe. Cryotherapy is applied until the echogenic sphere has replaced all the visible metastasis with a margin fully including the edges of the tumour to prevent recurrence. On follow up the metastasis forms a 'lollipop'-shaped defect with a cyst-like hypoechoic area representing the site of the treated tumour which has become necrotic with a tubular fluid density stem representing freezing around the probe shaft. Operative sonography can also be used to guide segmental resection by allowing visualisation of portal vein branches which can then be injected with dye. This leads to staining of the liver segment giving an accurate demarcation of its vascular boundaries on the liver surface. This technique can be further refined by the insertion of a 6-F balloon catheter into the supplying portal vein under intraoperative ultrasound guidance. Inflation of the placed balloon will create a relatively bloodless field for operation. Laparoscopic ultrasound is also valuable and has the advantage over abdominal sonography in that the probe can be used to 'palpate' the surface of the liver aiding diagnosis of haemangiomas which compress, unlike solid tumours which do not.

2.1.11 HEPATIC INFECTIONS AND ABSCESSES

Focal hepatic infections

Focal hepatic infection of the liver parenchyma is an uncommon but potentially fatal condition and thus a high index of suspicion is required if it is to be diagnosed sufficiently early to allow successful treatment. Hepatic infection occurs more frequently in adults than children and may complicate any infective process. The majority of infections are pyogenic and reach the liver either via the hepatic artery during septicaemia, via the portal vein from abdominal infection or via the biliary tree in ascending cholangitis.

Pyogenic liver abscess

Pyogenic liver abscesses are uncommon in children. The majority of these cases occur in children under the age of 5 years and are usually secondary to umbilical vein catheterisation, appendicitis, surgery, renal infection or immune deficiency such as chronic granulomatous disease of childhood. In older children the infection is often with *Staphylococcus* spp. whilst in adults 50 per cent of infections are caused by anaerobic bacteria reflecting the frequent spread of infection from the bowel. *Escherichia coli* is the most frequently isolated organism in adults, especially in the elderly, diabetics, cirrhotics and patients with congestive cardiac failure. In adults liver abscesses develop as a complication of several pathological processes which may be subdivided into several groups.

1. Primary or secondary cholangitis, the latter may be related to benign or malignant biliary obstruction. In Asia, Africa and South America hepato-biliary roundworm infestation is a common cause of liver abscesses.
2. Portal venous spread – the most frequent of this being from append-icitis, diverticulitis, inflammatory bowel disease, proctitis, infected haemorrhoids, pancreatitis and necrotic colonic carcinomas. Amoebic and other enteral infections of the bowel may also spread to the liver via the portal vein. This is particularly important in developing countries where hepatic infection is frequently caused by protozoal and helminthic organisms. Sonography has shown that portal venous involve-ment by infection is not as rare as believed prior to the development of sonography and CT, and partial or complete portal vein thrombosis is an uncommon but by no means rare finding in patients with intra-abdominal sepsis.
3. Systemic spread may occur from other sites of infection, septicaemia or bacterial endocarditis.
4. Direct extension from adjacent organs such as a perforated abdominal viscus, pneumonia, pyelonephritis and a subphrenic abscess.
5. Blunt or penetrating abdominal trauma.
6. Secondary infection in an existing liver mass lesion, for example simple cyst, haematoma, hydatid cyst, infarct, hepatocellular carcinoma or a necrotic metastatic deposit. However the source of the abscess is often not found.

The patient presents with hepatomegaly, pain, fever, nausea, vomiting, diarrhoea and pleuritis. There is usually leucocytosis with abnormal liver function tests and anaemia. In elderly, alcoholic and immune compromised patients liver abscesses may be occult and, since abscesses filled with debris may appear echogenic or solid, they may mimic solid tumours. No patient should be allowed to die from a presumed liver tumour unless the diagnosis has been proven, since occasionally large masses prove to be unexpected abscesses at autopsy particularly in debilitated patients and alcoholics. Liver biopsy guided by sonography undertaken during a single breath hold with a 16 gauge needle is a relatively safe procedure. Provided the patient's clotting is normal the authors discharge straightforward biopsy cases 4 hours post-procedure. Sonography allows the biopsy needle to avoid vessels and performing the biopsy during a single breath hold prevents laceration of the liver edge leaving only a very small defect in the liver surface. The majority of liver abscesses affect the right lobe (80 per cent), 10 per cent are multiple. Rarely abscesses may occur in the falciform ligament or ligamentum teres. A liver abscess may rupture into the subphrenic space, the abdominal cavity or the pericardium. Amoebic abscesses which occur most commonly high in the right lobe under the right hemidiaphragm may rupture through the diaphragm into the thorax.

Mortality is high and reaches almost 100 per cent if the condition is unrecognised or untreated. Sonographic appearances are very variable reflecting not only the nature and extent of infection but also the stage of abscess formation. Initially as the infection involves the liver appearances are normal, then subtle parenchymal changes occur, usually indicated by a reduction in the echogenicity. As the tissue inflammation progresses an area of increased or decreased echogenicity forms which may be quite heterogenous. Pyogenic liver abscesses are usually spherical or ovoid in shape. The walls are usually thick or irregular but may be well defined. Necrosis and pus formation at the centre of the abscess gives rise to an anechoic or hypoechoic area with few internal echoes, an irregular wall and variable distal acoustic enhancement. Established abscesses may contain debris, fluid–debris levels or uncommonly septae. A hypoechoic rim may surround the outer margin of the abscess. As a fibrous reaction occurs around the abscess an increasingly echogenic wall forms which may calcify in long-standing cases giving very high level echoes with or without distal acoustic shadowing. Gas-forming organisms may give rise to intense echoes arising in the centre of the abscess rather than within the wall (20 to 30 per cent). If the abscess is successfully treated with antibiotics but without surgical or radiological drainage then follow up will show reduction in the size of the anechoic collection with increasing organisation of the echogenic wall which may leave a scar. If in doubt an ultrasound-guided biopsy may be performed. The authors routinely aspirate abscesses provided that there is no evidence of hydatid or amoebic infection, as this allows accurate diagnosis of the organism with antibiotic sensitivity testing. Aspiration of the abscess also speeds recovery by removing the bulk of the debris, pus and organisms from the infective focus. Aspiration without drain insertion is relatively straightforward for a skilled operator but carries the risk of spreading the infection to peritoneum or pleura if an intercostal route is used.

Fungal liver abscess and other opportunistic infections

Focal fungal abscess is quite uncommon representing only 2 per cent of liver abscesses. The majority of cases affect the immune-compromised patient particularly patients with AIDS, organ transplants and patients undergoing chemotherapy for malignant disease. *Candida* spp. is the most frequently encountered systemic fungal infection in the immune-compromised, the liver is usually involved by haematogenous spread from the lung. Patients may present fever, abdominal pain and hepatomegaly. Clinical diagnosis may be difficult as only 50 per cent of patients have positive blood cultures with proven systemic infection. The abscesses may be single but are more often multiple. The sonographic appearance is variable, the most common being multiple uniformly hypoechoic lesions. Early in the course of the development of liver abscesses a 'wheel-within-a-wheel' appearance may be seen. Three concentric rings cause this pattern: an outer hypoechoic ring, an inner echogenic ring and a central hypoechoic nidus. The central nidus is related to focal necrosis in which fungal elements are found, the outer rings are caused by adjacent inflammatory reaction and surrounding oedema. A target appearance, indistinguishable from metastases is less common. The target appearance coincides with the return of the neutrophil leucocytosis to normal. The differential diagnosis includes metastases, lymphoma, sarcoid, septic emboli and Kaposi's sarcoma. The lesions may eventually become echogenic because of the development of scar tissue and calcification. The spleen is not infrequently involved with candida abscesses at the same time as the liver. Diffuse liver abscesses with *Pneumocystis carinii*, atypical mycobacterium, *Aspergillus* spp. and *Staphylococcus* spp. in AIDS patients may give rise to a mottled hypoechoic appearance similar to metastases. Numerous small echogenic foci have been reported in the liver, spleen and kidneys with *P. carinii* and cytomegalovirus. Primary hepatic actinomycosis indistinguishable from other liver abscesses has been reported in AIDS patients. The liver in the majority of AIDS patients has a bright appearance assumed to be due to fatty infiltration.

2.1.12 PARASITIC INFECTIONS OF THE LIVER

Hepatic amoebiasis

The protozoan *Entamoeba histolytica* is a common parasite in Asia, Africa, South and Central America and is said to affect 10 per cent of the world population. The parasite enters the body by ingestion of its cystic form. These cysts may pass through the stomach as the cysts are resistant to acid. The amoebae then colonise the large bowel particularly and secrete proteolytic enzymes which cause mucosal ulceration. Some amoebae penetrate the bowel wall and reach the liver via the portal venous system and/or lymphatics. Patients may be asymptomatic or present with abdominal pain and diarrhoea. The male to female ratio is 4 : 1. Amoebae may lie dormant in the liver for many years and there is often a significant delay between the initial bowel infection and the clinical presentation of an amoebic liver abscess. Amoebic liver abscesses are usually often solitary and peripherally located usually at the superior aspect close to the diaphragm. The right lobe is affected in 72 per cent and the left lobe in 13 per cent of patients (the remaining cases are multiple). The abscesses are usually thick walled and may contain necrotic liver tissue. They may rupture into the subphrenic or subhepatic spaces, while rarely rupture may occur into the pleural space. A sympathetic right-sided pleural effusion may be present with a subcapsular right lobe abscess. Approximately 6 per cent of amoebic abscesses rupture into the pleura and peritoneum thus aspiration should be considered if an abscess shows significant enlargement. With successful treatment abscesses resolve leaving an area of focal scarring though old amoebic abscesses may occasionally calcify. Sonography cannot accurately differentiate amoebic and other liver abscesses because bacteria super-infect 20 per cent of cases. Serological tests may be useful in differentiating amoebic from pyogenic abscesses. Sonography reveals solitary round or oval lesions with irregular margins that lack an obvious wall. They are generally hypoechoic with low echogenicity contents, hyperechoic areas and distal acoustic enhancement. The wall may appear nodular in 60 per cent of patients while 30 per cent of amoebic abscesses may have a multiseptate appearance. Low level echoes within the abscess are frequently found. About 10 per cent may be predominantly hyperechoic. With treatment the abscesses may clear in 6 weeks to 2 years although the abscesses may become sterile within weeks leaving a fluid area. With resolution of the abscess cavity a scar or sterile cyst is formed. Without treatment the mortality is nearly 100 per cent, with treatment the mortality drops to 10 per cent.

Ultrasonic characteristics of liver amoebic abscesses
Five characteristics have been described

1. absent wall or wall echoes
2. round or oval shape
3. hypoechoic mass with homogenous low level echoes
4. most abscesses are subcapsular
5. most enhance with good through transmission deep to the abscess.

Only 30 per cent of abscesses demonstrate all five features.

Hydatid liver disease

Hydatid disease is prevalent throughout the world particularly in sheep-raising areas. There are two main forms that affect humans – *Echinococcus granulosus* and *Echinococcus multilocularis.*

E. granulosus is a small tapeworm 3 to 6 mm long that lives in the intestine of a definitive host – usually a dog but in the less common sylvatic form the principal host may the wolf or fox. The life cycle of *E. granulosus* requires two hosts – a dog and grazing cattle or sheep, where the cattle serve as an intermediate host for the cystic form of the disease. Man may accidentally become infected through contact with infected dogs or other canines, or by ingesting food or water contaminated with canine faeces.

Once within man or the intermediate host, the outer coat of the egg is dissolved by gastric juice. The eggs hatch in the proximal small intestine. The larvae then migrate through the intestinal mucosa and enter the mesenteric venules and lymphatics. The liver acts as an effective filter for the larvae and is the most common organ involved (70 per cent of cases). If the liver barrier is overcome the larvae may enter the lungs via the inferior vena cava, this occurs in 15 to 30 per cent of cases. If the larvae escape the lungs they may become lodged in virtually any organ of the body but most notably the peritoneum, spleen, kidney, brain, bones, heart or pericardium and muscles. Once the larvae are lodged in the capillaries they provoke an inflammatory reaction and most are overcome by the host reaction and destroyed. Others may grow taking several years to reach a large size. The growth rate is usually 0.25 to 1 cm per year. The hydatid cyst in the liver has three layers made up of both host and parasitic tissue. The outer layer is formed by host inflammatory reaction. This is the pericyst, a fairly tough protective zone several millimetres thick. As the cyst grows in size and matures more and more host tissue and compressed host vessel and ductal elements are incorporated into the pericyst. This layer of compressed vessels explains the peritumoural blush on angiography and contrast enhancement on MRI and CT. The middle layer or ectocyst is 1 to 2 mm thick and is formed by a laminated chitin-like substance secreted by the parasite, which may calcify. The innermost layer or the germinal layer represents the live parasite. The germinal layer gives rise to brood capsules which may remain attached to the cyst wall, harbouring thousands of scolices, or which may detach and become free floating hydatid sand. The majority of smaller cysts are an incidental finding in endemic areas, being well encapsulated they have little effect on the health of the host. In some endemic areas over 95 per cent of the adult population show positive serology for hydatid disease. Another incidental finding is eosinophilia which may occur in 20 to 50 per cent of patients. Patients with larger cysts may present with pain, jaundice or biliary colic if the cyst ruptures into the biliary tree. Urticaria and anaphylaxis may follow a spontaneous rupture. It is said that symptoms usually occur in cysts larger than 10 cm. The right lobe of the liver is more often affected than the left, 20 per cent are multiple. The sonographic appearance of hydatid cysts depends upon the stage of evolution and maturity and the presence or absence of complications. A simple fluid-filled cyst is the earliest appearance of a hydatid cyst and is indistinguishable from a simple cyst. Cysts with undulating membranes occur because of endocyst rupture (sonographic 'waterlilly sign'). The appearance of cysts within a cyst occurs because of the presence of daughter cysts within a mother cyst. A multilocular cyst with echogenic matrix may form, which may appear as solid. If the echogenic matrix predominates then the cyst may appear solid. A complex mass with both solid and cystic elements which may mimic other liver mass lesions. The cyst may be densely calcified with distal acoustic shadowing. The presence of a heterogenous mass with areas of increased and decreased echogenicity may represent a secondary infection of the cyst. In these circumstances ultrasound diagnosis of a hydatid cyst is not always possible. The presence of air within the lesion may make the mass very echogenic. Solid cysts may occur demonstrating the 'ball of wool' sign, 'spin' sign, 'whorl' sign or 'congealed waterlilly' sign. Approximately 17 per cent of intra-abdominal cysts are solid. As the physical characteristics of the hydatid cyst fluid change from a watery to a viscid gel, it becomes echogenic. The intact folds of the germinal layer trapped within the viscid matrix give rise to the appearance of curvilinear structures which no longer move with changing patient posture. A 'spin' or 'whorl' sign representing collapsed parasitic membranes is considered strong evidence of hydatid disease even in the presence of negative serology. An echofree peritumoural collar and echofree spiral have been described as signs suggestive of hydatid disease. These signs correspond to peripherally placed daughter cysts and fragmented in-folded membranes respectively. It is possible that such an appearance may be related to degenerating and dead *E. granulosus*. The presence of a fat–fluid level in a hepatic hydatid cyst may be a sign of rupture into the biliary tree. With rupture into the biliary tree the contents of the cyst may become echogenic with or without posterior acoustic enhancement with a wall defect communicating with a biliary radical. The common bile duct may be dilated with echogenic material. Hydatid cysts are usually round or oval, well defined and usually have a demonstrable wall. Though diagnosis is straightforward in typical cases many hydatids have a non-specific appearance and serological tests for hydatid liver disease should be performed for further evaluation. Although the sensitivity of serological tests is variable (sensitivity 60 to 85 per cent) depending upon the type of test used, false positive tests occur. A biopsy should be avoided because of the risk of dissemination and anaphylaxis. However recently percutaneous drainage under ultrasound guidance, with or without medical therapy, has been advocated. At the present stage of knowledge surgery remains the treatment of choice perhaps supplemented by medical therapy.

Echinococcus multilocularis *infection*

Infection with the tapeworm *Echinococcus multilocularis* (alveolaris) is a less common but far more aggressive disease than that caused by *E. granulosus*. The definitive hosts are dogs, foxes, wolves and cats while field mice and other small rodents are the natural intermediate hosts. The geographic distribution includes south and central Europe, Siberia, Russia, Alaska and Canada, however it has been reported in Australia, South America, India and the United Kingdom. In the Arctic sled dogs are the usual source of infection while in agricultural regions the infection is usually related to ingestion of fruit or vegetables contaminated with canine faeces. The liver is the most common organ affected although widespread haematogenous dissemination is not uncommon. The cyst of *E. multilocularis* is multiloc-ulated rather than unilocular. The larva causes an invasive and destructive growth because humans cannot develop a pericyst. The infection therefore behaves like a malignant tumour and is extremely difficult to eradicate sur-gically. Presentation is with hepatomegaly, right upper quadrant mass and signs of portal hypertension, jaundice, ascites and splenomegaly. It is diffi-cult to differentiate between hepatocellular carcinoma and alveolar hydatid disease clinically and on imaging, since *E. multilocularis* causes echogenic solid-looking lesions. The disease runs a chronic course but ultimately is usually fatal. Sonography reveals a geographic, solid but ill-defined and echogenic single or multiple mass with propensity of spread to the hepatic hilum. Fine echogenic areas may give the resulting mass a 'hail-storm' appearance. The resulting mass may have a nodular appearance with cystic and necrotic areas. Calcification in the lesion is common (68 per cent). This appears punctate, usually 2 to 4 mm in diameter, typically spherical with central radiolucency on the conventional abdominal radiograph. Hepatomegaly occurs in 42 per cent of patients. Infection may be associ-ated with portal hypertension, portal vein thrombosis, inferior vena cava thrombosis, and splenic or retroperitoneal disease.

Schistosomiasis

The fresh water snail acts as an intermediate host in schistosomiasis. Cer-cariae penetrate the skin and reach the liver, gut and bladder via the blood stream. Here they promote a granulomatous reaction causing hepatic fibro-sis and cirrhosis. Schistosomiasis has been dealt with in the section on diffuse liver disease (see pp. 46-47).

Clonorchiasis

Clonorchis sinensis (the Chinese or Oriental liver fluke) is the most important liver fluke that infects man. It is prevalent in China, Japan and Indochina. It is an important pathogen causing cholangiohepatitis in the Far East. Snails and freshwater fish serve as intermediate hosts, infection in man usually occurs after eating raw fish (including dried, salted or pickled fish). The parasitic cysts are digested by gastric juice releasing the larvae which subsequently enter the common bile duct via the ampulla of Vater. The larvae migrate to the small intrahepatic ducts where they mature. After mat-uration the fluke returns to the common bile duct to lay its eggs. The infes-tation is often asymptotic but in severe infestation cholangiohepatitis and liver failure may occur. The complications of liver fluke infestations such as biliary calculi, liver abscesses, suppurative cholangitis with biliary dilatation or bile duct stenosis, periportal echogenicity and the development of hepatocellular carcinoma may all be detected on ultrasound. These ultrasound findings have all been described in the appropriate sections.

Chronic granulomatous disease

Chronic granulomatous disease of childhood is an X-linked recessive immune deficiency disorder associated with a congenital defect in leukocyte function. The polymorphonuclear leukocytes are unable to inactivate phagocytosed catalase-positive bacteria. This deficiency results in recurrent purulent infections with granuloma formation. The organisms involved include *Staphylococcus aureus*, *Serratia marcescens*, *Aspergillus* spp. and Gram negative cocci such as *Escherichia coli*. Children present with chronic infections of the skin, lymph nodes, lungs and liver. Pyoderma, chronic diarrhoea and perianal fistulae and abscesses are common. The condition is more common and appears to be more severe in boys. Sonography of the liver may reveal hepatomegaly with single or multiple liver abscesses and calcification. Early diagnosis is essential to institute effective antibiotic therapy.

Lepromatous leprosy

Leprosy is caused by *Mycobacterium leprae*, an acid-fast bacillus. The pathological response and clinical presentation depend upon the nature and extent of the host's response to the infection. With well-developed cell-mediated immunity, tuberculoid leprosy develops, but with failure of cell-mediated immunity lepromatous leprosy ensues. Lepromatous leprosy is a systemic disease with multiple organ involvement. The testis, bones, lymph nodes, liver, spleen and the kidneys are most often affected. Liver damage can be severe where poorly defined hypoechoic masses develop. Acid-fast bacilli are invariably present in aspirates from lepromatous lesions. The lepromin test is usually negative. There are conflicting reports on the influence of AIDS on leprosy. No convincing data has emerged to suggest an association.

2.1.13 TUBERCULOSIS OF THE LIVER

Calcified granulomas are not infrequently seen in the liver and spleen in regions where tuberculosis is endemic. Tuberculous granulomas can calcify irrespective of site and the liver, and particularly the spleen, may show multiple small calcific foci. Miliary tuberculosis often affects the liver but the miliary granulomas are not normally visible on imaging. However occasionally a 'starry sky' appearance can be seen in the liver. Tuberculous liver abscess is rare and only 444 cases have been reported in the world literature since 1930. Diagnosis is often delayed as the abscess may mimic a pyogenic or amoebic abscess. Diagnosis is usually made at laparotomy. Presentation is pyrexia of unknown origin and weight loss, but most patients are afebrile. The chest radiograph may be normal or show evidence of present or past tuberculosis. Sonography may show honeycomb liver with hypoechoic liver and splenic masses. The same lesions appear low attenuation and low density on CT.

2.1.14 HEPATIC VASCULAR ANATOMY

The liver receives blood via the hepatic artery and portal vein. Venous drainage is via the hepatic veins and via small veins directly from the caudate lobe to the inferior vena cava (hence the caudate lobe is relatively spared in the Budd–Chiari syndrome hepatic vein occlusion). Just over 70 per cent of hepatic blood flow is supplied by the portal vein but venous blood is only 80 per cent saturated with oxygen and portal venous blood supplies only 50 to 60 per cent of the hepatic oxygen requirement. The remaining oxygen is supplied by hepatic arterial blood which accounts for 25 per cent of the flow. This dual blood supply makes hepatic infarcts uncommon except in hepatic surgery which may directly affect the hepatic vasculature. In the absence of other diseases the hepatic artery may be occluded without major consequences. Portal and hepatic venous flow is essential for normal hepatic function. An exception seen with increasing frequency is the insertion of hepatic arterial lines for chemotherapy. If the hepatic artery is occluded chemotherapeutic agents given via the hepatic artery will tend to concentrate within the hepatic arterial branches and cause intense local necrosis eventually giving rise to biliary strictures. The portal vein branches, hepatic artery branches and bile ducts form portal triads running together in a collagenous sheath. They have echogenic margins and radiate from the porta hepatis branching as they pass into the liver. The hepatic veins run upwards and medially through the liver to the inferior vena cava. Unlike the portal veins the hepatic vein branches do not have visible walls. The calibre of the hepatic veins increases towards the diaphragm whilst the calibre of portal veins reduces. The portal vein is an isolated vascular unit as it is separated from both arterial blood flow and the inferior vena cava by capillaries. It shows a monophasic low velocity flow though there is often slight variation with respiration and pulsation of adjacent arteries. Hepatic veins drain via the inferior vena cava to the right atrium. They show triphasic flow. The hepatic arteries show a low resistance arterial pattern.

Portal venous anatomy

The portal vein forms behind the neck of the pancreas by the union of the splenic and superior mesenteric veins. It runs to the porta hepatis in the free edge of the lesser omentum and receives the cystic, pyloric, accessory pancreatic, superior pancreaticoduodenal and other small veins too small to visualise. Generally the portal vein enters the porta hepatis and divides into the right and left main branches. The right main branch divides into anterior and posterior branches supplying the anterior and posterior segments of the right lobe. The left main branch runs horizontally to the left before turning vertically to give rise to the medial and lateral segmental branches. Several variations of the portal venous anatomy have been described both at ultrasonography and cadaveric dissection (see Figure 2.7). These are uncommon and are seen in 1 of 100 patients.

1. Absence of the normal left main portal vein branch origin and the horizontal part of the left main portal vein. A branch of the right anterior portal vein radical supplies the left lobe of the liver.
2. Absence of the right main portal trunk, immediately after entering the porta hepatis the portal vein turns to the left without giving off any normal right portal vein branches. The right hepatic lobe is smaller than normal and is supplied by multiple small veins of varying sizes.
3. Lack of the right main portal vein trunk but with the presence of its branches. The anterior and posterior right portal vein branches arise by trifurcation of the main portal vein trunk.
4. The right posterior portal vein branch arises from the main portal vein trunk. The main portal vein then continues into the liver and bifurcates (Figure 2.7).

Portal vein congenital defects
Duplication.
Anomalous pulmonary venous drainage.
Atresia.
Abnormal ventral position.
Various fistulas.
Aneurysms.

Doppler studies of hepatic vessels

Flow studies of the hepatic vessels can give important information about the haemodynamic effects of hepatic parenchymal disease. Examination is not always straightforward as the liver can be quite mobile during respiration but breath holding can facilitate the demonstration of blood flow and hepatic waveforms particularly in the hepatic veins. Examination is

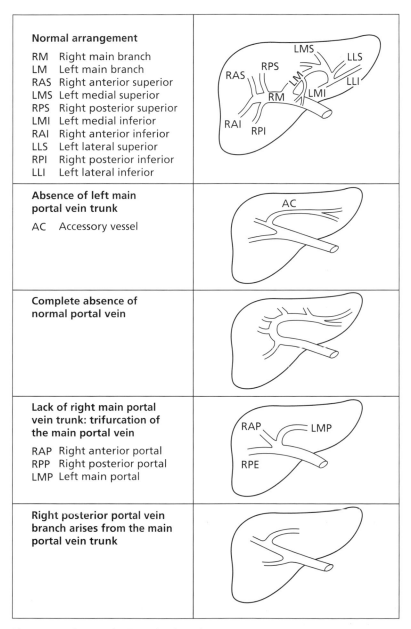

Normal arrangement RM Right main branch LM Left main branch RAS Right anterior superior LMS Left medial superior RPS Right posterior superior LMI Left medial inferior RAI Right anterior inferior LLS Left lateral superior RPI Right posterior inferior LLI Left lateral inferior	
Absence of left main portal vein trunk AC Accessory vessel	
Complete absence of normal portal vein	
Lack of right main portal vein trunk: trifurcation of the main portal vein RAP Right anterior portal RPP Right posterior portal LMP Left main portal	
Right posterior portal vein branch arises from the main portal vein trunk	

Figure 2.7 The portal vein and its branches.

undertaken with as small an angle as possible between the axis of the ultrasound beam and the long axis of the vessel, although generally fairly good Doppler signals can be obtained with an angle of less than 70 degrees. This is usually straightforward as the hepatic veins are running posteriorly to the inferior vena cava whilst the portal vein curves forwards as it passes through the porta hepatis. The blood flow waveform from the left hepatic vein frequently shows an artefact from transmitted cardiac pulsation, thus when the hepatic veins are examined the middle and right veins are usually assessed. The hepatic artery is small and usually has to be examined on suspended respiration. Doppler analysis of vascular flow patterns is a valuable adjunct to real time 2D scanning. Colour flow analysis is a valuable means of differentiating vessels from other fluid-filled structures. Power Doppler analysis is particularly valuable at demonstrating low flow rates in small vessels. Vascular indices, which are used in flow analysis, are 'time averaged mean velocity' and the 'pulsatility index'. The pulsatility index is low if the vascular bed is of low resistance and can accommodate sudden pressure waves. A high resistance or low compliance vascular bed will show a high pulsatility index.

Portal vein waveforms

The portal vein normally shows continuous forward flow with minor modulation by respiration and transmitted arterial pulsation (Figure 2.8). The rate of blood flow is greatest at the centre of the vessel and least at its margins. Average flow across a segment of the vessel is therefore used to overcome the internal variation with respiration and transmitted cardiac pulsation. Time averaged velocity is usually of the order of 12 to 14 cm/s in adults. Flow within the portal vein changes rapidly in response to eating. Blood flow to the small bowel begins to rise within 2 minutes of taking the first mouthful of food. Time averaged blood flow velocity in the portal vein may rise to 25 cm/s after a meal and, with minor increase in vessel diameter, flow volume may increase by 4 to 5 times. Increased mesenteric arterial flow may also increase the degree of transmitted arterial pulsation seen. The majority of patients with mild hepatic parenchymal disease show a normal portal vein blood flow. As hepatic disease becomes more severe the first detectable flow abnormality is a reduced increase in flow seen after a meal (Figure 2.9). The splenic and superior mesenteric veins may then begin to distend and the change in vessel calibre with respiration, which is seen in some normal patients, is lost. In severe hepatic parenchymal disease the portal vein blood flow is reduced and there is a rough correlation between the degree of reduction in portal flow velocity and the severity of hepatic parenchymal disease (providing the studies are performed on strictly fasting patients). As portal venous flow is further compromised, forward flow may only be seen during systole with reversed flow during diastole. Eventually

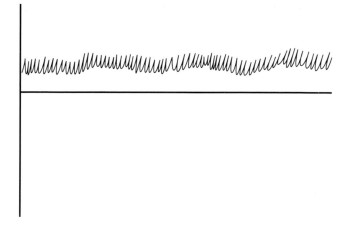

Figure 2.8 Portal venous flow. Normal portal vein Doppler flow trace. Time averaged mean velocity (TAV) in a fasting patient is 12–14 cm/s. After eating, portal venous flow increases by 4–5 ×. The vein dilates and the TAV rises to 25 cm/s. Transmitted arterial pulsations become apparent.

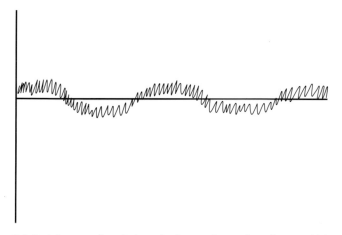

Figure 2.9 Portal venous flow in hepatic disease. Severe liver disease – high resistance to flow – 'balanced flow' forward flow only occurs during systole in the mesenteric arteries. Mild to moderate liver disease – the portal vein Doppler trace is normal. As liver disease progresses i) the first change to occur is a reduction in the normal flow increase after eating, ii) the time averaged mean velocity (TAV) is reduced with a rough correlation between the degree of liver disease and the reduction in TAV, iii) the 'balanced flow pattern' is seen. When disease is very severe reversed flow in the portal vein becomes persistent (but this can show a day-to-day variation).

flow within the portal vein may be continuously reversed but it should be remembered that the rate and direction of flow may vary from day to day particularly in cases of acute exacerbation of chronic liver disease. Serial examinations therefore give a better picture than single scans. (NB reduced portal flow velocity is associated with an increased risk of thrombosis.)

Portal venous shunts

The creation of artificial shunts between the portal venous and peripheral venous circulation is becoming increasingly common as a treatment for portal hypertension. Doppler ultrasound may be used to assess patency and show the direction of flow within the portal vein and shunt. If the walls of an artificial shunt prevent direct analysis of blood flow within it, then analysis of flow at the ends of the shunt usually allows adequate assessment of shunt function. Surgically created shunts include

1. portacaval (end–side of the main portal vein to inferior vena cava)
2. mesocaval
3. splenorenal (Warren).

The latter two shunts are used more frequently to leave the portal vein intact for transplant. Colour Doppler is valuable for evaluation of shunts.

Assessment of the patency of transjugular intrahepatic portosystemic shunts

Transjugular intrahepatic portosystemic shunts (TIPS) are percutaneously placed shunts via the jugular vein. TIPS is becoming popular as a means of decompressing the portal venous system as a definitive procedure or as a prelude to liver transplantation.

Sonographic evaluation Doppler ultrasound is a sensitive and relatively specific means of evaluating TIPS malfunction. Sonographic evaluation of the shunt is usually obtained within 24 hours after shunt placement to establish baseline velocities within the portal vein, hepatic veins and shunt. Baseline flow values are essential for accurate assessment of shunt function. Follow up studies are usually carried out at three-monthly intervals unless the clinical setting dictates the need for a more urgent examination. The main object for Doppler study of TIPS is to document flow in the shunt and search for stenosis. Successful shunt placement should double portal vein flow velocity and should result in antegrade flow if the flow was previously reversed. Shunt malfunction is suggested by a peak shunt flow velocity of either less than 90 cm/s or greater than 190 cm/s because of either reducing flow through the centre of the shunt or very high flow rate through a tight stenosis (sensitivity and specificity for a shunt malfunction are 84 per cent and 70 per cent respectively). Changes from the baseline are a decrease in peak flow of 40 cm/s or more, or an increase in peak flow velocity of 60 cm/s or more (sensitivity 71 per cent, specificity 88 per cent).

Direct observation of shunt thrombosis is possible with duplex/colour Doppler. Echo-enhanced (contrast enhanced) color Doppler ultrasound can also be helpful in the assessment of TIPS.

Complications of transjugular intrahepatic portosystemic shunts detectable with ultrasound

Early complications – intraperitoneal haemorrhage, shunt thrombosis, neck haematoma, compromise of hepatic blood supply (portal vein thrombosis, hepatic artery occlusion, hepatic infarction), failed stent deployment (inadequate stent expansion, stent retraction, stent fracture), biliary obstruction.

Delayed complications – shunt stenosis (1. pseudointimal hyperplasia, 2. hepatic vein stenosis).

Portal hypertension

Portal hypertension refers to elevated pressure in the portal venous system, which in most cases is related to increased impedance of blood flow through the liver as a result of cirrhosis. Traditionally the causes of portal hypertension (Figure 2.10) are subdivided into prehepatic, hepatic and posthepatic.

Prehepatic causes
1. Splanchnic arteriovenous fistula.
2. Splenic vein thrombosis.
3. Portal vein thrombosis.

Intrahepatic causes
1. Cirrhosis.
2. Malignant disease in the liver.
3. Nodular regenerative hyperplasia.
4. Idiopathic portal hypertension.
5. Sarcoidosis.
6. Schistosomiasis.
7. Myeloproliferative disorders.

Posthepatic causes
1. Inferior vena cava obstruction.
2. Budd–Chiari syndrome.

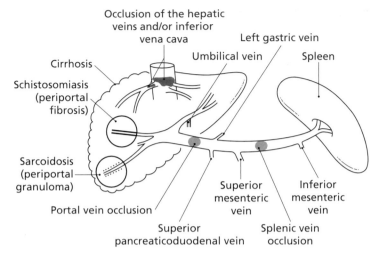

Figure 2.10 Causes of portal hypertension.

3. Veno-occlusive disease.
4. Cardiac disease.

Sonography of portal hypertension

Portal vein diameter is measured in a supine position, in quiet respiration, the patient having been starved for at least 4 hours. Measurements are made at the point where the portal vein crosses the inferior vena cava. In a normal individual the portal vein diameter is up to 13 mm (16 mm in deep inspiration), measurements over 13 mm under standard conditions indicate portal hypertension with a specificity of 100 per cent but a low sensitivity of 45 to 50 per cent. The sensitivity can be increased to 81 per cent by measuring splenic vein and superior mesenteric vein diameters. An increase in diameter by 20 to 100 per cent in deep inspiration is normal. An increase of less than 20 per cent is associated with portal hypertension.

Differential diagnosis of a dilated portal vein

Portal hypertension.
Splenomegaly and increased splenic blood flow regardless of the cause.
Acute portal vein thrombosis.
Post-prandial increase in portal vein diameter.

Portal flow direction and velocity

Normally blood flow in the portal vein is hepatopetal (towards the liver) during the entire cardiac cycle. The mean velocity of 15 to 18 cm/s shows variation with the cardiac cycle. In portal hypertension velocity fluctuations disappear giving rise to a continuous flow. With a further increase in portal venous pressure the blood flow direction becomes to and fro (biphasic) and finally the direction is reversed (hepatofugal).

Differential diagnosis of hepatofugal portal venous flow

Portal hypertension.
Budd–Chiari syndrome.
Side-to-side portocaval shunts.
Surgical or spontaneous splenorenal shunts with cirrhosis.
Tricuspid regurgitation (tricuspid flow reversal).
Severe congestive cardiac failure.

Differential diagnosis of reversal of hepatofugal to hepatopetal portal flow

Eating.
Drugs that increase portal flow.
Static flow without Doppler signal, occurs occasionally.

Pulsatile portal vein flow

A pattern similar to that seen in patients with impaired right heart function can occasionally be seen in patients with cirrhosis or portal hypertension. Patients with right-sided cardiac dysfunction with pulsatile portal vein flow invariably have an abnormal liver function.

Differential diagnosis of pulsatile portal vein flow

Tricuspid regurgitation.
Aortic–right atrial fistula.
Fistula between the portal vein and hepatic vein.
Portal hypertension.
Rarely a false positive finding.
Congestive heart failure.

Decreased volume flow in the portal vein

In mild to moderate portal hypertension volume flow in the portal vein is maintained. A reduction in volume flow occurs with advanced cirrhosis when intrahepatic obstruction to portal flow is severe as indicated by hepatofugal flow and extensive portosystemic collaterals.

The congestive index

Portal hypertension may be recognised by the 'congestive index'. This is the ratio of the portal vein area (cm^2) divided by the mean portal flow velocity (cm/s). This ratio reflects the physiological changes that occur in portal hypertension, that is portal vein dilatation associated with diminished flow velocity. In a normal individual the ratio should not exceed 0.7.

Splenomegaly

The size of the spleen does not correlate well with the level of portal hypertension, however if splenomegaly is absent portal hypertension is unlikely. The spleen is best measured in the coronal plane. A cephalocaudal measurement of over 13 cm suggests enlargement.

Splenic interface sign

Linear reflective channels are observed in the splenic parenchyma in a variable number of patients with portal hypertension. These channels could be explained by dilatation of intrasplenic venous sinuses with increased collagen in their walls and periarterial fibrosis. These pathological changes are known to occur in portal hypertension. This sign is seldom found in splenomegaly unrelated to portal hypertension. The vascular nature of these channels are readily confirmed by colour Doppler.

Ascites

Uncomplicated portal hypertension does not usually cause ascites. Ascites usually occurs secondary to underlying liver disease with liver cell failure.

Arterialisation of the hepatic blood supply

Hepatic arteries are enlarged and appear tortuous. As portal venous flow to the liver decreases arterial flow increases. Increased arterial flow occurs with the development of large collaterals and hepatofugal flow.

Differential diagnosis of an enlarged hepatic artery

Occluded or interrupted portal vein.
Surgical portosystemic shunt.
Reversal of flow in the portal vein.
Newborn infants receiving parenteral nutrition.
Hereditary haemorrhagic telangiectasia.
Cirrhosis or hepatic diseases associated with alcohol.
Vascular hepatic tumours.
Primary hepatic artery dissection.

Portosystemic venous collaterals

The demonstration of portosystemic venous collaterals indicates the presence of portal hypertension.

Sonography of portosystemic venous collaterals

Umbilical vein Umbilical vein collateral flow is an important feature of portal hypertension because it carries a specificity of virtually 100 per cent. An artery or vein with a diameter of up to 2 mm may normally be present within the ligamentum teres. Thus the mere demonstration of a blood vessel within the ligamentum teres does not equate to portosystemic venous collaterals. The diagnosis of portosystemic venous collaterals requires the demonstration of venous flow away from the liver. The enlarged umbilical vein is usually solitary originating from the left portal vein, which courses inferiorly through the falciform ligament and along the anterior abdominal wall to the umbilicus.

Coronary vein The diameter of a normal coronary vein is up to 4 mm, whereas a diameter of greater than 7 mm is evidence of an abnormal portal–systemic gradient (greater than 10 mmHg). As the coronary vein may be seen in some normal individuals its mere presence does not indicate portal hypertension. A coronary vein is seen as a prominent cephalad-directed vessel that joins with the portal vein near the termination of the superior mesenteric vein.

Splenosystemic collaterals These communications can form as a result of splenic vein occlusion as well as portal hypertension. The demonstration of splenic vein occlusion by ultrasound is straightforward as it is possible in most subjects to trace the splenic vein to the portal vein. With splenic vein occlusion, collaterals may be identified in the pancreatic bed or the gastroesophageal area.

Short gastric and gastroesophageal veins Tortuous vessels near the upper pole of the spleen and gastroesophageal junction are seen primarily on coronal images. Large portosystemic collaterals at the oesophageal-gastric junction may be mistaken for neoplastic masses if Doppler examination is omitted.

Right gastric veins These vessels are cephalad directed, and seen along the inferior border of the left lobe of the liver on longitudinal scans.

Splenorenal veins Tortuous inferiorly directed vessels from the splenic hilum to the left kidney, primarily seen on coronal images. The left renal vein may be dilated.

Retroperitoneal varices Retroperitoneal portosystemic collaterals (varices) may mimic other masses on both CT and ultrasound, such as carcinoma of the pancreas or other retroperitoneal tumours. Colour Doppler evaluation may show the mass to be full of flow colours and often associated with other signs of portal hypertension.

Banti syndrome (non-cirrhotic idiopathic portal hypertension)

This is a common cause of portal hypertension in India and Japan but is rare in the United States and Europe. The syndrome is characterised by signs of portal hypertension but the liver function tests tend to remain normal. Signs of hypersplenism are often present.

Sonography Ultrasound shows a liver that looks normal, patent hepatic veins and a patent portal vein that is associated with multiple portosystemic collaterals.

Portal vein thrombosis

Portal vein thrombosis is being recognised with increasing frequency at ultrasonography. Reduced portal blood flow because of hepatic parenchymal disease and abdominal sepsis are the major causes. Transient portal vein thrombosis is being recognised with increasing frequency partly because of the great increase in the use of ultrasound in the evaluation of patients with abdominal inflammation such as appendicitis. A tumour within the portal vein may have an appearance identical to thrombosis but is far less common; it is most frequently related to a hepatocellular carcinoma. Though this gives rise to serpiginous filling defects within the portal vein lumen, flow usually persists the tumour without complete occlusion. Adults who show acute portal venous thrombosis secondary to abdominal sepsis may show complete recovery and vessel recanalisation with successful treatment of the underlying sepsis. In children the portal vein may recanalise by the development of multiple small collateral channels seen as a partly echogenic band of small vessels running to the porta hepatis (cavernous transformation). These show reduced flow velocity of 2 to 7 cm/s. Non-visualisation of the portal vein is strongly suspicious of occlusion. The portal vein may then be seen as a band of high level echoes at the porta hepatis.

Causes of portal vein thrombosis

Idiopathic causes.
Causes secondary to a tumour – hepatocellular carcinoma, cholangiocarcinoma, pancreatic carcinoma, gastric carcinoma.
Traumatic causes.
Iatrogenic causes – umbilical vein catheterisation.
Abdominal sepsis – pancreatitis, perinatal omphalitis, appendicitis, diverticulitis.
Cirrhosis – especially in the young.

Sonographic features of portal vein thrombosis

Clot exhibits variable echogenicity. It is usually of moderate echogenicity but if recently formed it may be hypoechoic. Patent vessels may show increased intraluminal echogenicity because of erythrocyte rouleaux formation making slow-flowing blood slightly echogenic. Increased or decreased echogenicity within the lumen of portal vein in isolation is not sufficient to either diagnose or exclude portal vein thrombosis. Portal vein thrombosis eliminates the venous flow signal normally obtained from the lumen of the portal vein during either pulsed or colour flow Doppler. Colour flow Doppler can show flow around a thrombus that partially blocks the vein, however if flow is sluggish Doppler signal may not be detected. There may be colour flow in other small vessel collaterals. Incomplete occlusion may occur (common with neoplastic invasion) or thrombolytic recanalisation. The two cannot be differentiated on ultrasound. Cavernous malformation, spontaneous shunts and splenorenal and portosystemic collaterals may be seen. The underlying cause may be evident, for example hepatocellular carcinoma, metastases, cirrhosis and pancreatic neoplasms. The incidence of portal vein thrombosis is said to be low in portal hypertension. Portal vein thrombosis may complicate sclerotherapy. The 'string sign', thickening of the portal vein with narrowing of its lumen, is assumed to be caused by portal phlebitis; this is considered to be a precursor of portal vein thrombosis in patients with acute pancreatitis. The portal vein thrombus may calcify. The portal vein diameter is greater than 15 mm in 38 per cent of portal vein thrombosis cases.

Cavernous transformation of the portal vein

Cavernous transformation of the portal vein occurs with long-standing portal vein thrombosis because of the development of multiple small vessels in and around the recannalising portal vein. A leash of fine serpiginous vessels is seen in place of the portal vein. The application of colour or pulsed Doppler shows blood flow in these periportal collaterals around the thrombosed portal vein or replacing the vein. Time averaged mean velocity of blood flow in the recannalising portal vein is usually 2 to 7 cm/s. Cavernous transformation of the portal vein has been recorded as giving the appearance of a subhepatic 'sponge-like' mass. This appearance has also been reported in cases of pancreatic haemangiosarcoma. Bile duct varices, also called the 'pseudo-cholangiocarcinoma sign' are not infrequently observed by endoscopic retrograde cholangiopancreatography (ERCP) in portal hypertension because of cavernous transformation of the portal vein. It has been documented that this sign disappears following TIPS procedure.

Portal vein aneurysms

Portal vein aneurysms are rare. They are thought to be either congenital or secondary to portal hypertension. On ultrasound they appear as anechoic masses that connect with the portal venous system. Using colour and pulsed Doppler evaluation turbulent venous flow is shown within the aneurysm.

Portal venous gas

Gas within the portal venous system may occur secondary to bowel ischaemia, infarction, necrotising enterocolitis and other inflammatory conditions which reduce mucosal integrity or increase intraluminal pressure. Portal venous gas may be life threatening, it may suggest bowel infarction or bowel gangrene, and is often fatal in adults. The prognosis may not be so grim in children with necrotising enterocolitis. Gas may enter the portal vein by direct extension through the intestinal wall or by invasion of the portal vein by gas-forming organisms. Prior to ultrasonography the demonstration of gas in the portal venous system by plain film radiography was usually associated with a 100 per cent mortality. However, microbubbles of gas seen in the portal vein in patients with bowel inflammation and ischaemia carries a far better prognosis and although uncommon is not particularly rare if the portal vein is observed carefully in these patients.

Causes of portal venous gas
Intestinal infarction or gangrene – arterial or venous thrombosis and embolism.
Inflammatory bowel disease – ulcerative colitis, necrotising enterocolitis.
GI obstruction – oesophageal atresia, duodenal atresia and imperforate anus.
Iatrogenic causes – double contrast barium enema, injection of air during endoscopy, umbilical vein catheterisation.
Intra-abdominal abscess – septicaemia with gas-forming organisms.
Miscellaneous causes – gastric ulcer, diabetes mellitus and erythroblastosis fetalis.

Sonographic features of portal venous gas
Microbubbles are seen as intensely hyperechoic foci within the portal blood, that move with the flow. The high-amplitude echoes are usually seen in the non-dependent portions of the liver. The gas is rapidly carried peripherally within the intrahepatic portal vein branches and tends to collect in the uppermost branches (left lobe and anterior segment of the right lobe). Collection of gas is then seen as highly echogenic lines which may shadow. Doppler analysis may produce a 'pinging sound' and strong reflection with overloading of Doppler signal. Spectral analysis produces tall bidirectional spikes (because of the reflection from gas) superimposed upon a normal portal venous flow pattern. Differential diagnosis is from air in the biliary tree, which tends to be near the porta hepatis. Fat globules from an intrahepatic entrapment of umbilical vein catheter infusate may superficially resemble air within the liver. This will occur in a different clinical setting and usually in infants. Ultrasound shows layers of fat globules in fluid.

Hepatic artery

In most cases the liver is supplied from the coeliac axis. The coeliac axis, the most superior of the abdominal visceral arteries, arises from the anterior aortic surface and trifurcates 1 to 3 cm from its origin. The coeliac axis and its two major branches (the hepatic and splenic arteries) are readily identified at sonography. The common hepatic artery has a variable origin, arising from the coeliac axis in 72 per cent of cases, but less commonly from the superior mesenteric artery (4 per cent), the left gastric artery or directly from the aorta. In 11 per cent of individuals the right hepatic artery arises from the superior mesenteric artery and in 10 per cent the left hepatic artery arises from the left gastric artery. The common hepatic artery is the portion of the artery between its origin to the point where it gives off the gastroduodenal artery. The proper hepatic artery is the part of the hepatic artery between the origin of the gastroduodenal artery and the last artery supplied to the left lobe of the liver; the artery then proceeds as the right hepatic artery. The proper hepatic artery is not present if the left lobe arteries arise at the level of the gastroduodenal artery. The hepatic arterial system is well visualised on ultrasound from the anterior approach, using the liver as the acoustic window. The common hepatic artery is best visualised on transverse scans where it is readily traceable from its origin from the coeliac trunk. The proper hepatic artery is placed anteromedial to the portal vein seen with advantage on transverse or oblique scans. The right hepatic artery is anterior to the right portal vein, usually being seen at the porta hepatis lying between the portal vein posteriorly and the common hepatic duct (common bile duct) anteriorly. The left hepatic artery can also be traced with careful scanning within the substance of the liver running in a superior direction from the porta hepatis. There are no absolute measurements of hepatic artery size. As a rough guide a hepatic artery may be deemed enlarged when a 'double duct' sign is seen at the porta hepatis in the presence of a normal common bile duct.

Hepatic arterial waveforms

The normal liver has a relatively low vascular resistance as a result of which the hepatic artery shows fairly high-velocity forward flow throughout the cardiac cycle. The hepatic arterial waveform normally has a pulsatility index between 1 and 2. Patients with quite severe liver disease frequently show little change in the hepatic artery pulsatility or waveforms but a reduction in portal venous flow may be compensated for by an increase in hepatic artery flow. Increasing diastolic flow in these cases will result in a reduction in the pulsatility index. The flow patterns seen in adult liver disease do not necessarily occur in children who may show a completely different picture. Increasing vascular resistance in the cirrhotic paediatric liver may result in reduced diastolic flow hence increasing the pulsatility index. When liver disease is severe diastolic flow may be reversed and the pulsatility index may be as high as 10 (Figure 2.11). This pattern of hepatic artery flow is particularly common in children with secondary biliary cirrhosis such as occurs after partially successful treatment of biliary atresia. The progressive increase in the pulsatility index in these cases can be used as a means of monitoring disease progression.

Hepatic arterial blood flow changes in liver tumours

The majority of tumours of the liver have little effect on hepatic artery flow, though highly vascular tumours can result in increased flow and a reduction in the pulsatility index. Doppler examination does not usually aid diagnosis in these cases but can give a rough guide to the response to therapy. However on colour flow Doppler several patterns have been described in a variety of liver tumours.

1. 'Basket' network – a fine blood flow network surrounding the tumour nodule in 75 per cent of hepatocellular carcinomas.
2. Vessels running into and branching within the tumour in 13 per cent of hepatocellular carcinomas.
3. 'Detour' pattern – a dilated portal vein meandering around the tumour nodules in hepatic metastases.
4. 'Spot' pattern – colour-stained dots or patches in the central region of the tumour. Contrast enhanced colour Doppler ultrasound correlates well with angiographic findings when evaluating tumour vascularity. This non-invasive technique may be useful in diagnosing hypervascular hepatocellular carcinomas.

Hepatic artery aneurysm and pseudoaneurysm

Hepatic artery aneurysm is the fourth most common site of intra-abdominal aneurysm after aortic, iliac and splenic artery aneurysms. Most patients are asymptomatic prior to rupture, 80 per cent of patients experience a catastrophic rupture into the peritoneum, the biliary tree, gastrointestinal tract or portal vein. In most asymptomatic patients (60 per cent) diagnosis is often made from vascular calcification, or if the aneurysm is large it may produce symptoms from pressure effects. Rarely hepatic artery aneurysm may present with obstructive jaundice from pressure effect on the common bile duct or spontaneous rupture causing haemobilia, the latter itself may cause mild jaundice. The routine use of ultrasound has increased the likelihood of picking up asymptomatic hepatic aneurysms. Atherosclerosis,

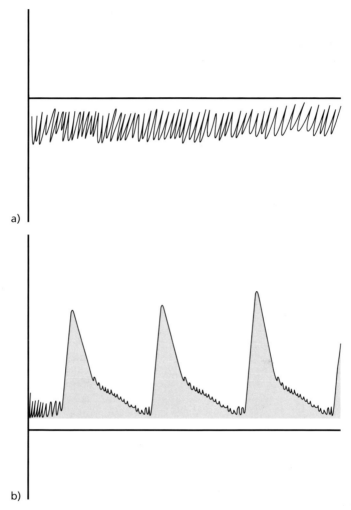

a)

b)

Figure 2.11 Portal vein flow. a) Very severe liver disease, continuous flow reversal. b) Hepatic arterial flow trace. Low resistance arterial system with relatively high diastolic flow, pulsatility index 1–2. NB – hepatic arterial flow may remain normal in liver disease but as the portal venous flow decreases arterial flow may be increased, increased diastolic flow leads to a reduction in the pulsatility index which may be less than 1.

infection and trauma account for most of these aneurysms. Hepatic artery aneurysms have been reported as a complication of gallbladder surgery. The approximate age at presentation is 38 years with a male to female ratio of 2/3 : 1. Extrahepatic aneurysms are four times more common than intrahepatic aneurysms. It is essential to diagnose these aneurysms because of their high mortality of up to 82 per cent at spontaneous rupture. Hepatic artery aneurysm can develop secondary to pancreatitis.

Sonography

Using colour and pulsed Doppler evaluation turbulent arterial flow can be shown within the anechoic liver mass.

Hereditary haemorrhagic telangiectasia (Osler–Weber–Rendu disease)

This is a hereditary autosomal dominant condition characterised by multiple skin and mucous membrane telangiectasia and visceral arteriovenous malformations. Any organ in the body may be involved, but the lungs and liver are more commonly affected. Approximately 60 per cent of cases are symptomatic by 16 years of age. Clinical presentation is usually with skin telangiectasis, epistaxis or sequelae of pulmonary arteriovenous malformation or liver dysfunction.

Sonography

There is a wide spectrum of vascular abnormalities ranging from minimal to severe. Ultrasound diagnosis of hepatic vascular malformation in hereditary haemorrhagic telangiectasia is difficult in mild cases. Doppler ultrasound with the clinical history allow easy differentiation of hereditary haemorrhagic telangiectasia from other causes of enlargement of hepatic artery. Differential diagnoses from dilated intrahepatic bile ducts is based on the co-existence of intrahepatic parallel channels with a dilated hepatic artery and a normal sized common bile duct. The coeliac axis may be enlarged. In more severe stages of hereditary haemorrhagic telangiectasia the findings might immediately suggest arteriovenous malformations. Because of its non-invasive nature sonography is ideal for screening patients with hereditary haemorrhagic telangiectasia.

The spectral waveforms show high velocity flow (even aliased or turbulent) in the hepatic artery and its branches as in arteriovenous anastamosis. Hepatic artery to portal vein shunts cause pulsatility of portal flow with phasic or continuous reversal. Hepatic artery to hepatic vein shunts may cause significant changes in the Doppler waveforms of the hepatic vein only in severe stages of the disease. Doppler findings can easily confirm the presence of hepatic vascular malformations and arteriovenous shunts and the haemodynamic significance of the shunts. Signs of portal hypertension may be present. The liver echogenicity may be altered usually to a heterogeneous echopattern.

Primary dissecting aneurysm of the hepatic artery

Dissection of the peripheral arteries without dissection of the aorta is rare. In descending order the frequency of primary dissection affects the renal, intracranial, pulmonary, superior mesenteric, coronary and hepatic arteries. A primary dissection of the hepatic artery is extremely rare (13 cases are reported in the literature), it leads to death in most instances and few are diagnosed before surgery or post mortem. Presentation is with right upper quadrant pain associated with biochemical liver abnormalities.

Sonography

A primary dissecting aneurysm appears as a tubular fluid-filled structure in the porta hepatis anterior to the portal vein. Doppler interrogation can then establish arterial flow in a dilated hepatic artery. The presence at ultrasound of an intimal flap or double lumen can confirm the diagnosis.

The hepatic veins

Superior veins (right, middle and left) drain most of the liver, they are normally up to 1 centimetre in diameter and pass obliquely back and upwards to the inferior vena cava. Small veins drain the caudate and adjacent part of the right lobe direct to the inferior vena cava. Separate caudate lobe venous drainage may allow preservation of caudate lobe function in hepatic vein obstruction (Budd–Chiari syndrome). Flow in the hepatic veins is complex as it is directly affected by flow and pressure changes in the right atrium and inferior vena cava (Figure 2.12). Throughout the greater part of the cardiac cycle flow is towards the heart, that is away from the ultrasound probe on the anterior abdominal wall. Forward flow towards the heart is reduced during right atrial systole as the pressure of right atrial contraction is carried back to the inferior vena cava and hepatic veins. Following right atrial systole there is a brief increase in hepatic vein flow, followed by a pressure wave caused by sudden tricuspid valve closure at the start of ventricular systole. The pressure wave caused by tricuspid closure may result in transient reversal of normal hepatic vein flow. The reversal of flow indicates that the liver is soft and compliant and can accommodate transient flow reversal. Hepatic parenchymal disease may increase hepatic rigidity, reducing compliance and preventing flow reversal. There is a rough correlation between the degree of flattening of the hepatic vein waveform and the degree of severity of hepatic parenchymal disease. Cardiac disease may affect the hepatic venous waveform generally increasing the waveform pulsatility but the effect depends upon the nature of cardiac disease and presence or absence of hepatic parenchymal disease. Hepatic disease increasing hepatic rigidity will reduce the effect of cardiac disease on the hepatic venous waveform. Prolonged or sudden severe inferior vena cava or hepatic venous congestion may cause hepatomegaly and jaundice. When the hepatic parenchyma is abnormally rigid, abnormal cardiac waveforms may be masked by reduced hepatic compliance.

Normal hepatic vein diameters

The maximum diameter of the main trunk right hepatic vein is

- 6.2 ± 1.43 mm in healthy men
- 5.6 ± 1.66 mm in healthy women.

Budd–Chiari syndrome

Budd–Chiari syndrome or hepatic venous occlusion is a spectrum of disease ranging from occlusion of a single hepatic vein to complete occlusion of the three major hepatic veins. Budd–Chiari syndrome is often clinically evident by hepatomegaly, ascites, abdominal pain and non-specific abnormalities of liver function tests. Budd–Chiari syndrome may be acute or chronic. The acute form is usually secondary to inferior vena cava or main hepatic vein thrombosis. The chronic form is related to fibrosis of the intrahepatic veins, presumably related to inflammation. There are two clinical conditions which may have similar manifestations

1. severe right-sided heart failure
2. hepatic veno-occlusive disease, this is characterised by inflammation of the post-sinusoidal venules resulting in their occlusion.

Causes of hepatic vein thrombosis

Idiopathic – 66 per cent.
Hypercoagulability states, especially polycythaemia rubra vera.
Paroxysmal nocturnal haemoglobinuria.
Collagen vascular disease.
Hepatic tumours especially hepatocellular carcinoma.
Renal and adrenal carcinoma.
Congenital hepatic webs.
Radiation.
Bone marrow transplantation.
Trauma.
Cardiac causes – right-sided failure, constrictive pericarditis.
Benign inferior vena cava obstruction with or without obstruction of the hepatic veins
    is the most frequent cause of Budd–Chiari syndrome in South Africa, Japan and

Korea. Two types exist – type I: membranous or web, type II: segmental obliter-ation of variable length. There is an increased risk of hepatocellular carcinoma.

Sonography

Colour flow Doppler shows abnormalities of the anatomy or flow. Visuali-sation of part or all of a hepatic vein on the right (regardless of apparent intraluminal echoes) but no flow or inappropriately directed flow on colour flow Doppler. No visualisation of part or all of a hepatic vein on either real time ultrasound or colour flow Doppler.

Discontinuity between the main hepatic vein and inferior vena cava

Reversed flow in hepatic veins – 'bicolour' hepatic veins

Intrahepatic collaterals:

- Intrahepatic veins that communicate with systemic vessels via sub-capsular collaterals
- Collateral vessels that shunt blood from occluded veins to non-occluded veins or to enlarged inferior hepatic veins or caudate lobe veins.
- Large collaterals that drain directly into the inferior vena cava
- Collateralisation is suggested when reversed flow is found which may be seen before and after shunting.

Portal vein changes:

- Flow may be hepatopetal or hepatofugal
- Portal flow dynamics may change between examinations

Inferior vena cava changes:

- No flow in inferior vena cava
- Reduced flow
- Very slow flow
- Balanced bi-directional flow
- Thrombus within the inferior vena cava
- Compression of the caudate lobe
- Long or localised segment narrowing
- Sonography easily depicts the echogenic membrane or fibrous cord in the inferior vena cava which is a common cause of chronic Budd–Chiari syndrome
- Sonography is not an accurate means of measuring the pressure gra-dient in the inferior vena cava, but the choice of appropriate decom-pressive shunt (mesoatrial versus portocaval or mesocaval) is dependent on the presence of pressure gradient within the inferior vena cava. Venography is likely to remain an important part of evalu-ation of Budd–Chiari syndrome in any patient in whom surgical decompression is being considered.

Veno-occlusive disease of the liver

This may be regarded as a variant of Budd–Chiari syndrome. Unlike classical Budd–Chiari syndrome there is no occlusion of the inferior vena cava or the major hepatic veins. The basic pathophysiology is related to the occlusion of the post-sinusoidal venules by an inflammatory process. Veno-occlusive disease is said to occur in up to 25 per cent of patients treated with bone marrow transplantation and usually occurs in the first 3 weeks after the procedure. An early diagnosis is desirable as veno-occlusive disease has a mortality of 83 per cent and may respond to treatment.

Sonography

Earlier work suggested that it is possible to establish a diagnosis using ultrasound, by showing an increase in the resistive index in the hepatic artery and decrease or reversal of flow in the portal vein. However latter work has been disappointing reflecting the non-specificity of the above mentioned signs. Thus at the present stage veno-occlusive disease remains a clinical or histological diagnosis.

Hepatic vein waveform in chronic liver disease

Duplex ultrasound of the hepatic veins may be useful for studying liver disease associated with fibrosis and steatosis. In patients with well-compensated liver disease flattening of the Doppler waveform suggests the presence of cirrhosis.

Splenic venous flow in chronic liver disease

Patients with chronic liver disease and Doppler ultrasound findings of splenic venous flow that exceeds portal venous flow usually have porto-systemic varices which tend to be large and have a high incidence of bleeding.

Passive hepatic congestion

Compromise of liver venous drainage causes passive hepatic venous congestion. It is not an uncommon complication of congestive heart failure and constrictive pericarditis, wherein the elevated central venous pressure is transmitted from the right atrium to the hepatic veins. Passive hepatic congestion is often accompanied by hepatomegaly. Hepatocytes are extremely sensitive to ischaemic injury even over short periods. A variety of heart-related circulatory disorders might inflict ischaemic injury on the liver.

Sonography

The inferior vena cava is distended associated with dilated hepatic veins. The normal variation of the inferior vena cava calibre with respiration is lost. Ascites may occur. The portal or splenic veins may show a variable degree of dilatation. Hepatomegaly may occasionally be associated with mild to moderate splenomegaly. There is variable echogenicity of the liver from echopoor to bright. In acute venous congestion the 'starry sky' appearance may occur. Pleural or pericardial effusions are often present. While scanning the liver cardiomegaly and cardiac rhythm abnormalities may be obvious.

Distension of inferior vena cava and hepatic veins

In central venous congestion the mean inferior vena cava diameter may increase from 8.8 ± 1.26 mm to 13.3 ± 1.74. The variation in the calibre of the vein with respiration is also diminished. Distension of the hepatic veins can be seen on cross section providing evidence of passive hepatic congestion.

Hepatic venous and inferior vena cava reflux

On intravenous administration of ultrasonic contrast, via an arm vein, contrast may reflux from the right atrium during right ventricular systole entering the inferior vena cava and hepatic veins directly from the right atrium in a retrograde manner without taking its normal course through the right ventricle. This can cause retrograde enhancement of the hepatic veins.

Abnormal hepatic venous and inferior vena cava flow

The inferior vena cava and hepatic veins normally show a triphasic flow pattern (Figure 2.12). In patients with elevated central venous pressure this triphasic wave pattern is lost. Colour Doppler may show a mixed flow pattern. In long-standing cardiac cirrhosis a unidirectional low velocity continuous flow may supervene.

Increased portal venous pulsatility

Apart from a minor increase in portal venous flow during expiration flow tends to be continuous. In patients with passive venous congestion the

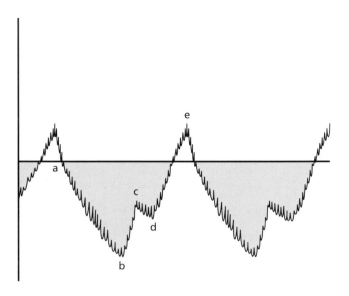

Key	
a–b	Flow from liver to the inferior vena cava
b–c	Pressure wave of right atrial systole reduces forward flow into the inferior vena cava
c–d	Flow into the inferior vena cava increases as atrial systole ends
d–e	Pressure wave from right ventricular systole and tricuspid valve closure reverses inferior vena cava and blood passes back into hepatic veins

Figure 2.12 Hepatic venous flow pattern.

elevated right atrial, inferior vena cava and hepatic pressure is transmitted into the portal vein via the sinusoids. This results in a pulsatile portal venous blood flow.

Differential diagnosis of hepatic vein distension

Congestive cardiac failure.
Tricuspid atresia or stenosis.
Tumour within the right atrium, inferior vena cava or invaded hepatic veins.

Clot within the hepatic venous system.

Constrictive pericarditis.

Inferior vena cava stenosis or web.

2.1.5 INTRAOPERATIVE ULTRASOUND

Intraoperative ultrasound can make a significant contribution to hepatic cancer surgery by aiding tumour characterisation, showing vascular invasion and allowing guided intraoperative biopsy. Intraoperative ultrasound allows biopsy of the liver via a sheath or port preventing seeding of tumour cells to the peritoneum or abdominal wall. The biopsy track within the liver can be planned such that any seeding of tumour cells within the liver will occur only within the segment(s) which will be resected. If the tumour can be resected under these controlled conditions then biopsy at laparotomy or percutaneous biopsy at laparoscopy need not render a curable liver mass inoperable. Intraoperative ultrasound at laparoscopy has the advantage that the appearance of the liver surface can be compared with the sonographic appearance of the liver parenchyma, and the liver surface can be palpated with the ultrasound probe. Haemangiomas, for example, are soft and can be compressed whilst Doppler evaluation will show refilling of the vascular spaces of the haemangioma as compression is removed. Intraoperative ultrasound is essential to liver surgery as a means of showing the margins of the tumour and any areas of vascular invasion. As the transducer probe is placed on the liver surface a high frequency probe can be used thus ensuring a high quality image. Intraoperative ultrasound will also show tumours more clearly than MRI and CT and thus new lesions may be found at surgery changing the staging of tumours and altering the level of resection necessary. Intraoperative ultrasound allows identification of portal vein branches within the liver. These can be cannulated and injected with indigo carmine. This process stains the liver segment within minutes, the stain becoming visible on the liver surface, facilitating the liver segment to be marked by means of electric cautery on the liver surface. The technique can be further refined by the placement of a 6F balloon catheter under ultrasound guidance in the portal vein branch, the balloon is subsequently inflated to create a bloodless field during surgery.

2.1.6 LIVER IMAGING: ULTRASOUND CHECKLIST

Liver Parenchyma:
1. Size
2. Outline
3. Overall echogenicity

- Increased
- Decreased
- Diffuse abnormal echogenicity
4. Focal echogenicity
    - Echogenic
    - Echopoor
    - Echolucent
5. Intra-hepatic bile ducts
    - Dilated ducts?
    - Pneumobilia?
6. Portal vein
    - Dilated?
    - Thrombosed?
    - Cavernoma?
7. Focal masses
    Single?
    Multiple?
        Echogenic?
        Echopoor?
        Mixed?

Gallbladder:
    Non-visualisation/contracted gallbladder?
    Double Gallbladder?
    Gallstones?
    GB thickened?
    Ultrasonic Murphy's sign?
    Distended GB?
    Echogenic GB wall?
    Polyps?
    Signs of perforation?

2.2 BILIARY SYSTEM

2.2.1 BILE DUCT ANATOMY

The right and left hepatic ducts unite at the porta hepatis to form the common hepatic duct which enters the free edge of the lesser omentum. It is joined by the cystic duct forming the common bile duct. The main left and right bile ducts lie anterior to the left and right portal veins. The hepatic artery branch usually lies anterior to the right portal vein but is often posterior to the left portal vein. In the liver the bile ducts run with portal vein and hepatic artery branches in a common sheath called the portal triad. The

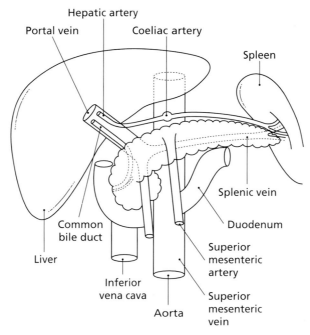

Figure 2.13 Anatomic relations at the porta hepatis.

common bile duct is approximately 8 cm long (Figure 2.13). It lies in the free edge of the lesser omentum, usually situated anterolateral to the portal vein. It then passes behind the superior part of the second part of the duodenum and traverses the head of the pancreas to the end at duodenal papilla. Behind the duodenum the common bile duct lies anterior to the portal vein with the gastroduodenal artery on its left side. Behind the head of the pancreas the common bile duct lies on the inferior vena cava, at this point it receives the common pancreatic duct and turns to the right to enter the duodenum. Just below the porta hepatis the right branch of the hepatic artery is usually seen passing between the common hepatic duct anteriorly and the portal vein posteriorly. The main variations of the hepatic duct confluence have been shown in Figure 2.14.

Common bile duct dimensions

The upper limit of normal for the common bile duct is 5 mm, 6 to 7 mm is regarded as equivocal and greater than 7 mm is usually pathological, although bile duct diameter does increase in elderly patients and post-

Typical anatomy RA Right anterior RP Right posterior LH Left hepatic	57%	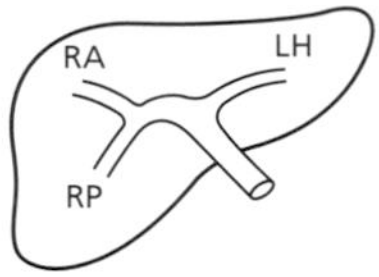	
Triple confluence	12%	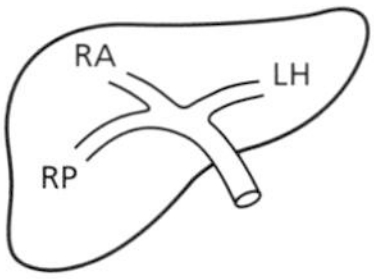	
Ectopic drainage of right sectorial duct into the common hepatic duct	20%	a) 16% 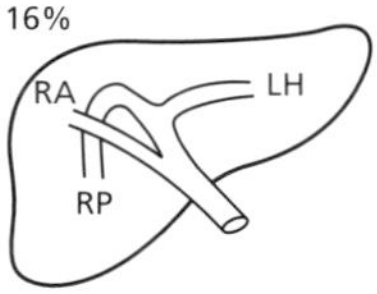	b) 4% 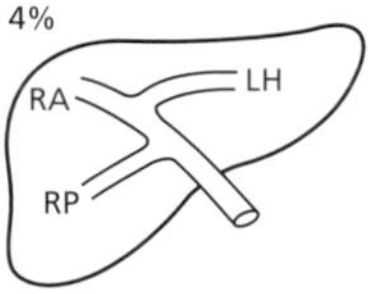
Ectopic drainage of right sectorial duct into the left hepatic ductal system	6%	a) 5% 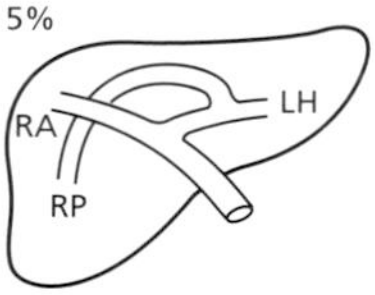	b) 1% 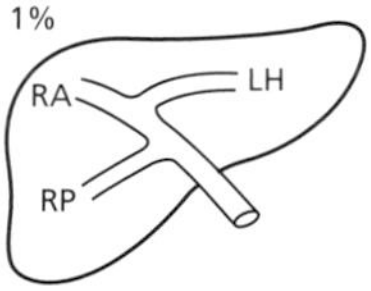
Absence of hepatic duct confluence	3%	a) 2% 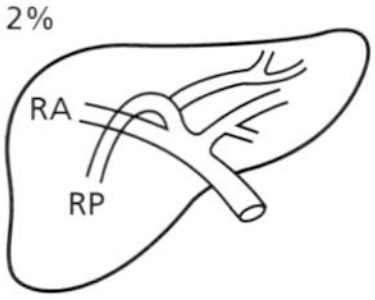	b) 1% 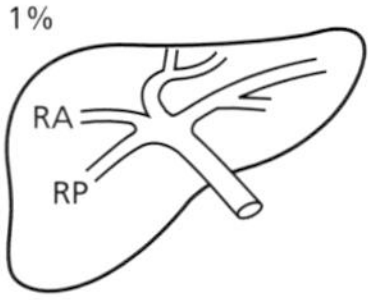
Absence of right hepatic duct and ectopic drainage of the right posterior duct into the cystic duct	2%	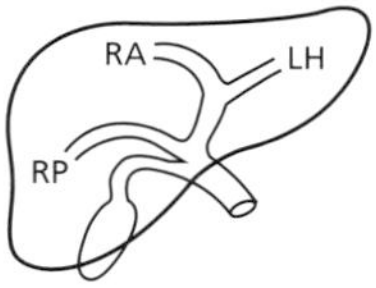	

Figure 2.14 Main variations of the hepatic duct confluence (Couinaud 1957).

cholecystectomy. The normal bile duct is 4 mm or less in 95 per cent of the adult population. In 98 per cent the common hepatic duct is 5 mm or less at the porta hepatis, while at the head of the pancreas the common bile duct normally shows slight narrowing. The intrahepatic duct just proximal to the common hepatic duct measures 2 to 3 mm. The cystic duct lies posterior to the common bile duct in 95 per cent and anterior to the common bile duct in 5 per cent of individuals. The cystic duct runs in in a common sheath with the common bile duct before their lumens unite, thus cholecystectomy leaves a variable length of cystic duct *in situ*. Stones can form in the cystic duct remnant compressing the common bile duct and thus causing jaundice (Mirrizzi syndrome).

Common bile duct diameter in children

In neonates and infants less than 1 year old the common bile duct diameter is less than 1.6 mm. In children and early adolescence the normal common bile duct is less than 2.5 to 3.0 mm. The common bile duct is distensible and responsive to fluctuation in prandial bile flow. The size increases slowly with age at a pace equal to the hepatic artery and half that of the portal vein. The duct is larger (slightly!) in children with contracted gallbladder, in contrast to the findings in adults.

Often there is discrepancy between the common bile duct diameter measurement between ERCP and ultrasound. This has been attributed to a variable cross section of the common bile duct, which is oval in 70 per cent of patients. The standard ultrasound technique involves measuring the anteroposterior diameter of the common bile duct. The anteroposterior diameter for oval and round ducts is similar, but the transverse diameter of an oval duct is greater. Thus there will be a discrepancy between ERCP and ultrasound when anteroposterior diameters are measured on ultrasound and conventional transverse diameters are measured on ERCP. Also, ERCP involves the injection of contrast during which the biliary system is stretched by the pressure of injection. Since transverse common bile duct measurements on ultrasound correlate better with disease than conventional anteroposterior diameters, transverse measurements can be useful in confirming or excluding bile duct dilatation when anteroposterior diameters are larger than normal. Post-cholecystectomy common hepatic duct and common bile duct dimensions are generally slightly greater than prior to surgery. Normal postcholecystectomy common hepatic duct mean diameter is 0.52 cm, and common bile duct 0.62 cm, at the porta.

Patients with gallstones also tend to have larger extrahepatic bile ducts though this does not always mean that there are gallstones within the bile ducts at the same examination.

2.2.2 SONOGRAPHIC EVALUATION OF THE BILIARY SYSTEM: TECHNIQUE

All examinations involving the biliary tree should be performed in a fasting state to allow optimal images of the gallbladder. Patients should be starved for 6 hours for optimal gallbladder distension and also to keep bowel gas to a minimum. If possible gallbladder examinations should be carried out early in the morning as bowel gas is at a minimum at this time. The gall-bladder lies under the liver usually directed to the right with the neck directed to the common bile duct beneath the porta. However, the position is quite variable and the gallbladder will change position with patient movement. Scanning is carried out in transverse, longitudinal and oblique planes. The most important rule in gallbladder evaluation is to remember to turn the patient from side to side when scanning or small stones may be easily missed if they lie hidden behind mucosal folds. Free movement of a stone within the gallbladder is the best way of confirming the presence of a stone and excluding a polyp. With careful scanning the cystic duct may be visualised in 51 per cent of patients. The Trendelenburg position may aid cystic duct filling if it is not visible on supine scanning. The cystic duct is posterior to the common bile duct in 95 per cent and anterior to the common bile duct in 5 per cent of individuals. The common bile duct should be examined in supine and both oblique and lateral decubitus positions. A knee–chest or Trendelenburg position may move calculi in the common bile duct to a more superficial position. A drink of water fills the pylorus and duodenum and may facilitate visualisation of the lower common bile duct. Ultrasound shows 75 per cent of calculi in the common bile duct. False negative diagnoses may occur when bowel gas obscures the distal common bile duct or when a calculus is lodged within a non-dilated duct. Soft pigment stone may also be misdiagnosed. Acoustic shadowing is less commonly seen in common bile duct stones than gallbladder stones, particularly those which have arisen after cholecystectomy reflecting the incidence of soft pigment stones without significant calcification in these cases.

False positive diagnoses may occur as a result of an echogenic gall-bladder neck or periampullary echoes. The overall accuracy of ultrasound detection of extrahepatic gallstones is over 80 per cent but high degrees of accuracy require careful scanning technique and meticulous attention to patient movement and positioning during scanning. Gallstones are common so any investigation of the gallbladder and biliary system should involve a full examination of the upper abdomen and gallstones frequently co-exist with other disease.

Modern ultrasound scanners show bile ducts adjacent to major portal vein branches in the liver, these should be no more than 20 per cent of the diameter of the adjacent veins. The umbilical vein portion of the left portal vein may be mistaken for a bile duct; the left portal vein branch runs horizontally, then runs out at an acute angle to form the umbilical portion. The left hepatic duct does not run at an acute angle but branches off to the left lobe, running superior to the umbilical portion of the portal vein.

2.2.3 BILIARY OBSTRUCTION

The upper limit of normal for the serum bilirubin level is around 17 mmol/L. Patients with elevated serum bilirubin do not become visibly jaundiced until the serum bilirubin level exceeds 30 mmol/L. Increased serum bilirubin may occur secondary to increased red cell breakdown, hepatocellular dysfunction or obstruction to biliary drainage. These groups are not clearly defined as any longstanding biliary obstruction may cause hepatocellular damage, which may cause persistent jaundice even after the biliary obstruction has been relieved. Jaundice is described in more detail in the following sections.

Dilatation of the biliary tree usually precedes biochemical evidence of biliary obstruction and jaundice, thus ultrasound is more sensitive than biochemistry at the detection of biliary obstruction. The degree of biliary dilatation depends upon the degree of obstruction, the speed of onset and the duration and compliance of the system.

In sudden complete obstruction dilatation may take a week to occur, but generally in patients with established jaundice lack of biliary dilatation excludes the diagnosis of major bile duct obstruction (excluding cases of sclerosing cholangitis). It should be remembered that lymphadenopathy at the porta hepatis may cause biliary obstruction without dilatation of the extrahepatic ducts but intrahepatic duct dilatation should be visible. A biochemical picture of obstructive jaundice may occur because of intrahepatic obstruction at a canalicular level. These cases will have obstructive biochemistry with normal calibre intra- and extrahepatic ducts. Biliary manometry has been performed at percutaneous transhepatic cholangiography showing an almost linear relationship between bile duct diameter and biliary pressure. The normal intraduct pressure is between 5 and 18 cm of water. This close relation between bile duct size and pressure makes ultrasound a reliable means for detection of extrahepatic biliary obstruction but sonography is less reliable at determining the level and cause of obstruction. When doubt exists about the state of the biliary system a repeat examination after a short delay may be invaluable. When the signs of biliary obstruction are equivocal, the response to a fatty meal or administration of intravenous chloecystokinin may be helpful; this causes gallbladder contraction, relaxation of the sphincter of Oddi and increased bile flow from the liver. Under normal circumstances the common bile duct shows little change in diameter, or there may be a reduction in diameter by up to 3 mm. With an obstructed common bile duct the diameter remains unchanged or may increase.

2.2.4 BILIARY DILATATION

Dilatation of peripheral radicles

The major intrahepatic bile ducts may be visible near the porta hepatis but the remaining intrahepatic ducts are not normally seen. When intrahepatic ducts are dilated they become visible and are seen as tubes which lie directly adjacent to the portal vein branches giving the double-barrel shotgun sign. Bile causes less attenuation of the ultrasound beam than blood in the adjacent veins and soft tissues, thus distal acoustic enhancement may be evident. Dilated ducts seen in transverse section have a double-barrel appearance because of the adjacent portal venous radicle.

Dilatation of the common hepatic duct

The point of union of the cystic duct and common hepatic duct cannot be exactly defined on ultrasound and thus the point of transition from common hepatic duct to common bile duct cannot be accurately demarcated. The common hepatic duct is seen anterolateral to the portal vein in the porta hepatis. The right branch of the hepatic artery is frequently seen passing between these two structures. The upper limit of normal for common hepatic duct diameter is 5 mm. Common hepatic duct dilatation is not always associated with intrahepatic bile duct dilatation particularly in early cases of biliary obstruction.

Dilatation of the common bile duct

The dilated common bile duct lies anterolateral to the portal vein. When examining the patient their right side should be raised to bring the common bile duct anterior to the portal vein.

Dilatation of the gallbladder

This is an unreliable sign of biliary obstruction as

- the normal gallbladder can show marked enlargement when a patient is fasting
- some patients with frank obstruction show only slight gallbladder distension
- a diseased gallbladder may be incapable of contraction or distension.

Signs of intrahepatic biliary dilatation

Only the major intrahepatic biliary radicles are normally visible. These are seen adjacent to the portal vein branches close to the porta hepatis. Visualisation of smaller bile ducts within the liver is always abnormal.

Signs of biliary dilatation

Parallel channel sign
In longitudinal section two anechoic tubes are seen side by side. The tube with the echogenic walls is a portal vein branch, the dilated bile duct does not have visible walls.

Double-barrel shotgun sign
In transverse section the dilated bile duct and adjacent portal vein branch are seen as two adjacent anechoic circles.

The presence of too many tubes
An arrangement of dilated bile ducts, giving the operator the impression that there are too many tubular structures in the liver, has been likened to a monkey-puzzle tree.

Dilated ducts are often beaded and tortuous
Dilated bile ducts cause less sound attenuation than adjacent blood-filled veins. Focal areas of acoustic enhancement may thus be seen behind dilated bile ducts. This may make assessment of liver parenchyma difficult. Any tubular structure with no visible walls and posterior enhancement in the liver should be regarded as a dilated duct unless proven otherwise. Application of colour or power Doppler may be helpful in differentiating a dilated duct from vascular structures.

2.2.5 JAUNDICE

Neonatal jaundice

In utero, bilirubin crosses the placenta and is excreted by the mother. After birth the infant must activate its own excretory mechanism. In the 2 to 3 days following birth the bilirubin level rises resulting in 'physiological jaundice'. This jaundice usually clears at the end of the first week of life. The bilirubin is largely unconjugated and the baby remains well. Jaundice may be more severe and prolonged in preterm infants, especially if complicated by hypoxia and hypoglycaemia, bowel obstruction and ileus (the latter conditions increase bilirubin reabsorption). Unconjugated bilirubin is lipid soluble. It is bound to albumin in blood but may cross the blood–brain barrier and cause severe neurological deficit. In a healthy full term infant bilirubin greater than 380 mmol/L is the threshold for severe neurological damage; the threshold is much lower in preterm and sick infants.

Jaundice in the first 24 hours of life may be related to congenital transplacental infections which include toxoplasmosis, rubella, cytomegalovirus, herpes simplex and syphilis. The majority of cases however are caused by excess haemolysis. Haemolytic disease of the newborn results from an incompatibility with maternal antibodies, the mother being sensitised by mismatched transfusion or from a previous pregnancy, for example the mother is Rh negative and the baby Rh positive. The antibodies cross the placenta causing haemolysis of foetal blood resulting in increased bilirubin production. After birth the bilirubin level rises rapidly causing severe jaundice in the baby. The baby may be severely anaemic associated with generalised oedema (hydrops fetalis) because of severe haemolysis *in utero*. Haemolysis may also be due to a lack of enzymes, for example glucose-6-phosphate dehydrogenase, or inherited red blood cell anomalies such as spherocytosis. Jaundice beginning between the second and fifth day may be pathological because of infection (for example *Escherichia coli* septicaemia), galactosaemia or haemolysis caused by birth trauma. Delayed jaundice may be secondary to breastfeeding, hypothyroidism, neonatal hepatitis, galactosaemia and biliary atresia, and it may occur in infants of diabetic mothers. Jaundice in the neonate can be subdivided into unconjugated and conjugated types though it is more convenient to classify it by medical and surgical causes from the management point of view. The causes of unconjugated hyperbilirubinaemia are physiological jaundice of the newborn, haemolysis and genetic anomalies of bilirubin metabolism (rare). The main causes of conjugated hyperbilirubinaemia are infection, metabolic abnormalities (alpha$_1$-antitrypsin deficiency, cystic fibrosis and hereditary tyrosinaemia), idiopathic, bile duct malformation or atresia and bile duct stasis due to total parenteral nutrition. The medical causes of jaundice are inherited metabolic disease, intrauterine infection, cystic fibrosis, alpha$_1$-antitrypsin deficiency, bacterial or viral sepsis and idiopathic neonatal jaundice. The surgical causes of jaundice in a neonate include biliary atresia or hypoplasia, choledochal cyst, spontaneous bile duct perforation, bile plug syndrome and intrahepatic ductal atresia or hypoplasia. See Figure 2.15 for the management of neonatal jaundice.

Ultrasonography

Ultrasonography is the initial imaging investigation of choice in jaundiced babies but can only exclude biliary atresia in normal cases. In those cases in which ultrasonography has failed to confirm the normality of the biliary system other investigations must be performed. Biliary atresias caused by an intrauterine insult to the bilary system may prevent normal development or lead to fibrous obliteration of an atretic duct system. It may be intra- or extra-hepatic and, rarely, the extent of the atresia may progress after birth. The normal bile ducts in neonates are too small to see and do not usually become dilated above an atretic segment. Biliary atresia is thus a diagnosis of exclusion. If a jaundiced neonate has a normal-looking liver and gallbladder and

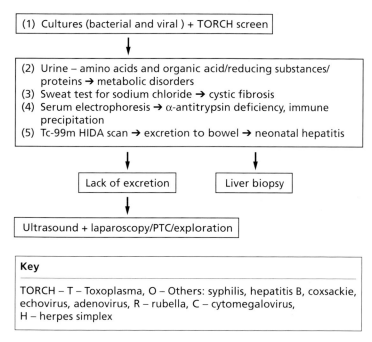

(1) Cultures (bacterial and viral) + TORCH screen

(2) Urine – amino acids and organic acid/reducing substances/
    proteins → metabolic disorders
(3) Sweat test for sodium chloride → cystic fibrosis
(4) Serum electrophoresis → α-antitrypsin deficiency, immune
    precipitation
(5) Tc-99m HIDA scan → excretion to bowel → neonatal hepatitis

Lack of excretion

Liver biopsy

Ultrasound + laparoscopy/PTC/exploration

Key

TORCH – T – Toxoplasma, O – Others: syphilis, hepatitis B, coxsackie,
echovirus, adenovirus, R – rubella, C – cytomegalovirus,
H – herpes simplex

Figure 2.15 Management of neonatal jaundice. Surgery in atresia must be early
to reduce the risk of biliary cirrhosis.

the gallbladder contracts well after a fatty meal the child does not have biliary atresia (the gallbladder can occasionally be seen in cases of biliary atresia, thus seeing a gallbladder does not exclude this disease). Unfortunately the main differential diagnosis in severely jaundiced babies is neonatal hepatitis and these babies may show poor bile flow such that the gallbladder (if seen) is poorly filled and shows little contraction following a fatty meal. Thus, if the normality of the biliary system has not been proven by sonography the diagnosis still rests between neonatal hepatitis and biliary atresia. In these cases an isotope (HIDA) scan is undertaken. If there is evidence of bile excretion to the bowel (delayed images may be necessary) the child does not have biliary atresia, but if no excretion is seen the differential diagnosis remains the same. These cases will require either liver biopsy, percutaneous transhepatic cholangiography or laparotomy. Some cases which have laparotomy will prove to have neonatal hepatitis with a normal biliary system rather than biliary atresia, since it is not always possible to show bile excretion in severe neonatal hepatitis. None the less it is important that children with biliary atresia have surgery within the first few weeks of birth or they will suffer severe liver damage leading to cirrhosis. As you cannot adopt a wait-and-see policy in these cases, some cases of neonatal hepatitis will necessarily come to laparotomy to exclude biliary atresia.

Jaundice in children

Jaundice in children is usually hepatocellular, obstructive jaundice is comparatively rare although we are seeing gallstones in children with increasing frequency. Gallstones seen in neonates usually reflect bile stasis, particularly if the child was ill at birth, and these stones often resolve spontaneously over the next year. The causes of obstructive jaundice include biliary atresia, neoplasms especially rhabdomyosarcoma and lymph nodes at the porta hepatis, biliary calculi, acute pancreatitis and choledochal cyst. After the neonatal period ultrasound is the imaging of choice in children presenting with jaundice. In medical jaundice ultrasound examination usually does not show bile duct dilatation. In surgical jaundice bile duct dilatation will usually be apparent except in very young children. The cause of the obstruction may also be seen, for example choledochal cysts, calculi, etc.

Jaundice in adults

Jaundice in adults may be the result of haemolysis giving rise to an isolated rise in bilirubin while the rest of the liver function tests are either normal or show borderline abnormalities. There are a group of familial non-haemolytic hyperbilirubinaemias with accumulation of unconjugated bilirubin in Gilbert's and Crigler–Najjar syndrome and conjugated hyperbilirubinaemia in Dubin–Johnson and roter syndromes. Jaundice in familial non-haemolytic hyperbilirubinaemias is usually biochemical and imaging studies are normal. There are a group of conditions which cause hepatocellular damage or intrahepatic bile stasis with no biliary dilatation. These conditions include acute viral hepatitis, drug-induced hepatitis, alcohol abuse (large tender liver), hepatic metastases, benign recurrent cholestasis, primary biliary cirrhosis (positive antimitochondrial antibody) and primary sclerosing cholangitis (associated with inflammatory bowel disease). The function of ultrasound in these patients is to exclude large duct obstruction and surgically curable causes of jaundice. Ultrasound should be able to distinguish obstructive from non-obstructive jaundice with 95 per cent accuracy. With lesions at the porta hepatis the accuracy of ultrasound is near 100 per cent. False negative examination may occur with intermittent bile duct obstruction (usually from calculi) or primary sclerosing cholangitis as fibrosed bile ducts may not be able to dilate (in clinical practice this is quite uncommon). Jaundice if obstructive can be further evaluated with radionuclides (Tc-99m HIDA) CT, ERCP, magnetic resonance

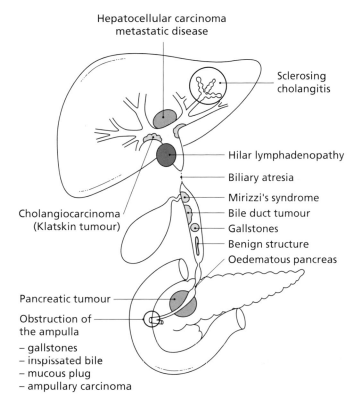

Figure 2.16 Causes of obstructive jaundice.

scanning and PTC (percutaneous transhepatic cholangiogram). Sonographic guidance makes entry into a dilated system easier when performing PTC thus speeding the procedure and reducing complications. Obstructive jaundice is common amongst adults and has multiple causes (see gamut).

The clinical presentation of intrahepatic cholestasis and large duct obstruction are similar as the basic fault lies in defective delivery of bile to the duodenum. The history is usually that of jaundice, itching or both. The stools are pale and the urine dark.

Causes of obstructive jaundice in adults (see Figure 2.16)

Benign causes – traumatic or iatrogenic stricture, biliary calculi, pancreatitis both acute and chronic, pancreatic pseudocyst, sclerosing cholangitis, recurrent pyogenic cholangitis, oriental cholangiohepatitis ascariasis, liver flukes, aortic aneurysm, liver cyst, duodenal diverticulum, benign tumours, common bile duct sludge (particularly in patients with AIDS and cystic fibrosis), bile duct papilloma or adenoma, migration of inferior vena cava umbrella.

Malignant causes – pancreatic carcinoma, ampullary carcinoma, duodenal carcinoma, cholangiocarcinoma (Klatskin tumour), primary hepatocellular carcinoma (at hilar location), biliary papillomatoses.

Metastases – gastric, pancreatic, colon, lung, breast and lymphoma.

Bile duct obstruction is often associated with infection especially *Escherichia coli*, *Klebsiella* spp., enterococci and *Proteus* spp.. The risk of infection is twice as great with calculi as with malignancy. Thus, when undertaking cholangiography antibiotic cover should be given.

2.2.6 CONGENITAL BILIARY ATRESIA

Biliary atresia is an uncommon condition affecting 1 in 20 000 live births, but it should always be considered in cases of neonatal jaundice as the complications of delayed diagnosis are severe. Biliary atresia is now thought by some to be an active postnatal process, possibly caused by an intrauterine insult, it is not a static anatomic defect but has a changing spectrum. This accounts for difficulties in differentiation of infection and biliary atresia. Biliary atresia may take one of several forms

1. diffuse extrahepatic biliary atresia (commonest) most probably caused by chronic cholangitis *in utero*
2. Focal atresia, probably as a result of intrauterine vascular insult, this form is more amenable to treatment
3. intrahepatic ductal atresia, which may be related to intrauterine infection such as by reovirus.

Microscopically there is proliferation of bile ducts in all the portal triads. An association has been reported with polysplenia and trisomy 18 in 15 per cent of cases. In classical biliary atresia, microscopic ductules lose their patency at the porta hepatis by the age of 3 months, but usually much sooner. Therefore if treatment is to be effective surgery should be performed early, hopefully within 1 month of the onset of jaundice. The success rate of Kasai operation depends upon the stage of disease, when performed at less than 60 days of age the success rate is 90 per cent, it is 50 per cent when surgery is carried out between the age of 60 and 90 days. The success rate falls dramatically to 17 per cent when surgery is delayed beyond the age of 3 months (although the above success rates are published in the literature it is the authors' experience that, although surgery may successfully relieve the obstruction irreversible liver damage will have occurred by 30 days and early diagnosis and surgery are essential).

Diagnosis of congenital biliary atresia

Diagnosis is achieved with a combination of Tc-99m HIDA, ultrasound, laparoscopy and cholangiography. On ultrasound initially the liver shows slight enlargement. Hepatic echogenicity may be normal or may be heterogeneous and increased. The presence of a visible gallbladder (20 per cent) reduces the likelihood of biliary atresia but does not exclude it. Gallbladder contraction after a fatty meal is presumptive evidence of biliary drainage, but it may not occur. Thus in cases of neonatal hepatitis absence of gallbladder contraction does not shorten the differential diagnosis. Although sonography is valuable in assessment of the biliary system, dilated ducts are not evident in extrahepatic biliary atresia and Tc-99m HIDA isotope scan is a valuable means of demonstrating biliary drainage. Severe cases of neonatal hepatitis may also show abnormalities of biliary drainage because of bile stasis and all such cases should have further assessment of the biliary system by laparoscopy or cholangiography. Bile formation occurs from the twelfth week of intrauterine life. The earlier that atresia occurs *in utero* the greater the liver damage that occurs before birth. Thus, despite early diagnosis and intervention some cases have irreversible liver damage at presentation.

2.2.7 IDIOPATHIC NEONATAL HEPATITIS

This diagnosis is arrived at by a process of exclusion when infection, metabolic disorders, etc. have been ruled out. A liver biopsy, which is a part of the diagnostic work-up, reveals giant cell transformation with the bile ducts usually free of bile. However in severe neonatal hepatitis this causes cholestasis and may mimic biliary atresia. Elements of both biliary atresia and neonatal hepatitis may co-exist. Neonatal hepatitis may resolve spontaneously.

Sonography

The diagnostic pathway has been described under the management of jaundice. An ultrasound scan may be normal but the gallbladder may not be visualised. The bile ducts are of normal calibre. Hepatic echogenicity is often normal at presentation but may be increased in long-standing cases. The differential diagnosis is from biliary atresia.

2.2.8 SPONTANEOUS PERFORATION OF EXTRAHEPATIC BILE DUCTS

This is a rare cause of jaundice in the neonate. The commonest site of perforation is the confluence of the cystic and hepatic ducts. The age range affected is usually 5 weeks to 3 years with no apparent gender predilection. The pathogenesis is unknown but transient obstruction of the common bile duct from a mucous plug, inspissated bile or cholelithiasis has been implicated. The possibility of congenital narrowing has also been raised. The clinical presentation is with jaundice, failure to thrive and abdominal distension.

Sonography

Sonography may reveal ascites (biliary) and loculated subhepatic and porta hepatis fluid collections. The porta hepatis fluid collection is usually clear bile with posterior acoustic enhancement and may thus mimic a choledochal cyst. Tc-99m HIDA may demonstrate diffuse leakage into the peritoneal cavity. A collection of the radionuclide may occur at the porta hepatis at the site of the bile 'pseudocyst', again mimicking a choledochal cyst.

2.2.9 CHOLEDOCHOCOELE

Choledochocoele is a cystic dilatation of the intraduodenal part of the common bile duct with herniation of the common bile duct through the ampulla, it is akin to a ureterocoele in the bladder. It may be congenital or acquired. The congenital type is said to originate from a small diverticulum distal to the common bile duct found in 5.7 per cent of the normal population. A stenosis of the terminal part of the lumen of the common bile duct associated with intrinsic weakness of the wall of the duct has also been implicated. The acquired choledochocoele may result from stenosis of the duct following the passage of a calculus. Patients may present either as children or young adults with right upper quadrant pain and jaundice. They may give a history of several episodes prior to the diagnosis being reached.

Sonography

Choledochocoeles can be difficult to see on ultrasound as they may be surrounded by gas in the duodenum. They often contain calculi and sludge. If the common bile duct is dilated this may be seen on ultrasound. The imaging procedure of choice is cholangiography which may show a localised dilatation of the intraluminal part of the common bile duct. On ERCP the smooth club-like intraduodenal filling defect with a sack-like dilatation may sometimes be seen. The differential diagnosis includes cholelithiasis, choledochal cysts and pancreatitis.

2.2.10 CHOLEDOCHAL CYST

Choledochal cyst represents a congenital cystic dilatation of the biliary system. The cystic duct and the gallbladder are not usually affected. An

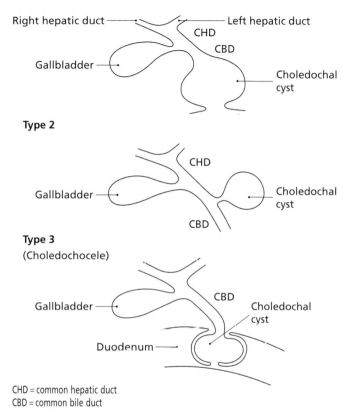

CHD = common hepatic duct
CBD = common bile duct

Figure 2.17 Choledochal cysts.

anomalous junction of the pancreatic duct and common bile duct proximal to the sphincter is the most probable cause. This arrangement allows a build up of high pressures within the pancreatic duct that allows reflux of enzymatic fluid into the common bile duct weakening its walls. These cysts may be classified into different types by their anatomy (Figure 2.17).

1. Localised cystic dilatation of the common bile duct. Common hepatic duct, cystic duct and the gallbladder are normal, this is the commonest form.
2. Choledochal cyst is a diverticulum arising from the common bile duct.
3. Choledochocoele (see above).
4. Dilatation of the whole of the common bile duct and common hepatic duct.

There is an association with dilatation, stenosis or atresia of other parts of the biliary system, gallbladder anomalies, failure of union of the left and right hepatic ducts and polycystic liver disease. Occasionally the pancreatic duct and accessory bile ducts may drain directly into the choledochal cyst. Eight per cent of cases are associated with Caroli's disease. Choledochal cysts usually present with an abdominal mass, pain, fever or jaundice. The latter is only present in 42 per cent of cases and only 25 per cent give a classic history. The incidence of cysts is greatest in children but may occur in adults and may be associated with gallstones, pancreatitis or even secondary biliary cirrhosis. There is an increased incidence amongst females and orientals.

Sonography

The cysts are seen as anechoic fluid-filled structures in the right upper quadrant though their communication with the biliary tree may not be apparent. There may be an abrupt change of calibre at the junction of the dilated to the non-dilated bile ducts. The remaining biliary system may be dilated but despite this choledochal cysts may be indistinguishable from other upper abdominal cysts. The diagnosis may be confirmed with Tc-99m HIDA, which normally accumulates within the cyst (but not always).

Differential diagnosis of choledochal cyst

Hepatic cyst.
Pancreatic pseudocyst.
Enteric duplication cyst.
Renal cyst.
Adrenal cyst.
Hepatic artery aneurysm.
Spontaneous perforation of the bile ducts.
Omental or mesenteric cyst.
Hydronephrotic kidney.

2.2.11 CAROLI'S DISEASE

This is a rare syndrome in which there is non-obstructive saccular dilatation of the intrahepatic bile ducts. This is associated with an increased incidence of gallstones and cholangitis. Some cases are also associated with medullary sponge kidneys, renal tubular ectasia, congenital hepatic fibrosis, autosomal recessive renal polycystic disease and rarely choledochal cysts. Caroli's disease is thought to be a form of congenital biliary ectasia but usually presents in adults. It is more common in females than males. Secondary biliary cirrhosis and portal hypertension may occur but are uncommon. There is an increased incidence of cholangiocarcinoma in patients with Caroli's disease. Clinical presentation in the second or third decade is usually with cramp-like upper abdominal pain.

Sonographic features

Sonography shows irregular dilatation of intrahepatic bile ducts without an obvious extrahepatic cause such as nodes at the porta. Small intraduct stones, sludge and gallstones may also be evident. Portal vein radicles may appear entirely surrounded by dilated bile ducts, which may show 'bridge' formation across the lumina. There may be intraluminal bulbar protrusions.

2.2.12 BILE PLUG SYNDROME

Bile duct obstruction by inspissated bile is a rare but correctable cause of conjugated hyperbilirubinaemia in infancy. The condition is associated with cystic fibrosis, erythroblastosis fetalis and total parenteral nutrition. Sonography may reveal a dilated common bile duct and intrahepatic ducts associated with sludge in the common bile duct and gallbladder. Differential diagnoses at this age include biliary atresia, neonatal hepatitis and choledochal cysts (especially debris-filled) may mimic a bile plug syndrome.

2.2.13 CHOLANGITIS

Acute cholangitis

Acute cholangitis represents an acute infection or inflammation of the bile ducts that may be related to previous iatrogenic bile duct stricture, bile duct stones, primary sclerosing cholangitis, percutaneous or endoscopic bile duct drainage, parasitic infestation and malignant bile duct strictures. Presentation is usually with right upper quadrant pain, pyrexia, rigors and jaundice. Blood cultures are positive in over 90 per cent of cases and usually yield *Escherichia coli*, *Klebsiella* spp., *Pseudomonas* spp. or enterococci. Acute cholangitis may take one of two forms

1. a non-suppurative form in which the patient remains non-toxic and the bile is usually clear
2. a suppurative form which occurs in less than a quarter of the patients, it is usually associated with either bile duct calculi or bile duct or pancreatic malignancy.

Prognosis is poor if the biliary system is not decompressed, with 100 per cent mortality. Mortality is over 50 per cent even with treatment.

Sonography

There are no specific sonographic features but ultrasound may reveal the predisposing factors such as gallstones, neoplasm or parasites (for example ascaris) associated with bile duct dilatation. Biliary sludge may be present or there may be features of pneumobilia. Occasionally common bile duct strictures are seen.

Sclerosing cholangitis

Sclerosing cholangitis represents a chronic inflammation of the biliary system. Presentation is with intermittent jaundice or vague non-specific symptoms such as general debility, abdominal pain, pruritis or fever. Recurrent pancreatitis may be the presenting symptom in 14 per cent of patients. Over half the patients give a history of previous biliary surgery. Secondary biliary cirrhosis, portal hypertension or cholangiocarcinoma may complicate sclerosing cholangitis.

Sonography

Sonography may reveal brightly echogenic portal triads, low reflectivity peri-portal collar or features of portal hypertension in long-standing cases. Bile duct dilatation is usually minimal because of fibrosis from pericholangitis. Bile duct wall thickening has been reported but this also occurs in cholangiocarcinoma and suppurative cholangitis. The differential diagnoses include a cholangiocarcinoma, primary biliary cirrhosis and acute cholangitis, the latter may usually be excluded on the basis of presenting history.

Primary sclerosing cholangitis

Primary sclerosing cholangitis represents a chronic non-specific inflammation of the biliary system of unknown aetiology, although a hypersensitivity reaction has been implicated. There are no predisposing factors and diagnosis is only made if the following conditions are excluded: gallstones, malignancy, previous biliary surgery, primary biliary cirrhosis, inflammatory bowel disease or retroperitoneal fibrosis. Presentation is with progressive jaundice of obstructive type. The role of sonography is to rule out secondary causes of cholangitis.

Secondary sclerosing cholangitis

This form of sclerosing cholangitis is secondary to other diseases which are mostly autoimmune in nature. Most cases are associated with inflammatory bowel disease, 1 to 4 per cent of patients with inflammatory bowel disease will develop the condition. It occurs most frequently with ulcerative colitis.

An association has been described with retroperitoneal fibrosis, chronic active hepatitis, Reidel thyroiditis, hypothyroidism and Peyronie's disease.

Recurrent pyogenic cholangitis

Recurrent pyogenic cholangitis is synonymous with oriental cholangitis or cholangiohepatitis, biliary obstruction syndrome and intrahepatic pigment stone disease. It is a progressive disease of uncertain aetiology. Many believe that there is an association with parasitic infestations such as ascariasis, clonorchiasis and *Trichuris trichiura*. There is also the belief that dead parasites act as nidus for developing biliary calculi. Clinical presentation is with recurrent attacks of cholangitis with abdominal pain, jaundice (77 per cent), rigors, nausea and vomiting. The liver function tests reveal an obstructive type picture. Hepatomegaly is invariable. The age at presentation is usually between 20 and 50 years with no gender predilection. In recurrent pyogenic cholangitis both the intrahepatic and extrahepatic bile ducts are dilated and contain soft pigment stones, debris and pus.

Sonography
The common bile duct is invariably dilated, dilatation is not always related to the location of calculi. There is intrahepatic biliary dilatation in 66 to 79 per cent of cases. In 50 to 90 per cent of patients intrahepatic calculi are detected. Most, but not all, calculi shadow. Isoechoic stones may be easily missed. Pneumobilia may obscure gallstones. Non-shadowing extrahepatic calculi are more easily seen than intrahepatic calculi because of bile duct dilatation and surrounding bile. Bile duct strictures are seen in 22 per cent of patients. There may be periportal echogenicity, portal vein occlusion, calculi within the gallbladder, hepatomegaly, splenomegaly and other evidence of portal hypertension (for example varices). Pyogenic liver abscesses, cholangiocarcinoma, segmental hepatic atrophy, biloma and pancreatitis may complicate recurrent pyogenic cholangitis. The differential diagnosis is from Caroli's disease.

2.2.14 AIDS-RELATED CHOLANGIOPATHY

AIDS-related cholangitis is usually related to opportunistic infection of the biliary tree. Cytomegalovirus and *Cryptosporidium* cholangiopathy may occur at any stage of HIV. *Mycobacterium tuberculosis* usually affects the early to intermediate stage of immunocompromise when the CD4 lymphocyte count is 200 to 750/mm^3. Protozoon, fungal and *Mycobacterium avium* intracellulare infections occur when the CD4 counts are severely depressed (less than 200/mm^3). Cytomegalovirus is found in two-thirds of autopsies. Co-infection with *Cryptosporidium* sp. and *Candida albicans* is common. Clinical presentation is with nausea, vomiting, jaundice and right upper quadrant pain. The liver function tests may reveal obstructive type biochemistry.

Sonography

Sonography may reveal a dilated gallbladder with sludge. The gallbladder may show mural thickening and both the intra- and extrahepatic bile ducts may be dilated. Echogenic nodules may occur at the lower end of the common bile duct caused by oedema of the papilla of Vater. Asymptomatic reversible gallbladder thickening has been described in patients receiving interleukin-2 infusion therapy for AIDS. Biliary obstruction has also been associated with non-Hodgkin's lymphoma, primary biliary lymphoma and Kaposi's sarcoma in AIDS patients. Differential diagnoses include acalculus cholecystitis, papillary stenosis and sclerosing cholangitis.

2.2.15 PRIMARY BILIARY CIRRHOSIS

Primary biliary cirrhosis is an idiopathic cholangitis affecting the interlobular and septal bile ducts. There is a progressive destruction of these ducts associated with portal fibrosis and regenerative liver parenchymal nodules. Primary biliary cirrhosis primarily affects females, with a male to female ratio of 1 : 9. The age of onset is usually in the late forties to early fifties. Clinical presentation is insidious with pruritis followed by jaundice and skin pigmentation. Serological blood tests show positive antimitochondrial antibodies in 65 to 100 per cent of patients associated with increased levels of immunoglobulin M in 95 per cent of patients. Liver function tests usually reveal an obstructive type of biochemistry. Other disorders said to be associated with primary biliary cirrhosis include thyroid disease, scleroderma, the sicca complex, renal tubular acidosis and hypertrophic pulmonary osteoarthropathy.

Sonography

Ultrasound examination may be completely normal in the early stages. Even with advanced disease the extrahepatic bile ducts are normal. Nearly half the patients have hepatomegaly. The tortuous small intrahepatic ducts with narrowing and calibre variation seen on ERCP in 50 per cent of patients are rarely seen on ultrasound. Cholelithiasis is present in 39 per cent of cases obscuring the underlying cirrhosis. The changes in the intrahepatic ducts are probably related to distorted hepatic architecture due to cirrhosis and may be used as a sign that cirrhosis has supervened. However the abnormal intrahepatic cholangiographic findings of primary biliary cirrhosis are not related to its clinical severity. In advanced stages the signs of portal hypertension such as portal vein dilatation, varices, ascites and splenomegaly may be apparent. Lymphadenopathy at the porta hepatis and in the hepatoduodenal ligament is a feature of primary biliary cirrhosis and may be visualised on ultrasound. Changes in the size of the lymph nodes in the hepatoduodenal ligament may reflect inflammation and cholestasis in primary biliary cirrhosis and thus may be used as a prognostic indicator. There is no association between lymph node size and histologic stage.

2.2.16 HEPATOBILIARY ASCARIASIS

Ascaris lumbricoides infests one quarter of the world's population. The parasite is 15 to 35 cm long and colonises the gastrointestinal tract where it may cause intestinal obstruction, volvulus or even perforation. Most age groups are affected but it is predominantly a disease of children and young adults. There is slight female preponderance. The worm lives mainly in the jejunum. Most gastrointestinal infestations are asymptomatic, serious complications may occur when the ascaris migrates up the bile ducts where it may cause acute cholecystitis, ascending cholangitis, liver abscess, pancreatitis or obstructive jaundice. However not all biliary invasions are symptomatic. Migration of the worms into the biliary tree is as frequent a cause of biliary pathology as calculus disease in endemic areas. Migration into the gallbladder is rare. Pregnancy and anomalous origin of the cystic duct arising directly from the ampulla of Vater increases the incidence of round worm migration into the gallbladder. The incidence of increased migration in pregnancy may be related to hormonal changes and smooth muscle activity resulting in stasis and common bile duct dilatation. The clinical features associated with biliary ascariasis include recurrent biliary colic, pyogenic cholangitis, vomiting of round worms, hepatomegaly and acute cholecystitis. Some features are vague such as biliousness, others present with obstructive jaundice. Fragments of the adult worm or their ova may form a nidus for the development of biliary calculi. In areas where the worms are endemic, ascariasis is a common cause of 'acute abdomen' in children second only to acute appendicitis, with 37.7 per cent presenting with symptoms of biliary disease.

Sonography

A single or multiple tubular structure 2 to 4 mm wide with a central echolucent line (representing the alimentary canal of the worm) can be detected within the dilated common bile duct. There may be features of associated pancreatitis, liver abscesses or intestinal obstruction. Sludge within the gallbladder is common and air within the bile ducts and liver is not unusual.

The roundworms may get impacted in the larger intrahepatic ducts where they appear as immobile echogenic serpiginous tubes with a central echolucent canal. When the roundworms enter the gallbladder, they appear as mobile echogenic intraluminal tubes with a characteristic zigzag movement on real time sonography. A round to oval non-shadowing mass may occasionally be seen representing a dead macerated worm associated with or without biliary dilatation. In the latter instance the differential diagnosis includes a sludge ball, non-shadowing gallstone, and cholangiocarcinoma. The pure intraluminal location makes the diagnosis of a cholangiocarcinoma less likely. Biliary ascariasis should be included in the differential diagnoses when such masses are seen in young people in endemic areas. Only a single case of biliary ascariasis associated with cholangiocarcinoma detected by sonography has been reported in the English literature.

2.2.17 MUCINOUS BILIARY PAPILLOMATOSIS

Mucinous biliary papillomatosis is a rare cause of biliary obstruction. It appears in the fifth to seventh decades of life and occurs three times as often in men as in women. It has an indolent course, high recurrence rate, and a risk of malignant transformation. The disease is considered to be a low-grade malignancy that has a significant rate of recurrence but not widespread metastasis. Patients usually present with obstructive jaundice, epigastric pain, haemobilia and anaemia. A small number of mucinous biliary papillomatosis cases are asymptomatic, presenting as a biochemical abnormality of liver function tests. Several associations have been reported namely, cholelithiasis, chronic gallbladder disease, choledocholithiasis, gallbladder dysplasia, choledochal cyst, gallbladder papilloma, gallbladder adenoma, ampullary carcinoma and *Clonorchis sinensis* infestation. A common link may be recurrent cholangitis. Death occurs as a result of secondary biliary cirrhosis and liver failure and can be as early as 5 to 6 years after presentation. Diagnosis is important for early intervention.

Sonography

The imaging findings in mucinous biliary papillomatosis reflect the gross macroscopic appearance of a doughy or jelly-like loose tumour found in the bile ducts. Sonography shows a non-shadowing expansile solid mass of intermediate echogenicity that is fairly well defined and demarcated from the surrounding bile duct wall. Such a mass may represent the tumour alone or a combination of tumour and mucoid sludge. Proximal bile duct dilatation is often present and calculi within the gallbladder and/or common bile duct may be identified. ERCP or percutaneous cholangiography reveals single or multiple polypoid filling defects within the bile duct(s) with proximal bile duct dilatation. ERCP may also show excessive mucous or blood within the common bile duct and duodenum. CT shows a solid intra-luminal bile duct mass with proximal biliary dilatation. The wall of the bile duct remains well defined. Endoluminal masses within the biliary tract are rare but have a wide differential diagnosis that includes various carcinomas and adenomas, biliary metastasis, granular cell myoblastoma, lipoma, fibroma, carcinoid, carcinosarcoma, sludge ball, non-shadowing gallstone, ascaris, blood clot, neuroma, granuloma and material from a ruptured hydatid cyst. Most of these masses are single, whereas more than 90 per cent of mucinous papillary adenomas are multiple. Cholangiocarcinoma is often scirrhous, brightly echogenic, ill defined and diffusely infiltrative, with apparent loss of the involved bile duct wall. An identical appearance to that of biliary papillomatosis has been described in mucinous cholangiocarcinoma with CT but not ultrasound. Mucin secretion is also a feature of mucinous cholan-giocarcinoma and mucinous cystadenocarcinoma. However, their gross and histological features differ from those of mucinous biliary papillomatosis.

2.2.18 PNEUMOBILIA

Pneumobilia is the presence of air within the biliary tree. This is usually caused by air ascending from the duodenum but may be rarely due to cholangitis. Ascending air is seen most frequently after ERCP and sphinc-terotomy but may also occur after the passage of gallstones or distortion of the lower common bile duct by local inflammation, tumour or duodenal ulceration. Air within the bile ducts is seen as densely echogenic lines with shadowing along the course of the biliary system. The air is not carried peripherally to the same extent as portal venous gas.

Causes of gas in the biliary tree

Following ERCP.
Sphincterotomy.
Following surgery – biliary–enteric anastamosis.
Biliary fistula – passage of stone (90 per cent), gastric/duodenal ulcer, gastric/colonic carcinoma, bile duct carcinoma, gallstone ileus, following cholecystectomy, carcinoma gallbladder, Crohn's disease.
Trauma.
Duodenal diverticulum (ruptured).
Emphysematous cholecystitis.
Cholangitis.
Patulous ampulla.
Rupture of hydatid cyst into the bile ducts.
Hepatobiliary ascariasis.

Tracheobiliary fistula – a rare congenital anomaly presenting with respiratory distress in the newborn.

Effect of drugs on the sphincter – magnesium sulphate, atropine, nitroglycerine and dopamine.

2.2.19 BILIARY TUMOURS

Biliary tumours – benign

Benign biliary tumours are a rare cause of biliary obstruction. These tumours include papilloma, adenoma, hamartoma, cystadenoma, lipoma, fibroma and neurofibroma. Most of the benign tumours within the common bile duct and other bile ducts are exceptionally rare. Granular cell tumours are rare, generally benign, tumours but they do have a slight malignant potential. Benign tumours are usually small at diagnosis, usually less then 3 cm. Biliary tree granulosa cell tumours are more commonly recorded in young Afro-Americans. Benign biliary granulosa cell tumours are usually cured by resection.

Sonography

Benign bile duct tumours usually cause biliary obstruction with biliary dilatation. If there is sufficient bile around the tumour it may be apparent within the dilated duct. The bile duct wall usually remains well defined with no evidence of invasion into the adjacent hepatic parenchyma. Bile duct obstruction by a benign tumour may be complicated by cholangitis which can cause changes in echogenicity around the portal tracts. Papillomas and solid adenomas appear as solid intraluminal filling defects of low to moderate echogenicity without shadowing and may thus mimic sludge. Biliary cystadenoma (see pp. 64–65) presents as a large bulky multiloculated thin-walled cystic mass, associated with intraluminal nodules and papillary infoldings that normally do communicate with the bile ducts. Biliary cystadenoma has to be differentiated from hydatid cysts, cystic neoplastic disease, abscess and a liquefied haematoma.

Further imaging (ERCP, MRCP [magnetic resonance cholangiopancreatography] and CT) can be useful in defining the lesion. Brush biopsy and bile collected during ERCP may be examined cytologically but tissue diagnosis is often difficult without recourse to resection. Granulosa cell tumours present as echogenic tumours within the biliary tree that may shadow and are hence indistinguishable from gallstones.

Biliary tumours – malignant

The clinical and sonographic features of cholangiocarcinomas, Klatskin (cholangiocarcinomas at the porta hepatis) tumours and cystadenocarcinoma have already been described (see pp. 84–86). Extrahepatic cholangiocarcinoma usually occurs in the sixth to seventh decade with a female to male ratio of 3 : 2. The predisposing factors are the same as for intrahepatic cholangiocarcinoma.

Metastases to the bile ducts are rare but can occur with melanoma and colon primaries. Primary non-Hodgkin's lymphoma of the bile ducts is rare but has been recorded, the presentation may be indistinguishable from cholangiocarcinoma or sclerosing cholangitis on imaging although intrahepatic mass lesions may suggest metastases from a cholangiocarcinoma or lymphoma.

Carcinoid of the bile ducts is exceptionally rare and only a dozen or so cases have been reported in the world literature. Sonography, CT and cholangiography show a tumour within the ducts with some extraluminal extension. Biliary botryoid sarcoma (embryonal rhabdomyosarcoma) is a rare childhood tumour that may involve the liver or biliary tree. On imaging it is not possible to differentiate between other intraluminal tumours and botryoid sarcoma. However in children presenting with biliary obstruction from a mass, botryoid sarcoma should be included in the differential diagnoses.

Periampullary tumours

Periampullary carcinomas can arise in one of several locations around the lower common bile duct. Adenocarcinoma (90 per cent) arising from the epithelium of the lower common bile duct and the main pancreatic duct, pancreatic acini, ampulla or rarely the duodenal mucosa. The incidence of periampullary tumours is increasing with a possible relationship to smoking. Diabetes is found in 40 per cent of cases because of pancreatic dysfunction. Other periampullary tumours include pancreatic carcinoma, carcinoid, duodenal wall adenoma and smooth muscle tumours.

Ampullary tumours

Ampullary tumours arising from the glandular epithelium of the ampulla of Vater may be benign or malignant. There is an association between these tumours and Gardner syndrome, familial polyposis coli and colonic carcinoma. Patients present with intermittent jaundice, epigastric pain, weight loss, intestinal bleeding and occasionally signs and symptoms of cholangitis.

Sonography

Sonography may be entirely normal in the initial stages. When obstruction is established biliary dilatation may be apparent. The pancreatic duct may be dilated depending upon the actual location of the ampullary tumour. The tumour itself is visible in a minority of patients. Endoscopy may show the tumour protruding through the orifice or a prominent papilla or a submucosal mass. The most promising imaging is endoscopic ultrasound that has an 87 per cent staging accuracy. Differential diagnosis includes impacted stone, sludge, ascaris, duodenitis, pancreatitis, choledochocoele and peri-ampullary tumours.

2.2.20 HAEMOBILIA

Haemobilia or haemorrhage into the biliary tract is relatively rare to uncommon and usually reflects trauma, inflammation or occasionally tumour. The presence of coagulopathy makes the patient particularly prone to haemobilia. Trauma is the most frequent cause accounting for over 50 per cent of cases. Trauma may be iatrogenic related to TIPS procedure, percutaneous liver biopsy and cholangiography or biliary drainage procedures. Other rare causes include vascular–biliary fistula, neoplasms involving the bile ducts, biliary papillomatosis, ascariasis, ectopic gastric mucosa ulcerating into the biliary tree, liver abscess or hydatid cyst rupture into the bile ducts. Spontaneous haemobilia has been described. Haemorrhage into a choledochal cyst has been reported in a haemophilic child who presented with abdominal pain, mass and obstructive jaundice.

Sonography

Sonography appearance depends upon the acuteness and age of the bleed. An acute bleed is echogenic, non-shadowing and mass like. The thrombus may stick to the gallbladder or bile duct wall mimicking a tumour. However the clot may be mobile within the lumen. When the clot begins to lyse the appearance of the clot changes with one or more concave borders. Biliary dilatation may occur. With further lysis a multiloculated mass appears with or without linear strands. Duplex or colour Doppler confirms the presence of an avascular mass. The differential diagnoses at this stage include biliary neoplasms, biliary papillomatosis, parasitic infestations and gangrenous cholecystitis. Diagnosis of haemobilia should be sought in the appropriate clinical setting. The diagnosis of blood within the intrahepatic ducts is difficult as blood clot tends to be isoechoic to the liver parenchyma. When clot retracts within the common bile duct it may lead to underestimation of the common bile duct size. Post-procedural haemobilia may be difficult to diagnose. The differential diagnosis of blood within the biliary tree includes sludge, pus, non-shadowing calculi, biliary papillomatosis and biliary parasitic infestations.

Echogenic bile

Haemorrhage into the bile ducts.
Sludge – bile stasis with precipitation of cholesterol and calcium bilirubinate crystals.

Pus.
Non-shadowing calculi.
Neoplasm.
Biliary papillomatosis.
Pneumobilia.
Previous biliary atresia*.
Post-liver transplant*.
Cystic fibrosis – inspissated bile*.
Familial immune deficiency*.

Bile duct narrowing

Malignant stricture – for example cholangiocarcinoma.
Inflammation.
Sclerosing cholangitis.
Recurrent pyogenic cholangitis.
Erosion from a stone.
Mirizzi syndrome.
Radiation therapy.
Papillary stenosis.
Biliary atresia.
Perforated duodenal ulcer.
Primary biliary cirrhosis (usually intrahepatic ducts).
Extrinsic compression.
Benign causes – pseudocyst, abscess, pancreatitis, portal vein aneurysm, hepatic artery aneurysm, peribiliary cysts (mucinous hamartoma of the bile duct).
Malignant causes – hilar lymphadenopathy, pancreatic carcinoma, ampullary carcinoma, periampullary tumours, duodenal carcinoma, mucinous biliary papillomatosis.
Congenital causes – for example choledochal cyst.
Trauma – post-operative, blunt or penetrating trauma, hepatic embolisation and hepatic artery chemotherapy.

Thickened bile ducts

Adenomatous hyperplasia, inflammatory cell infiltrate and periductal fibrosis account for the majority of cases of bile duct wall thickening.

Other causes include –

Hepatic clonorchiasis (see pp. 101–102, 167)

Sclerosing cholangitis (primary) - thickening is more severe and is associated with bile duct dilatation focal and discontinuous.

---

* All these patients may have signs of cholangitis.

AIDS-associated cholangitis, this may produce echogenic nodules in the distal common bile duct because of oedema of the papilla of Vater, probably infective in origin (see pp. 147–148) associated findings are acalculus cholecystitis, papillary stenosis or biliary dilatation and hepatomegaly with diffuse hyperechogenicity. *Fasciola hepatica* results in biliary dilatation and bile wall thickening. The vermiform structures within the gallbladder resemble Clonorchiasis.

Oriental cholangiohepatitis (see p. 146)

Biliary ascariasis, (see pp. 149–150)

Peribiliary cysts (hepatic hilar cysts, mucinous hamartoma of the bile duct), these cysts are associated with a variety of disorders. Pathologically they represent obstructed small periductal glands. They are usually asymptomatic and an incidental finding. However rare cases of biliary obstruction due to large perihilar cysts have been reported. Recognition is important to avoid misdiagnosis of dilated ducts, cystic neoplasm or abscess. Most of these cysts have been reported on microscopy, but occasionally these cysts are large enough to be seen on ultrasound. Sonography reveals small peribiliary cysts, sometimes septate coursing anterior to the portal vein. Colour or power Doppler will exclude collateral vessels. Associations: extrahepatic portal venous obstruction/idiopathic portal obstruction, systemic infections/septicaemia, cirrhosis (50 per cent), ascending cholangitis (31 per cent), obstructive jaundice (38 per cent), adult polycystic disease, normal livers (5 per cent). Bile duct varices, these may be secondary to enlarged vasa vasorum of the portal vein wall and newly developed periportal veins or both as a consequence of portal vein obstruction. There are serpentine vessels in the wall/lumen of the bile ducts, anechoic beading confirmed on duplex/colour/power Doppler. A network of tiny vessels in the wall of the common bile duct may be merely seen as thickened bile ducts, therefore colour/power Doppler is mandatory whenever a thick duct wall is seen.

Acute portal vein thrombosis, as bile duct may be mistaken for portal vein.

Infiltrating tumours (see pp. 74, 168)

Low reflectivity periportal collar, tramline appearance along the portal tract with target appearance on cross section that may be secondary to one of the following causes:

1. Periportal lymphoedema associated with malignant lymphadenopathy.
2. Sclerosing cholangitis.
3. Primary biliary cirrhosis (stage 2/3)
4. Cryptogenic cirrhosis.
5. Lymphoproliferative disorders after bone marrow transplantation.
6. Following liver transplantation.

2.2.21 BILLIARY COMPLICATIONS AFTER HEPATIC TRANSPLANTATION

1. Biliary obstruction, anastamotic with choledochojejunostomy and malignant anastamotic stricture.
2. Bile leaks, anastamotic or T-tube dislodgement.
3. Arterial thrombosis, loss of arterialisation predisposes to biliary complications, bile duct obstruction and/or leakage.
4. Diffuse biliary abnormality narrowing, stretching and separation of intrahepatic ductal branches. These findings are non-specific being seen with acute rejection, preservation injury, infarction and hepatitis. Biliary complications occur in 31 per cent of paediatric and 22 per cent of adult recipients, 1 day to 4 years after transplantation.

2.2.22 CAUSES OF BILIARY DISORDERS

Biliary obstruction in the newborn

Extrahepatic biliary atresia.
Intrahepatic biliary atresia with or without lymphoedema.
Bile duct hypoplasia.
Bile duct plug syndrome.
Choledochal cyst.
Cystic fibrosis.
Biliary or hepatic neoplasm.
Periductal lymphoedema.
Gallstones, these are quite uncommon but gallstones are being seen with increasing frequency in babies who are ill at birth and spend time on a Special Care Baby Unit, often with prolonged periods of intravenous and tube feeding.

Biliary dilatation without jaundice

Early obstruction.
Post-obstruction – for example recent passage of a stone.
Common bile duct surgery.
Gallstones – either within the gallbladder or within the common bile duct but without acute obstruction.
Post-cholecystectomy.
Intraluminal sludge ball – for example in severe haemolysis, AIDS.
Only part of the biliary system is obstructed (intrahepatic).
Worms and other parasites.
Intestinal hypomotility.

Normal variant – this diagnosis should be made with extreme caution after exclusion of other causes and prolonged follow up.

Age – common bile duct calibre increases with age and the upper limit of normal may be 0.75 cm at 75 years.

Morphine in a neonate, failure of relaxation of the sphincter.

Biliary obstruction without apparent dilatation

Sudden severe biliary obstruction.

Biliary fibrosis – for example post-sclerosing cholangitis, this may prevent dilatation of obstructed ducts.

Cholangitis.

Small calculi.

Pancreatitis.

Haemobilia.

Ducts filled with debris.

Cholangiocarcinoma – tumour encasement.

Metastases – tumour encasement.

Previous surgery in this area (fibrosis).

Technical difficulties giving poor visualisation.

Common hepatic duct dilatation (the upper limit of normal is 4 mm in young adults)

Post-cholecystectomy – upper limit of normal is 7 mm.

Choledochal cyst or choledochocoele.

Calculus.

Choledochal diverticulum.

Mirizzi syndrome – common hepatic duct obstruction – a stone impacted in the cystic duct.

Oriental cholangiohepatitis – there may be a large amount of sludge in the bile duct with or without stones.

Primary or secondary cholangitis.

Cholangiocarcinoma.

Any cause of common bile duct dilatation – for example carcinoma of the head of the pancreas.

Compression by lymph nodes.

AIDS.

Dilated pancreatic duct and common bile duct

Carcinoma of the head of the pancreas.

Ampullary tumour.

Periampullary tumour.
Ampullary stricture.
Impacted calculus.

Intraluminal common bile duct masses

Calculus, shadowing or non-shadowing.
Blood (see causes of haemobilia, pp. 154–156).
Sludge and debris.
Air bubbles (see causes of pneumobilia, pp. 151–152).
Haematoma – submucosal, trauma, instrumentation.
Food or faeces (see causes of enterobiliary fistula, p. 151).
Pus.
Mirizzi syndrome.
Fibrosis.
Cholangitis.
Abscess, extrinsic compression.
Pseudo-calculus – contracted distal common bile duct sphincter.
Parasites – *Ascaris lumbricoides* alive or macerated, *Clonorchis sinensis*, *Fasciola hepatica*, hydatid rupture into the biliary tree.
Neoplasms – ampullary carcinoma, adenocarcinoma, cholangiocarcinoma, intraductal hepatoma, papilloma/adenoma, metastases (melanoma, colon), carcinoid, hamartoma, embryonal rhabdomyosarcoma, mucinous biliary papillomatoses, granular cell tumour.

2.2.23 GALLBLADDER ANATOMY

The gallbladder stores and concentrates bile while the ducts function as a transfer system. Bile duct flow is affected by hepatic secretory pressure, tone in the sphincter, the rate of gallbladder fluid absorption and gallbladder contraction. Anatomically the gallbladder is a pear-shaped musculomembranous sac lying in a fossa under the liver. The fundus of the gallbladder lies close to the anterior abdominal wall and the hepatic flexure of the colon. The surface marking of the gallbladder fundus is in the region of the costal cartilage. At this point it is covered by peritoneum and its proximity to the hepatic flexure of the colon may obscure it. The body of the gallbladder is adjacent to the duodenum, which indents it and mimics gallstones or a gallbladder mass. The mucosa of the gallbladder neck is thrown into folds giving an echogenic appearance which may also mimic gallstones. A small pouch projects from the right side of the gallbladder neck. This is Hartmann's pouch which, when visible, is frequently associated with pathology, particularly dilatation. The gallbladder fundus is often 'folded over' and the gallbladder then assumes a double-barrel appearance. Pseudo-septation of the gallbladder fundus because of kinking, folding or sometimes a true septum, may sometimes be seen. This is called a Phrygian cap and is seen in 2 to 6 per cent of individuals.

Sonography of the gallbladder

The gallbladder is a pear-shaped or ellipsoid anechoic sac indenting the inferomedial aspect of the right lobe of the liver. A linear echogenicity representing fat in the main interlobar fissure is seen interposed between the gallbladder and the right main portal vein. The inner surface of the gallbladder mucosa is hyperechoic, the middle layer (submucosa and muscle) is hypoechoic while the serosal surface (pericholecystic fatty layer) is hyperechoic. There is a linear fold on the posterior gallbladder wall at the junction of the body and neck termed the junctional fold that is of no pathological significance. Sound waves from the neck of the gallbladder (spiral valve of Heister) may shadow and mimic a gallstone. The normal gallbladder wall thickness is never more than 3 mm. Provided the patient has been starved for 8 to 12 hours there should be virtually 100 per cent visualisation of the normal gallbladder. In a true fasting patient gallbladder nonvisualisation is pathological in 96 per cent of patients.

Gallbladder dimensions

The dimensions of the normal gallbladder are

- length 7 to 10 cm (the normal gallbladder is nearly always less then 13 cm long)
- diameter 2 to 3.5 cm (normally less than 4 cm)
- wall thickness 2 to 3 mm.

In the fasting patient the normal gallbladder seldom exceeds 4×10 cm, with a cystic duct length of 3 to 4 cm. Gallbladder size generally increases with age but the wall thickness is unaffected by age.

Average neonatal gallbladder dimensions are

- length 2.5 cm
- diameter 0.5 to 1.6 cm (mean 0.9 cm)
- wall thickness 1 mm.

2.2.24 GALLBLADDER DYNAMICS

Physiology and pathophysiology of gallbladder kinetics have gained considerable scientific interest recently. Assessment of gallbladder function has traditionally been carried out by oral cholecystography and radionuclide methods. There has been great interest in assessing gallbladder function non-invasively by ultrasound. Several methods have been developed, the gold standard is considered to be the 'sum of cylinders method'. The method is accurate but tedious and time consuming unless a computer programme is available. The authors prefer the ellipsoid method which is considered less taxing.

$$\text{Vol.} = 0.52 \times W \times H \times L$$

Gallbladder contraction varies widely in each person and therefore a single recording may be misleading.

Fasting gallbladder normal vol. 1.9 to 45.5 ml.

Residual gallbladder vol. 0.1 to 21.0 ml.

Normal range gallbladder contraction is 10 to 99 per cent

In 60 per cent of subjects gallbladder contraction falls in the 60 to 87 per cent range. A gallbladder contraction of 20 per cent is used as cut off for lithotripsy and oral dissolution therapy. In everyday practice a simple measurement of gallbladder area in a single plane is usually adequate for comparison of pre-prandial and post-prandial gallbladder sizes.

Non-visualisation of the gallbladder in a truly fasting patient is highly suggestive of gallbladder disease (at least 88 per cent of these cases have gallbladder pathology with gallbladder contraction). In some centres oral cholecystography is used as a further imaging modality in these cases. If ultrasound is repeated with more rigorous fasting the contracted gallbladder can often be identified.

2.2.25 GALLBLADDER ANOMALIES

Anomalous position or orientation of the gallbladder

Situs inversus – the gallbladder is in the left upper quadrant.

Gallbladder is related to the left lobe of the liver, this is rare.

Heterotaxia – intermediate situs with the gallbladder in the midline, associated with asplenia, polysplenia, pulmonary isomerism and congenital heart disease.

Anomalous orientation – horizontal.

Unusual location – intrahepatic, suprahepatic, lateral, anterior abdominal wall, retrorenal, within the thorax, within the falciform ligament or interlobular fissure and in the transverse mesocolon.

Wandering gallbladder – suspended on its own mesentery.

Normal impression – duodenum or colon.

Displaced gallbladder (intrinsic) – hepatocellular carcinoma, nodule, metastases, cyst etc. (see gallbladder compression sign p. 168).

Displaced gallbladder (extrinsic) – renal tumour or cyst, lymph nodes, pseudocyst, etc.

Agenesis of the gallbladder

This is a rare anomaly found in 0.04 to 0.07 per cent of autopsies. Agenesis may be associated with biliary atresia, imperforate anus and common hepatic duct and common bile duct anomalies. Rarely the gallbladder opens separately into the duodenum.

NB beware laparoscopic cholecystectomy may leave no scars.

Anomalies of gallbladder shape

The most common anomalous shape is because of the Phrygian cap (2 to 6 per cent) in which the gallbladder fundus is folded back on itself producing a kink in the fundus. The gallbladder may rarely appear as diverticulum with no cystic duct. Other anomalies of shape include a fishhook, a siphon, and an hourglass configuration.

Gallbladder duplication

True duplication is rare but has been reported to occur in 1 in 3000 to 4000 people with a male to female ratio of 2:1. Triplication is even rarer and may be an incidental finding at autopsy. In duplication each gallbladder may have separate cystic ducts or one cystic duct. A septate gallbladder may have an isolated transverse septum (true duplication has a longitudinal septum). A multiseptate gallbladder is extremely rare with multiple locules connected by small pores, this is particularly prone to bile stasis and calculus formation. A diverticulum of the gallbladder is extremely rare and usually located at the neck of the gallbladder, it is rarely symptomatic unless complicated by calculus disease.

Anomalous cystic duct insertion

The cystic duct may insert into the common bile duct or common hepatic duct high or low. The cystic duct is often intramural running for some distance in the wall of the common bile duct within a common sheath. Congenital stenosis of the cystic duct is extremely rare and may be complicated by calculus disease.

Heterotopic tissue within the gallbladder

Heterotopic gastric or pancreatic tissue has been described within the gallbladder wall, which may easily be confused with other pathology.

Visualisation of two gallbladders

True duplication.
Folded gallbladder.

Phrygian cap.
Pericholecystic fluid.
Focal adenomyomatosis.
Gallbladder plus diverticulum.
Gallbladder plus renal or omental enteric cyst, aneurysm, etc.

2.2.26 GALLSTONES

Gallstones are common affecting 10 to 20 per cent of the adult population, the incidence rising with increasing age. The peak incidence is in the fifth to sixth decade with a male to female ratio of $1:4$. Although most stones occur in adults they are not rare in children, particularly those who have had intravenous feeding (in these cases the gallstones may actually resolve). Chronic haemolysis such as hereditary spherocytosis and the haemoglobinopathies also predisposes to gallstone formation. Up to 27 per cent of children and 70 per cent of adults with sickle cell anaemia have gallstones. Ten per cent of gallstones contain sufficient calcium to be visible on conventional abdominal radiographs.

Diagnostic criteria for gallstones

Mobile echogenic structures with distal acoustic shadowing within the gallbladder lumen on images taken in two planes at right angles are virtually 100 per cent accurate for gallstones. Non-visualisation of the gallbladder lumen with echogenic structures with distal acoustic shadowing rising in the gallbladder fossa is 96 per cent accurate for gallstones in a diseased gallbladder. Gallstones 3 mm or more in diameter usually cause shadowing. The shadowing is 'clean' unlike the shadowing distal to bowel gas, which shows reverberation echoes. Reverberation artefact can also occur distal to gallstones but is usually more regular than distal to bowel gas and may indicate calcium content of the stone. Gallstones usually lie in the most dependent part of the gallbladder but can float in the bile particularly after cholecystographic contrast. It is important that a patient being examined for gallstones is turned from side to side during the examination or mucosal folds of the spiral valve of Heister may hide small stones which do not cause shadowing.

Causes of gallstones in a neonate (rare)

Total parenteral nutrition.
Frusemide (furosemide) therapy, also causes renal medullary calcification.
Prolonged fasting.
Phototherapy.

Rhesus/ABO blood incompatibility.
Gastrointestinal dysfunction.
Neonatal sepsis.

Causes of gallstones in children

Haemolysis – hereditary spherocytosis, sickle cell disease and thalassaemia.
Total parenteral nutrition, especially long-term intravenous feeding in premature babies.
Cystic fibrosis.
Bowel resection and disease of the terminal ileum.
Malabsorption.
Chronic hepatitis.
Any severe illness associated with prolonged fasting – these gallstones may resolve on recovery from the underlying illness.
Congenital biliary anomalies – choledochal cyst.
Leukaemia.
Cirrhosis.
Ellis-van Creveld syndrome.
Following radiotherapy for Wilms tumour.
Frusemide (furosemide) therapy.

The majority of children, like adults, have a known cause of gallstones.

Causes of gallstones in an adult

Haemolytic causes – congenital spherocytosis (43 to 85 per cent), sickle cell disease (7 to 37 per cent), thalassaemia, prosthetic heart valves, pernicious anaemia, mitral valve stenosis, aortic aneurysm, hypersplenism.
Metabolic causes – 'fat, female, fair, fertile and forty', diabetes mellitus, obesity, haemosiderosis, pregnancy, prolonged use of oestrogens or progesterones, hyperparathyroidism, cystic fibrosis, pancreatitis, hypothyroidism, muscular dystrophy, Crohn's disease, ileal resection and intestinal malabsorption, type IV hyperlipidaemia, surgical bypass for obesity.
Cholestasis chronic hepatitis, cirrhosis.
Congenital biliary malformation – Caroli's disease.
Parasites – ascariasis, liver flukes.
Drugs – methadone.
Biliary strictures – oriental cholangiohepatitis.
Genetic predisposition – native American tribes.

There is a higher incidence of intrahepatic gallstones in Chinese and Japanese.

Mimics of gallstones

Partial volume – usually due to impression by the duodenum.

Misidentification of gallbladder – fluid-filled bowel associated with gas, hepatic or renal cyst with debris or haemorrhage.

Non-visualisation of the gallbladder in a fasting patient in the presence of shadowing foci in the gallbladder bed is strong presumptive evidence of gallbladder disease. The WES (wall-echo-shadow) triad is useful in this situation. This complex consists of two parallel arcs of echogenic lines with an inter-spaced anechoic space. The echogenic lines represent the gallbladder wall and the leading edge of the gallstone separated by anechoic bile. The WES sign is useful in differentiating a contracted diseased gallbladder from other causes with similar appearance, for example porcelain gallbladder, emphysematous cholecystitis, air-filled bowel.

Reverberation echoes from folds in the gallbladder neck.

Respiratory motion artefact – usually not a problem with real-time scanners.

Shadows arising directly anterior or posterior to the gallbladder, for example rib.

Junctional mucosal fold.

Clips in the cholecystectomy bed – patients may be unable to relate to a previous cholecystectomy or may be unaware that their gallbladder has been removed.

Inspissated bile sludge – commonly seen in ill patients.

Any cause of intraluminal filling defect.

Pseudosludge – artefactual appearance of layering sludge caused by slice thickness and side lobe artefact. These artefacts can be reduced by appropriate focussing, centring the gallbladder in the field of view and optimising gain settings.

Adenomyomatosis and cholesterolosis are forms of hyperplastic cholecystoses. These conditions are usually asymptomatic but symptoms may occur because of associated gallstones. Adenomyomatosis is characterised by out-pouching of the gallbladder mucosa into the muscular layer of the gallbladder wall. These out-pouchings are called Rokitansky–Aschoff sinuses. These sinuses contain bile and may appear cystic. Cholesterol deposits often occur within these sinuses which appear as echogenic foci with trailing comet tail or V-shaped artefact. These reverberation artefacts are short and tapered as compared to the artefact behind air (emphysematous cholecystitis, bowel gas) which is long and straight with linear margins. In cholesterolosis, cholesterol deposits may vary in size from a few mm to 10 mm, they are echogenic but do not usually shadow. Emphysematous cholecystitis and porcelain gallbladder may cause patchy shadowing and occasionally present without associated gallstones. Air and calcification are echogenic and cause shadowing.

Echogenic bile is often associated with biliary stasis or bile duct obstruction, its echogenicity varies but there is usually no shadowing.

Polyps within the gallbladder vary in size and echogenicity but do not shadow, differentiation from adherent gallstones may be difficult.

Filling defects within the gallbladder

Metabolic

Gallstones – shadowing or nonshadowing

Tumefactive sludge and debris – postoperative, diabetes, patients on total parenteral nutrition, alcoholics, AIDS patients and cystic fibrosis patients.

Sonography

Well-defined masses of low amplitude echoes which may or may not be mobile within the gallbladder.

Cholesterolosis – strawberry gallbladder (multiple fixed mural plaques).

Cholesterol papilloma – 3 to 5 mm is usual, maximum is 10 mm, often multiple cholesterolosis is found in 23 per cent of cases at surgery.

Adherent gallstone.

Cholesterol crystals.

Reversible ceftriaxone pseudolithiasis – this has been reported with ceftriaxone a parenteral third generation cephalosporin used for treating bacterial infections. Since its release in 1984, 74 cases have been reported. The drug forms a complex with calcium in bile salt forming a precipitate that mimics gallstones on ultrasound. With discontinuation of treatment these 'stones' resolve spontaneously.

Artefact

Pseudosludge – A partial volume effect – anechoic bile and adjacent echogenic liver may result in low amplitude echoes that resemble layering sludge.

Pseudo-mass due to impression of the duodenum.

Anatomical variants – ectopic tissue

Mucosal junctional fold at the junction of the gallbladder body and neck.

Ectopic gastric, pancreatic, intestinal, hepatic and prostatic tissue in the gallbladder.

Inflammation or infection

Mucosal hypertrophy or hyperplasia.

Inflammatory polyp.

Pus – this may be seen in empyema of the gallbladder.

Enterobiliary fistula – food or faeces.

Epithelial cyst.

Mucosal retention cyst.

Tuberculosis – a normal gallbladder is highly resistant to tuberculosis, underlying cholelithiasis or cystic obstruction is essential for developing tuberculosis of the gallbladder. Four types of gallbladder tuberculosis are described depending upon whether the gallbladder is involved alone or in association with miliary or generalised abdominal tuberculosis. In the most usual type the gallbladder is involved in association with other abdominal organs. Sonography: shows an enlarged gallbladder with a variegated intraluminal soft tissue mass associated with a calculus. Other associated findings are ascites, mesenteric and retroperitoneal lyphadenopathy.

Xanthogranulomatous cholecystitis (XC): This is a chronic inflammatory condition associated with gallstones in 96 per cent of patients. The appearance may mimic a carcinoma of the gallbladder. Patients characteristically have gallstones, and complications such as gallbladder perforation and fistula formation are frequent. The possibility that an inoperable gallbladder tumour may in fact be xanthogranulomatous cholecystitis should always be considered, and may be confirmed with frozen sections.

Clonorchiasis

Liver flukes within the gallbladder may appear as floating discrete, non-shadowing echogenic foci which usually sink to the dependent part of the gallbladder, but may float with a change in patient position or tap with the ultrasound probe. The flukes are unlikely to be confused with gallstones as they are fusiform, weakly echogenic and nonshadowing. The gallbladder may distend with thick walls and gallstones may form. Clonorchiasis is associated with an increased incidence of hepatocellular and cholangiocarcinoma. Oriental cholangiohepatitis: is a recurrent pyogenic cholangitis associated with pigment stones but not all patients have stones (13–63 per cent). When stones are present they invariably shadow.

Ascaris lumbricoides: see page 148

Fascioliasis: is an infection by the sheep liver fluke, which is found worldwide. The parasite is characterised by leaf-like appearance with a thin central anechoic stria due to its alimentary canal.

Paragonimiasis: is an infection with the lung flukes of the genus paragonimus, which may occasionally affect sites other than the lungs for example brain, liver, peritoneum.

Schistosomiasis: see pages 46–67

Vascular

Tortuous artery/aneurysm
Gallbladder varices

Tumours: benign

Adenomyomatosis
Polyps: (1) Adenomatous (0.2 per cent) generally single 0.5–4 cm associated gallstones in 38 per cent. (2) Hyperplastic.

Sonography

Hyperplastic polyps are isoechoic with liver parenchyma. When gallbladder polyps are sessile over 10 mm in the maximum diameter or isoechoic with the liver they are highly likely to be malignant.
Papillomas: may have finger like projections, single or multiple <5 mm.
Fibroadenoma
Neurofibroma

Tumours: malignant

Carcinoma: predominantly affects females over the age of 50, gallbladder carcinoma is twice as common as cholangiocarcinoma, the other major malignancy of the biliary tree. The disease is usually at an advanced stage at presentation and the prognosis is poor, 90 per cent of patients are dead within a year regardless of treatment employed. The patients who tend to survive are those in whom cancer is discovered incidentally as a polyp on ultrasound.

Sonography of gallbladder tumour

The most common appearance is that of a mass in the gallbladder fossa, usually hypoechoic and usually associated with gallstones causing areas of shadowing. There is usually large bile duct obstruction and intrahepatic metastases are often present at diagnosis. These patients are usually inoperable at diagnosis. Gallbladder carcinoma may rarely present as focal gallbladder wall thickening, difficult to differentiate from other causes of focal gallbladder wall thickening. As mentioned earlier gallbladder cancer may present as a polyp, while this finding may be safely observed in younger patients, it must be regarded potentially malignant in older patients and investigated aggressively as at this stage there is potential for cure. See also pages 179–180.

Leiomyosarcoma: this is a rare neoplasm which has a non-specific clinical presentation that may present with features of acute cholecystitis or gallbladder empyema. Associated calculi have been observed. Sonography: is non-specific, irregularly thickened gallbladder wall and polypoid protrusion into the lumen has been observed. A solitary case of an echogenic mass obliterating the gallbladder lumen with a stone in the centre of the mass has been reported.

Metastases: melanoma, renal cell carcinoma, Kaposi sarcoma, lymphoma, leukaemia, breast, carcinoid, lung and oesopragus.

Extrinsic compression

Masses such as cysts and solid tumours may compress the gallbladder; see gallbladder compression sign.

Non-shadowing mobile intraluminal gallbladder mass

Calculi.
Tumefactive sludge.
Cholesterol crystals.
Pseudosludge – artefact.
Food or faeces.
Blood.
Pus.
Fibrinous debris or desquamated mucosa.
Ascaris lumbricoides.
Clonorchis sinensis.
Fasciola hepatica.

Low-level echoes within the gallbladder

Concentration of bile in the fasting patient may give rise to sludge formation. This is slightly echogenic but does not shadow and may form a bile or sludge level. The biochemical nature of sludge has recently been recognised to be predominantly aggregates of cholesterol crystals and liquid crystalline droplets, and in some cases of obstructive jaundice and symptomatic liver disease of bilirubin granules embedded in a gel matrix of mucous glycoproteins. Biliary sludge is often associated with biliary stasis such as with TPN, fasting, pregnancy and in mucous hypersecretion such as mucin-secreting bile duct tumours. In the majority of patients the presence of sludge is a transient phenomenon – as the patient's condition improves the sludge resolves. If the lumen of the gallbladder is completely filled with sludge with a similar echogenicity as the liver the gallbladder may not be seen, a process called hepatisation.
Cholesterol crystals – small but very echogenic.
Multiple small calculi.
Pus.
Abnormal mucus.
Parasites.
Milk calcium bile or limy bile – echogenicity is intermediate between sludge and calculi.

Structures mimicking the gallbladder

Duodenal cap and fluid-filled bowel loops.
Hepatic cysts.
Omental cysts.

Ligamentum teres abscess.
Choledochal cysts.
Solitary renal cysts.
Dilated cystic duct remnant after cholecystectomy.

Non-visualisation of the gallbladder

Post-prandial contraction.
Chronic cholecystitis – contracted fibrotic gallbladder.
Gallbladder obscured by gas, gallbladder obscured by or mistaken for bowel loop.
Ectopic gallbladder (see p. 161).
Post-cholecystectomy.
Congenital absence (0.03 per cent).
Porcelain gallbladder.
Gangrenous cholecystitis.
Carcinoma of the gallbladder.
Metastases involving the gallbladder or gallbladder bed.
Acute hepatic dysfunction, for example hepatitis – poor bile flow and non-specific gallbladder wall thickening.
Air in the gallbladder.
Technical factors – obesity, very thin patient with a superficial gallbladder.

Increased gallbladder wall thickness – anterior gallbladder wall thickness 3mm or more

Physiological
Fasting – 3.5 per cent of fasting patients show transient gallbladder wall thickening.
Poor distention (post-prandial).

Artefact
Oblique sections

Intrinsic causes
Acute cholecystitis
Chronic cholecystitis
Carcinoma gallbladder
Xanthogranulomatous cholecystitis
AIDS
Hyperplastic cholesterolosis
Gallbladder varices
Adenomyomatosis
Leukaemia – gallbladder infiltration
Gallbladder perforation
Gallbladder torsion

Oriental cholangiohepatitis

Hepatic clonorchiasis

Cholecysto-enteric fistula: gallbladder wall thickening, air within the biliary tree, echogenic material may be seen passing from gallbladder to bowel, the ultrasound 'halo sign' may be more specific

Focal obstruction to gallbladder lymphatic drainage for example nodes at the porta

Extrinsic causes: Liver

Hepatitis (80 per cent)

Cirrhosis

Acute alcoholic abuse – there is often quite severe gallbladder wall thickening after an alcoholic binge which can make the gallbladder difficult to define

Portal hypertension

Veno-occlusive disease

Congestive cholecystopathy – in chronic liver disease, hypoalbuminaemia is not an important factor, portal hypertension is the dominant factor causing gallbladder thickening in cirrhosis. Ultrasound demonstration of gallbladder wall thickening in chronic liver disease but without stones should suggest the presence of portal hypertension

Hepatoportal sclerosis

Infectious mononucleosis

AIDS

Extrinsic causes: systemic

Hypoproteinaemia/hypoalbuminaemia

Ascites

Acute pancreatitis

Acute myelogenous leukaemia

Sepsis

Graft versus host reaction – bone marrow transplantation

Brucellosis

Systemic venous hypertension

Right sided heart failure

Acute pyelonephritis: gallbladder wall thickening is secondary to adjacent inflammatory process, similar to that seen in pancreatitis and peptic ulcer disease

Renal failure

Myeloma

Appendicitis

Peptic ulcer disease

Infusion with interleukin-2 in HIV infection: Symptomatic gallbladder wall thickening during infusion of interleukin 2 can exactly mimic other forms of acalculus cholecystitis except that when associated with interleukin 2 the gallbladder wall thickness resolves after cessation of therapy. Surgical treatment is not required. A HIDA scan may be useful in clinical decision making.

2.2.27 CHOLECYSTITIS

Acute cholecystitis

Acute inflammation of the gallbladder is usually bacterial in origin but it may be sterile. The peak incidence is in the fifth to sixth decades with a male to female ratio of $1:3$. Patients usually present with acute right upper quadrant pain, fever, leucocytosis and mild abnormalities of liver function tests. However in the elderly, debilitated and diabetic patients symptoms may not be so obvious. The majority of cases are associated with the presence of gallstones, the inflammatory episode being precipitated by gallstone impaction in the cystic duct (90 per cent). In 85 per cent of patients the stone disimpacts spontaneously. Distension of the gallbladder by mucus causes venous congestion and eventually leads to arterial embarrassment and ischaemia. If the obstructed gallbladder does not become infected then distension by mucus leads to mucocoele formation. Infection in these cases causes acute cholecystitis. If medical treatment is given early in an attack 95 per cent of cases resolve but at least 50 per cent will have further attacks. Acute cholecystitis may be complicated by haemorrhage, empyema, reflux pancreatitis, gallbladder gangrene and perforation or rupture leading to peritonitis, biloma or pericholecystic abscess. Rupture into the liver may result in a liver abscess.

Sonography

1. Calculi in the gallbladder, Hartmann's pouch or cystic duct, the latter may be hard to detect.
2. Anterior gallbladder wall thickness greater than 3 mm.
3. Positive ultrasonic Murphy's sign (pain on compression of the gallbladder with the ultrasound probe).
4. Pericholecystic fluid in severe cases, this is a sign of actual or impending perforation.
5. Echopoor halo in or around the gallbladder wall (oedema).
6. Non-visualisation of the gallbladder in a truly fasting patient is strong evidence of gallbladder disease.
7. Acalculus cholecystitis, 5 per cent of these cases are not associated with gallstones.
8. Gallbladder distension, 93 per cent of patients with a gallbladder volume over 70 ml have acute cholecystitis.
9. Increased periportal echogenicity presumably due to a local inflammatory infiltrate.
10. Loss of definition of the gallbladder margins.
11. Intraluminal wall desquamation giving rise to a lace-like lumen.

12. Colour flow and power Doppler may reveal hypervascularisation of the gallbladder wall associated with gallbladder wall thickening on grey scale imaging.

13. Hypervascularisation has been reported without gallbladder wall thickening in acute cholecystitis.

14. In children acute cholecystitis may be acalculus, with increased gallbladder wall thickening, signs of hydrops, positive ultrasound Murphy's sign and increased diameter of the common bile duct with sludge.

15. Cystic duct obstruction is present in 95 per cent of cases of acute cholecystitis. This may be demonstrated by HIDA isotope scanning. In fasting patients HIDA excreted in the bile outlines the gallbladder. Lack of gallbladder visualisation is presumptive evidence of cystic duct obstruction and is 94 to 100 per cent accurate as a marker for acute cholecystitis.

False positive results at HIDA scan (i.e. lack of gallbladder visualisation)

Prolonged fasting (gallbladder full).

Total parenteral nutrition.

Inadequate fasting.

Acute pancreatitis.

Acute alcoholic hepatitis.

Cirrhosis.

Gallbladder hydrops.

Desquamative cholecystitis – rarely cholecystitis results in a desquamative process in the gallbladder wall, this give rise to a bizarre multiseptate appearance.

Mirizzi's syndrome – an obstruction of the common hepatic duct due to an impacted stone in the cystic duct remnant post-cholecystectomy, causing inflammation or pressure necrosis of the common hepatic duct. The pressure necrosis may lead to obstruction of the common bile duct and can eventually cause stricture or fistula formation. Sonography will reveal calculi and dilated intrahepatic ducts or common hepatic duct. Occasionally lymph node compression may give rise to a similar appearance.

Acalculus cholecystitis

Infection may occur in bile stasis without the presence of gallstones. Bile stasis usually occurs because of other intercurrent illness particularly with fever and dehydration. *Escherichia coli*, *Salmonella* spp. (typhoid) or parasites (*Giardia* spp.) may invade the gallbladder. Up to 30 per cent of cases are jaundiced but as the cystic duct is not obstructed gallbladder distension is less marked than when associated with gallstones. In children gallstones are uncommon and acute cholecystitis is often acalculus, but the association with gallstones rises with age. Gastroenteritis may result in dehydration, biliary stasis and hyperconcentration of bile, which in turn results in gallbladder inflammation.

Sonography
A thick gallbladder wall, often with striated oedema pattern, dependent sludge, pericholecystic fluid, sloughed mucosa and a positive ultrasonic Murphy's sign. Ultrasonically guided cholecystostomy can be used as a diagnostic and therapeutic procedure.

Causes of acalculus cholecystitis
Surgery.
Burns.
Gastroenteritis.
Trauma.
Parenteral nutrition.
Mechanical ventilation.
Blood transfusion.
Narcotics.
Diabetes mellitus.
Antibiotics.
Hepatic arterial embolisation.
Post-partum complications.
Vascular insufficiency.
Arteriostenosis or hypertension.
AIDS – cytomegalovirus, *Cryptosporidium* sp.

Causes of pericholecystic fluid

Acute cholecystitis.
Pericholecystic abscess.
Sub-acute gallbladder perforation.
Gangrenous infarction of the gallbladder.
Ascites.
Pancreatitis.
Peptic ulcer with or without perforation.
Liver abscess.
Peritonitis.
Ligamentum teres abscess.
Ruptured hepatic adenoma.
Ruptured ectopic gestation.
AIDS.
Low level echoes in the adjacent liver for example secondary to inflammation of the hepatic flexure of colon

The lack of associated findings of acute cholecystitis and a clinical setting not suggestive of acalculus cholecystitis should raise the possibility of other causes of pericholecystic fluid.

Emphysematous cholecystitis

In emphysematous cholecystitis ischaemia of the gallbladder wall is followed by infection with gas-forming organisms giving rise to gas in the gallbladder lumen or wall. Pre-existing diabetes mellitus is present in 30 to 50 per cent of patients with a male to female ratio of 5:1. Gas may be confined to the gallbladder but in 20 per cent gas is also seen in the rest of the biliary tree. Gallstones are not present in 30 to 50 per cent. Mortality is 15 per cent. There is propensity for gangrene formation and perforation but the clinical symptoms are deceptively mild. Emphysematous cholecystitis has been reported following chemoembolisation for palliation of hepatocellular carcinoma, atheromatous embolism during aortography and gallbladder hypoperfusion during cardiorespiratory resuscitation. When gas is prominent the gallbladder may be mistaken for a bowel loop because of the increased echogenicity and shadowing.

Sonography
Gas in the lumen of the gallbladder is hyperreflective with distal reverberation artefact in the gallbladder lumen. Intramural gas is characterised by hyperreflective foci within the gallbladder wall, with or without reverberation artefact. An 'effervescent gallbladder' with a large number of bubbles rising like gas bubbles in a glass of champagne from the dependent part of the gallbladder has been reported. The differential diagnosis is from other causes of pneumobilia.

Hyperechoic foci in the gallbladder wall

Cholesterol plaques
Rokitansky–Aschoff sinuses – containing stones or sludge
Intramural gas in emphysematous cholecystitis
Small adherent stones
Small polyps
Intramural microabscesses

Gallbladder perforation

Perforation occurs in 6 to 12 per cent of patients with acute cholecystitis. Acute perforation of the gallbladder causes peritonitis. Subacute perforation may result in a pericholecystic abscess. Chronic perforation indicates a fistulous communication between the gallbladder and some other viscus such as cholecystoduodenal (77 per cent), cholecystocolic (15 per cent) and cholestoantral (rare). The gallbladder fundus is the most common site of perforation because of its poor blood supply. Perforation can occur 2 days to several weeks after the onset of symptoms. Mortality is 19 to 24 per cent. The predisposing factors include cholelithiasis, infection, trauma, diabetes mellitus, malignancy angitis, atherosclerosis and steroids. Perforation follows an impaction of a calculus in the cystic duct followed by gallbladder distension, vascular insufficiency leading to ischaemia, necrosis and perforation.

Sonography

The following sonographic features have been described

1. pericholecystic fluid collection
2. free peritoneal fluid
3. irregular gallbladder wall thickening
4. gallbladder distension
5. gallstones
6. coarse intracholecystic echogenic debris
7. sonolucent band within the gallbladder wall
8. air in the biliary tree
9. complex mass in the gallbladder fossa
10. direct visualisation of gallbladder perforation (specific sign)
11. colour Doppler ultrasound visualisation of bile leak across the gallbladder wall.

Gallbladder torsion

Torsion of the gallbladder presents acutely as right upper quadrant pain, nausea, vomiting, fever and a palpable mass. Almost all patients are elderly with a male to female ratio of 1:3. The majority of patients who develop gallbladder torsion are from the 4 per cent of the population where the gallbladder is free-lying on a mesentery and not closely applied to the fossa of the liver. There are two anomalies associated with torsion

1. the gallbladder and cystic duct are mobile on a mesentery (either fully or partially)
2. the gallbladder is suspended freely from a pedicle.

Clinically and sonographically torsion may mimic acute cholecystitis. On sonography the lack of gallstones may suggest acalculus cholecystitis, however acalculus cholecystitis typically occurs in a critically ill patient unlike torsion which occurs *de novo*.

Sonography

Various sonographic features have been described

1. a square-shaped gallbladder with equal length and width
2. a 'floating gallbladder'
3. a stretched cystic duct and gallbladder neck seen as a conical-shaped structure comprising multiple linear echoes converging towards the tip of the cone
4. a positive ultrasonic Murphy's sign
5. a thickened gallbladder wall
6. a hypoechoic rim between the echogenic layers of the wall
7. signs of gallbladder perforation may be present.

Gallbladder injuries

The gallbladder may be lacerated, avulsed or contused in blunt abdominal trauma. Laceration is the most common trauma accounting for 3.2 per cent of abdominal injuries. Shearing-type trauma accounts for the majority of avulsions of the gallbladder.

Sonography
Hypoechoic thickening or echolucency of the pericholecystic or hepato-cholecystic space should raise the suspicion of gallbladder injury. This appearance may be related to vascular injury, blood dissection in the sub-mucosal tissues, bile leak or a combination of these factors.

Contusion and intramural haematoma appear as echogenic intramural masses which may change in echogenicity with time.

Hydrops of the gallbladder

Tense gallbladder distension is uncommon in the absence of gallstones, inflammation, lymphadenopathy at the porta hepatis or congenital malformation. The majority of cases occur in children as an inflammatory or non-specific reaction to hepatitis, gastroenteritis, leptospirosis, upper respiratory tract infection, scarlet fever or lymph node compression in mucocutaneous lymph node syndrome (Kawasaki's syndrome). Torsion of the gallbladder may also result in hydrops.

Sonography
Sonographically the appearances may be indistinguishable from a mucocoele of the gallbladder although the latter is usually larger and associated with cystic duct obstruction without ensuing infection. Lack of gallbladder drainage may be confirmed by pre- and post-prandial examination and may be due to transient cystic duct obstruction by sludge or pressure from an adjacent lymph node.

Empyema of the gallbladder

Acute cholecystitis is almost always the result of cystic duct obstruction from a gallstone, the exception being acalculus cholecystitis which occurs in a different clinical setting. The gallbladder usually distends with inflammatory cells mixed with bile and calculi. As the condition progresses the bile becomes infected. The cystic duct disimpacts in 85 per cent of patients in which case the inflammation in the gallbladder settles. If the cystic duct remains impacted the inflammatory process may progress to an empyema of the gallbladder eventually leading to perforation.

Sonography

Sonography may reveal calculi within the lumen of the gallbladder, occasionally the impacted calculus may be identified. The gallbladder may be distended and tender to pressure from the ultrasound probe. Within the gallbladder lumen there may be gravity-dependent layering of pus or debris and bile. Particulate matter may appear as medium to coarse bright echoes without shadowing.

Cholecystomegaly

Obstructive cholecystomegaly – cystic duct obstruction (if infected empyema), stones, pancreatic neoplasms, bile duct stricture, pancreatitis, mucocoele of the gallbladder.

Non-obstructive cholecystomegaly – prolonged fasting, post-surgery, intravenous feeding, vagotomy, diabetes mellitus, neuropathic, appendicitis in children, hypertrophic pyloric stenosis in children (a small proportion show bile duct distension due to the weight of the pyloric muscle mass resting on the bile duct), acromegaly, Kawasaki's syndrome, bed-ridden patients, AIDS, alcohol abuse, narcotic abuse.

Normal in 2 per cent of the population – gallbladder size is variable and is related to the length of fasting. In a normal physiological state the gallbladder wall is not usually thickened. The normal anteroposterior diameter is less than 4 cm and the horizontal diameter is less than 5 cm.

Small gallbladder

Chronic cholecystitis.
Cystic fibrosis (30 to 50 per cent).
Congenital hypoplasia.
Hepatitis.
Extracorporeal shock-wave lithotripsy (this may be a transient phenomenon).

Multiseptate gallbladder

Appearance of a normal gallbladder folded over.
Congenital multiseptate gallbladder with fine non-shadowing septations.

Desquamated gallbladder mucosa in acute cholecystitis.

Polypoid cholesterolosis – non-shadowing mural and intramural densities which do not bridge the lumen.

Adenomyomatosis – Rokitansky–Aschoff sinuses – these are within the wall and are usually quite small. Unless gross they will not be confused with a multiseptate gallbladder.

Acute hepatitis – the gallbladder wall is thickened, the gallbladder volume is reduced associated with increased bile echogenicity and, rarely, has a multiseptate appearance.

Chronic cholecystitis

The sonographic diagnosis of chronic cholecystitis is less reliable than acute cholecystitis. Lack of gallbladder visualisation in a truly fasting patient is virtually diagnostic of gallbladder disease but many cases simply show evidence of gallstones with or without gallbladder wall thickening. As gallstones are common these findings do not necessarily indicate that they are the cause of the patient's symptoms. ERCP may also be unhelpful as an abnormal gallbladder may distend during a contrast injection, yet it may not distend under physiological conditions. The most reliable sign of chronic cholecystitis is a shrunken gallbladder containing gallstones but care must be taken not to mistake a bowel loop for a contracted gallbladder in non-fasting patients.

Porcelain gallbladder

A porcelain gallbladder shows diffuse wall calcification and is found in 0.6 to 0.8 per cent of cholecystectomies. Gallstones are found in 90 per cent with the gallbladder often non-functioning. The walls are often inflamed and fibrotic. Calcified foci are seen diffusely throughout the mucosa, submucosa and serosa. There is an increased risk of gallbladder carcinoma in 20 per cent of cases. The porcelain gallbladder should therefore be removed.

Sonography

There is a curvilinear densely reflective area with distal shadowing. The differential diagnosis is from bowel loops, chronic cholecystitis, cholelithiasis and emphysematous cholecystitis.

2.2.28 CARCINOMA OF THE GALLBLADDER

Carcinoma of the gallbladder is not uncommon, it accounts for up to 3 per cent of primary malignancies. It is the commonest biliary malignancy and usually occurs in the sixth to seventh decade with a male to female ratio of $1:4$. Seventy-five per cent of cases have gallstones (although only 1 per cent of patients with gallstones develop gallbladder carcinoma). Eighty to ninety per cent of cases are adenocarcinoma, others are squamous, anaplastic carcinoma, etc. Tumour has usually invaded the gallbladder bed before the onset of symptoms. Local infiltration usually infers a poor prognosis. The carcinoma may be infiltrating causing diffuse thickening and induration of the gallbladder wall or fungating resulting in a mass which fills the gallbladder lumen and invades the wall. Gallbladder polyps over 2 cm in size have a 64 to 98 per cent chance of being malignant. Appearances may be indistinguishable from chronic cholecystitis and many cases are only diagnosed at surgery. At presentation the tumour may have invaded the liver, common bile duct or lymph nodes and average survival is only 6 months. Seventy-five per cent of metastases are to the liver and pancreaticoduodenal lymph nodes. There is an association with inflammatory bowel disease, chronic cholecystitis and familial polyposis coli.

Sonography

The following sonographic signs are seen

1. gallstones within a mass strongly suggest carcinoma of the gallbladder
2. localised diffuse gallbladder wall thickening
3. polypoid intraluminal mass
4. diffusely echogenic mass
5. extensive tumour spread causing obstructive jaundice
6. low echogenicity mass extending into the porta and liver
7. high velocity arterial flow signal in tumour mass on colour flow Doppler
8. colour flow signal in the gallbladder wall
9. in gallbladder cancer the Doppler velocity is 39.0 ± 12.4 cm/s and the resistive index is 0.62 ± 0.12 (controls are: 11.4 ± 2.5 and 0.75 ± 0.03 respectively)
10. spread from carcinoma of the gallbladder may cause lymphadenopathy in the region of the head of the pancreas, this may obstruct the common bile duct and mimic carcinoma of the head of the pancreas, up to 25 per cent of cases show calcification in the gallbladder wall or typical appearance of porcelain gallbladder.

2.3 PANCREAS

2.3.1 INTRODUCTION

The pancreas is a lobulated retroperitoneal organ. It has a relatively long slender configuration being 12 to 20 cm long depending upon the patient's build. It weighs 60 to 100 g but often shows atrophy in elderly individuals. It does not have a true capsule and merges with the retroperitoneal fat accounting for its lobulated contour, which is more evident on CT than ultrasound and becomes more prominent with age.

The pancreas, as with other abdominal organs, shows craniocaudal movement with respiration but, being retroperitoneal and limited above by the coeliac axis origin from the aorta it shows far less movement than the liver, spleen and kidneys. Movement between inspiration and expiration is usually less than 1 cm but has been recorded to be up to 3.5 cm. The pancreas lies on the posterior abdominal wall with its head in the 'C' of the duodenal loop. The body and tail extend obliquely upwards to the left, the pancreatic tail lying in the lienorenal ligament adjacent to the spleen and the upper pole of the left kidney. The head of pancreas has an uncinate process, which extends posteroinferiorly around the superior mesenteric vein at the portal vein origin. The uncinate process extends inferior to the main body of the pancreas thus it is important to scan the full extent of the pancreas or carcinoma of the uncinate process may be missed.

2.3.2 ANATOMICAL RELATIONSHIPS

The pancreas lies in the anterior pararenal space (Figure 2.18). The head lies within the curve of duodenal loop with the inferior vena cava and right renal vessels lying posteriorly. The common bile duct receives the main pancreatic duct as it passes through the pancreatic head and then drains into the second part of the duodenum at the ampulla of Vater. The gastroduodenal artery may be seen anteriorly at the pancreatic head and neck. The head of the pancreas is the most bulbous part of the gland which then narrows at the 'neck'. The union of the superior mesenteric and splenic veins forming the portal vein posteriorly marks the anatomical position of the pancreatic neck. The pylorus and gastroduodenal artery lies anteriorly. The lesser sac lies anterior to the body of the pancreas while the splenic vein runs along its posterosuperior surface. The tail of the

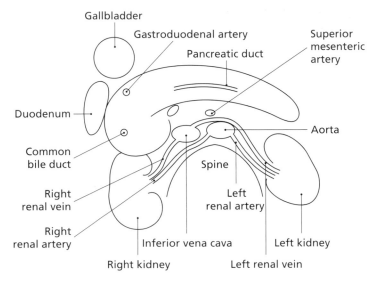

Figure 2.18 Anatomical relationships of the pancreas.

pancreas is related to the spleen, left adrenal and the upper pole of the left kidney.

2.3.3 EXAMINATION OF THE PANCREAS

The pancreas and retroperitoneum are easily obscured by bowel gas and are thus best examined in the morning when bowel gas is at a minimum. When the stomach is empty the pancreas may be examined by scanning directly through the pylorus. Alternatively the stomach and transverse colon may be displaced inferiorly either by inspiration or by pushing the abdomen out (which displaces the bowel inferiorly without over-inflating the lungs). If necessary the patient can drink water to fill the stomach thus providing an acoustic window. Water is initially echogenic after swallowing because of the presence of microbubbles but these disperse relatively quickly. Some workers have used metoclopramide, a pharmaceutical agent that speeds gastric emptying, to reduce gastrointestinal bowel gas. This can occasionally cause oculogyric crises (an uncommon and unpleasant idiosyncratic reaction) and thus has not gained widespread use during routine scanning. The distal body and tail of the pancreas may be examined by scanning obliquely through the spleen and upper pole of the left kidney using a left lateral or posterolateral approach.

2.3.4 SONOGRAPHIC APPEARANCES OF THE PANCREAS

The pancreas normally shows a homogeneous echopattern which is more echogenic than liver in 52 per cent of young patients and equally echogenic in 48 per cent. The gland becomes more echogenic with age and may become heterogeneous in echopattern.

Grading of pancreatic echogenicity

- Grade 1   pancreatic echogenicity is equal to the liver.
- Grade 2   pancreatic echogenicity is slightly greater than the liver.
- Grade 3   pancreatic echogenicity is clearly greater than the liver.
- Grade 4   pancreatic echogenicity is equal to the retroperitoneal fat.

In health echogenicity is related to age and body fat. However, the variation in echogenicity within the normal population is such that grading pancreatic echogenicity is of limited value. Grades 3 and 4 pancreatic echogenicity may be normal in adults and the elderly but this appearance is usually pathological in children and adolescents. In up to 10 per cent of very young children the pancreas may appear less echogenic than the liver whilst in preterm neonates and infants the pancreas may be quite echogenic. In these cases pancreatic echogenicity reduces as the gland matures.

Pancreatic duct

Using modern scanners the main pancreatic duct (Wirsung's duct) can be visualised in up to 85 per cent of patients. It is seen as a hypoechoic tube with fine echogenic walls. When the duct is collapsed it is seen as a fine echogenic line. The normal duct lumen is less than 2 mm in diameter though some series have reported normal ducts up to 3 mm in diameter in the pancreatic head. The main duct diameter increases with age. Duct dimensions are

- average duct diameter is 1.3 mm ± 0.3 mm
- average diameter in patients with gallstones is 1.4 mm
- average duct diameter in acute pancreatitis is 2.9 mm (the duct diameter reduces as the pancreatitis settles but it may not return to normal).

Pancreatic size

Average pancreatic anteroposterior diameter is

- head   2.5 to 3.5 cm
- body   1.75 to 2.5 cm
- tail   1.5 to 3.5 cm

The average gland size is variable depending upon the age and other characteristics of the population studied hence the variation in the results shown above. The pancreas may become infiltrated by retroperitoneal fat, particularly in obesity, changing its size and outline. Generally the gland size decreases with age while echogenicity increases. As with other organs actual measurements serve only as a guide to gland assessment and the overall impression of gland configuration and appearance is often more important. This can only be achieved with experience and overreliance on measurements in diagnosis will lead to errors (particularly when dealing with very variable patient groups such as children).

2.3.5 PANCREATIC BIOPSY

Pancreatic biopsy may be performed under ultrasound, CT or magnetic resonance guidance. The mode of imaging depends upon local preferences and the size and nature of the mass. It is usual to have a cytologist present at biopsy as immediate tissue analysis reduces the need for multiple biopsies. A fine needle aspiration biopsy is usually taken because of the risk of pancreatitis particularly with larger needles. The close relationship of the aorta, inferior vena cava and mesenteric vessels to the pancreas makes the risk of haemorrhage from a pancreatic biopsy significant.

2.3.6 PANCREATIC ANOMALIES

Annular pancreas

Annular pancreas is a congenital variant in which a ring of pancreatic tissue lies around the duodenum, 75 per cent of cases are associated with other congenital anomalies such as Down's syndrome, tracheo-oesophageal fistula, duodenal stenosis or atresia and imperforate anus. It may present in childhood or in adults with apparent enlargement of the pancreatic head and poor duodenal drainage, giving rise to duodenal dilatation. There is an increased risk of pancreatitis and peptic ulceration. The presence of duodenal dilatation and an apparently abnormal pancreatic head, particularly in young children, may suggest this diagnosis when pancreatic carcinoma is not expected.

Pancreas divisum

The pancreas forms from ventral and dorsal buds, which should fuse at around 8 weeks of life. Pancreas divisum results from failure of fusion of the pancreatic ducts of Wirsung and Santorini in 5 to 11 per cent of the population. The incidence is 1.3 to 6.7 per cent in ERCP series but it is found in 12 to 26 per cent of cases of recurrent pancreatitis. The diagnosis is best made on ERCP and not ultrasonography but it should be remembered as a cause of chronic pancreatitis.

Ectopic pancreas

Ectopic (aberrant) pancreatic tissue is relatively common, being found in 2 per cent of post-mortem examinations. It is rarely seen at sonographic examination but can give rise to nodules of tissue up to 3 to 4 cm in diameter. These show normal pancreatic histology and are usually located in the bowel affecting the stomach, duodenum, jejunum, Meckel's diverticulum and ileum in decreasing order of frequency. The sonographic appearance is non-specific and the diagnosis is made at biopsy.

Accessory spleen in the pancreas

Accessory spleen in the abdomen can be confused clinically and on imaging with neoplasms, 10 to 20 per cent are attached to the pancreatic tail where they may mimic tumours of the pancreas. An epidermoid cyst within an accessory spleen in the pancreas has been reported. If a question of accessory spleen is raised confirmation can be obtained by a radionuclide scan, using Tc-99m colloid or labelled denatured red cells.

Hypoechoic intrapancreatic fat

Fat is normally echogenic but hypoechoic fat within an intrapancreatic lipoma has been described. This phenomenon is extremely rare but has important clinical and imaging implications when it occurs as it may mimic other tumours of the pancreas. If the question is raised confirmation of an intrapancreatic lipoma may be obtained by CT.

Causes of pancreatic atrophy

Pancreatic atrophy is commonly seen in the elderly but may occur with other pathologies.

Pancreatic duct obstruction.
Cystic fibrosis.
Schwachman syndrome.
Haemochromatosis.
Viral infection.
Malnutrition.

2.3.7 PANCREATITIS

Acute pancreatitis

Acute pancreatitis is a relatively common clinical condition associated with a high morbidity and a significant mortality. Patients usually present with severe abdominal pain caused by pancreatic inflammation as a result of premature activation of proteolytic enzymes within the gland. The gland thus undergoes a process of autodigestion with further proenzyme activation. Inflammation and small vessel thrombosis occur. Severe inflammation may lead to vascular collapse and shock. Acute pancreatitis may be mild and self limiting or severe resulting in necrosis and suppuration. The diagnosis is usually made from the clinical history, physical examination and serum biochemistry (elevated serum amylase level) but presentation may be atypical and should be considered as a possible diagnosis in any case of abdominal pain. Up to 80 per cent of cases are secondary to other disease processes. Sonography is valuable in the assessment of underlying disorders and complications. In the United States 65 per cent of acute pancreatitis cases are alcohol related. This is more common in males than in females (6:1). In Europe biliary disease is the commonest association, 5 per cent of patients with gallstones will develop acute pancreatitis.

Causes of acute pancreatitis
Biliary disease, gallstones are present in 68 per cent of cases in the United Kingdom
Alcoholism – male to female ratio is 6:1
Trauma – including biopsy and ERCP
Adjacent inflammation
Sepsis
Viral infections – mumps and hepatitis
Hypercalcaemia
Pregnancy
Drugs – isoniazid, rifampicin, tetracycline, steroids, contraceptive pill, phenformin.
ERCP
Following surgery
Hereditary
Autoimmune disease – polyarteritis nodosa
Hyperlipidaemia
Pancreatic malignancy
Penetrating peptic ulcer
Dialysis
Ascariasis
Idiopathic (20 per cent)
Anatomical anomalies – annular pancreas, pancreas divisum

Complications of acute pancreatitis

The pancreas has only a thin fibrous sheath with no true capsule. Fluid from the inflamed pancreas easily penetrates the covering sheath to spread to adjacent areas, particularly to the lesser sac and retroperitoneum. Fluid, especially in the lesser sac, may be localised by blockage of the foramen of Winslow. Accumulation of fluid in the peritoneum results in pancreatic ascites. The pancreas is in the anterior pararenal space with the duodenum and ascending and descending colon. Fluid may extend into transverse mesocolon with the associated risk of venous thrombosis, mesenteric ischaemia and perforation. Encasement of the colon by inflammation may mimic colonic carcinoma. Inflammatory fluid can spread to the mediastinum via the oesophageal hiatus and crura. Pseudocysts due to tissue necrosis with osmotic influx of fluid develop in 20 per cent of cases. The cyst wall eventually undergoes fibrosis and may later calcify. Pseudocysts may be localised to the pancreas or extend into the abdomen or mediastinum and are usually unilocular. Pseudocysts may haemorrhage or rupture into adjacent structures, for example bowel and blood vessels. Haemorrhage may cause layering of fluids. Most pseudocysts (80 per cent) resolve spontaneously. Treatment is reserved for pseudocysts which enlarge or become infected. Fluid may be drained into the stomach by surgery or radiological drain insertion.

Cystic neoplasms and pancreatic duct dilatation may mimic a pseudocyst. An abscess may develop in a pseudocyst, other pancreatic fluid collections or tissue necrosis. Fluid in this instance may become echogenic and a fluid–fluid level may develop. The commonest infective organism is *Escherichia coli.*

Haemorrhage into the inflamed pancreas may occur with increasing pancreatic echogenicity. The haemorrhage may liquefy and look like other fluid collections. After the acute phase the pancreas may appear normal or atrophic and fibrosed. The gland size may increase or reduce. The pancreatic duct may dilate and eventually focal calcification may develop within the gland substance. This is seen most often in alcoholic pancreatitis.

Sonography

The pancreas may appear normal in 30 per cent of patients. Oedema and swelling may result in enlargement of the gland which may become hypoechoic or heterogeneous. In 67 per cent of patients the pancreas may be so echopoor that it is virtually indistinguishable from the contiguous splenic and portal veins. However the pancreas may show increased reflectivity in patients with severe inflammation due to haemorrhage or necrotising pancreatitis. The latter is related to blood products, tissue debris and soponification of fat by pancreatic enzymes in the pancreatic bed. In haemorrhagic pancreatitis there is usually considerable pancreatic enlargement and the echopattern is more heterogeneous. The adjacent soft tissues may be oedematous and echopoor. The margins of the pancreas may be indistinct.

Chronic pancreatitis

Recurrent or persistent attacks of pancreatitis lead to irreversible damage. This is particularly likely when the cause of the initial attacks persists. Thirty to sixty-five per cent of cases are associated with pancreatic calcification on the plain abdominal radiograph.

Sonography

The gland may appear normal even in the presence of advanced disease. In the early stages the gland is enlarged and hypoechoic with duct dilatation. The gland then becomes heterogeneous with areas of increased echogenicity and focal or diffuse enlargement. Pseudocysts may occur and focal hypoechoic inflammatory masses may mimic pancreatic neoplasia. Calculi and calcification within the gland give rise to densely echogenic foci which may shadow. The pancreatic and common bile duct may be dilated. In the late stages of the disease the gland becomes atrophic, fibrosed and shrinks. This results in a small echogenic gland with a heterogeneous echopattern. The pancreatic duct may remain dilated with a beaded appearance due to multiple stenosis.

2.3.8 PANCREATIC TRAUMA

Though the pancreas moves with respiration it is like other retroperitoneal organs, relatively fixed compared to the overlying bowel. The pancreas is thus prone to injury by blunt abdominal trauma when it is compressed against the spine. The pancreas is traumatised in 3 to 12 per cent of abdominal injuries as a result of seat belt or steering column impact. Up to 20 per cent mortality has been reported with pancreatic injuries as these are often associated with trauma to other organs such as the duodenum. Injury to the duodenum may give rise to an intramural haematoma obstructing the bowel lumen. There may be delayed retroperitoneal perforation of the duodenum. Injury to the pancreas may cause contusion or rupture. Rupture may be complete or incomplete but both frequently cause pancreatitis and fluid collections or pseudocyst formation. Pseudocysts usually form anteriorly but may be adjacent to any part of the gland and can occasionally be quite distant. Pancreatic lacerations are diagnosed by showing loss of contiguity but this may be masked by inflammation. Although ultrasound is excellent at showing fluid collections these patients are often immobile and often have gaseous distension, making CT a more suitable diagnostic tool. Moreover CT images the retroperitoneum.

2.3.9 PANCREATIC ASCARIASIS

Ascaris lumbricoides may migrate into the pancreatic duct and cause an acute pancreatitis. *A. lumbricoides* within the pancreatic duct can be diagnosed by the appearance of the 'four-line' sign. There are four bright echogenic lines, the outer pair corresponding to the duct walls and the inner pair to the body wall of the ascaris. This diagnosis should be considered in endemic areas or in visitors from endemic regions when a tubular structure is seen lying within the pancreatic duct in the appropriate clinical setting.

2.3.10 DIFFERENTIAL DIAGNOSIS OF AN ECHOGENIC PANCREAS

Pancreatitis in children

In nearly half the children with pancreatitis, the pancreas has increased reflectivity (grade 2) as compared to the liver. However, an equal number of children with pancreatitis have a grade 1 reflectivity, occasionally the reflectivity may be reduced initially and subsequently increase.

Acute pancreatitis in adults

Patients with acute pancreatitis usually have a hypoechoic gland due to the presence of interstitial oedema. However the pancreas may show increased reflectivity in patients with severe inflammation due to haemorrhage or necrotising pancreatitis because of high reflectivity from blood, tissue debris and saponification of fat in the pancreatic bed.

Chronic pancreatitis

See p. 188.

Cystic fibrosis

See p. 191.

Hereditary pancreatitis

Hereditary pancreatitis is inherited as an autosomal dominant condition. Patients present in the first decade of life and usually develop marked endocrine and exocrine deficiency. The appearances on imaging are no different from other forms of chronic pancreatitis. There is an increased incidence of pancreatic adenocarcinoma.

Non-alcoholic tropical pancreatitis

This is an idiopathic disorder usually presenting in the first and second decades. The patients are frequently diabetic and have extensive pancreatic calcification.

Shwachman–Diamond syndrome

This is a rare condition; the main features include pancreatic insufficiency, cyclic bone marrow depression, metaphyseal dysostosis and short stature. Associated findings include dental abnormalities, delayed puberty, renal dysfunction, disturbances in respiratory functions and hepatomegaly. The pancreas is echogenic because of fatty infiltration.

Johanson–Blizzard syndrome

This syndrome is extremely rare. The main findings include pancreatic insufficiency, nasal alar hypoplasia, deafness, teeth abnormalities, ectodermal scalp defects, psychomotor retardation, short stature, hypothyroidism and rectourogenital malformations. Cardiac anomalies have been described. The pancreas is echogenic because of fatty infiltration.

Fatty infiltration of the pancreas

Fatty infiltration of the pancreas from whatever cause, whether related to body habitus or metabolic disorder, gives rise to an echogenic appearance.

Lipomatous pseudohypertrophy of the pancreas

Lipomatous pseudohypertrophy of the pancreas is a rare disorder of unknown cause. It is characterised by massive replacement of the pancreas by fat. The condition may occur at any age and is associated with a variety of conditions which include obesity, diabetes mellitus, chronic pancreatitis, alcoholic liver disease, fibrocystic disease of the pancreas, Cushing's disease, steroid therapy, malnutrition, haemochromatosis and old age. The pancreas is enlarged with a heterogeneous bright echopattern.

Idiopathic fibrosing pancreatitis

Idiopathic fibrosing pancreatitis is an uncommon condition of unknown aetiology causing interstitial pancreatic fibrosis. This is associated with only marginal elevation of blood and urine pancreatic enzymes and there is a lack of pancreatic necrosis and autodigestion. Sonography shows diffuse pancreatic enlargement. Echogenicity is variable and may be normal to bright. The fibrotic process may constrict the common bile duct causing biliary obstruction and proximal biliary dilatation.

Cystic fibrosis

Cystic fibrosis is a relatively common condition which occurs with autosomal recessive transmission. One in twenty whites are carriers but the condition is rare in blacks and orientals. The cystic fibrosis gene is on the long arm of chromosome 7. There is a defect in mucous secretions involving the lungs, pancreas and hepatobiliary system resulting in the production of viscid secretions. There is a pronounced increase in pancreatic echogenicity, which is present in children. Duct blockage leading to atrophy and progressive fibrosis occurs in 85 to 90 per cent of patients with significant disease. Small cysts occur particularly in the pancreatic tail and as the gland atrophies there is a reduction in the anteroposterior diameter of the pancreas. The duct may be dilated and ductal calculi may be identified, but these changes are far less common than the generalised increase in pancreatic echogenicity which is almost universal from mid-childhood. Occasionally children with severe lung disease have relatively mild digestive problems and patients with severe digestive disorders can have relatively mild lung problems.

Sonography
Ultrasound is frequently used to assess changes in gland morphology but sonographic features do not correlate well with endocrine or exocrine pancreatic function. Pancreatic sonography is usually combined with evaluation of the liver, gallbladder, common bile duct, portal venous system and spleen and is more valuable in the assessment of liver disease and portal hypertension.

Causes of pancreatic calcification

Pancreatic calcification is usually seen as multiple small densely echogenic foci with distal shadowing.

Chronic pancreatitis - alcohol (commonest cause), gallstones, hereditary pancreatitis, idiopathic, chronic pseudocyst.
Haemorrhage – old haematoma, trauma, ruptured aneurysm.
Abscess.
Infarction.
Hyperparathyroidism – 20 per cent show pancreatic calcification, 50 per cent get chronic pancreatitis, may also show nephrocalcinosis.
Cystic fibrosis – fine granular calcification.

Haemochromatosis.

Kwashiorkor.

Neoplasia – adenocarcinoma (2 per cent), microcystic adenoma (sunburst cal-cification), macrocystic cystadenoma, cavernous lymphangioma, haemangioma, colonic carcinoma metastases.

2.3.11 CYSTIC PANCREATIC MASSES

Pancreatic pseudocyst

Fluid collections occur in up to 50 per cent of cases of acute pancreatitis. Pseudocysts are usually seen as anechoic fluid spaces but they may show internal echoes if they contain necrotic tissue or clot. Small fluid collections are often transient and fluid collections less than 5 cm in diameter may be treated conservatively. They may dissect tissue planes and thus can present at a distance from the pancreas. They have even been reported in the medi-astinum and scrotum. Without treatment some collections may become massive distending the lesser sac or filling the abdomen.

Aspiration of a pseudocyst increases the risk of infection and should only be carried out when clearly indicated. Surgical drainage requires organisa-tion of the pseudocyst wall so that it can hold sutures. Percutaneous drainage may also be performed under ultrasound guidance; the drain may be inserted through the stomach in a manner similar to marsupialization performed at surgery.

Pancreatic abscess

Pancreatic abscess is usually secondary to infection of a pseudocyst but may rarely occur as a result of direct spread from renal or colonic infection. Typically a pancreatic abscess occurs 2 to 4 weeks following an episode of acute pancreatitis. Sonographically the appearances may be similar to a pseudocyst. In general the appearance depends upon their age. In the acute phase the changes may be subtle with only loss of normal pancreatic contour associated with obliteration of the pancreatic outline and the peripancreatic vascular and other soft tissues spaces. These changes may be indistinguish-able from that found in severe acute pancreatitis. In the subacute and chronic stages when central necrosis occurs, an anechoic or complex cystic mass is usually seen. A debris level may be observed in the dependent portion of the abscess. There is usually good through transmission in these abscesses in the subacute or chronic phase except when gas is present within the abscess. In the presence of gas, the abscess may become very echogenic and may shadow. The walls of subacute or chronic pancreatic abscesses have variable features. The walls may be thick, irregular and well defined or the abscess may have no definable wall at all. The ultrasound findings are non-specific but in the appropriate clinical setting, a diagnosis of an abscess may be suggested and confirmed by percutaneous aspiration or CT.

Pancreatic cysts

Unlike the liver and kidneys, asymptomatic pancreatic cysts are uncommon. Pancreatic cysts may occur in combination with polycystic disease elsewhere, particularly those diseases with an autosomal dominant inheritance. The majority of pancreatic congenital cysts have been reported in infants and children. On sonography congenital cysts present as well-defined anechoic masses with good through transmission. The walls are smooth with no intramural excrescences or septations. Associated renal and hepatic cysts may be seen. Congenital cysts normally occur on the background of an otherwise normal-looking pancreas. Differential diagnosis is from cystic neoplasms, pancreatic pseudocysts and acquired cysts. Most congenital cysts occur in children while cystic neoplasms occur in adults. With pseudocysts there is often a previous history of acute pancreatitis and they are frequently seen on the background of inflammatory pancreatic disease. Congenital pancreatic pseudocysts have been described in neonates, sometimes reaching giant proportions.

Retention pancreatic cysts

Like pseudocysts, retention cysts are a complication of pancreatitis, usually a chronic calcific type occurring in alcoholic patients. Alcohol causes precipitation of protein within the pancreatic duct, causing protein plug blockage of the duct. Such blockage results in proximal duct dilatation forming a cyst. These cysts are usually small (1 to 2 cm in diameter) and asymptomatic, however rarely these cysts may acquire enormous proportions and no longer remain within the confines of the pancreas. Retention cysts have also been reported with ampullary stenosis and pancreatic carcinoma. Ultrasonography may reveal the underlying pancreatic abnormality (calcific pancreatitis) and small cysts in continuity with a dilated pancreatic duct. Stigmata of alcohol liver disease may be present.

Parasitic pancreatic cysts

Both *Echinococcus granulosus* and *E. multilocularis* cysts of the pancreas have been described although pancreatic involvement is exceptionally rare. *E. granulosis* cysts may be unilocular, multilocular or complex cystic. On imaging alone differentiation from other cystic masses is difficult. Serological tests may be useful in the appropriate clinical setting. *E. multilocularis* cysts, as elsewhere, show an echogenic infiltrative pattern. This diagnosis should be entertained in endemic regions when such pattern is seen.

Lymphoepithelial pancreatic cysts

Lymphoepithelial cysts of the pancreas are extremely rare. The pathological features of lymphoepithelial cysts are well-defined epithelial-lined cysts surrounded by a rim of lymphoid tissue. They present predominantly in middle-aged and elderly males with non-specific symptoms such as abdominal pain and diarrhoea. Ultrasound, particularly endoscopic sonography, is a sensitive means of diagnosing pancreatic cysts. Lymphoepithelial cysts are mainly cystic structures, but are not completely transonic and do contain some debris because of their keratin content. Cystic neoplasms and pseudocysts may have a similar appearance. As with some pseudocysts an elevated CEA (carcinoembryonic antigen) is found in lymphoepithelial cyst aspirates, therefore elevated CEA does not reliably predict malignancy.

Pancreatic dermoid cysts

Dermoid cysts within the pancreas are very rare but they do have some distinctive features such as cystic component teeth, fat inclusions and calcification. However it may not be always possible to differentiate these masses from neoplasms.

Pancreatic haematoma and traumatic pancreatitis

See pp. 186–188.

Von Hippel–Lindau disease

von Hippel–Lindau disease is an autosomal dominant condition with variable penetrance and delayed expression (reported in identical twins). Tumours or cysts occur in the central nervous system, genitourinary system, liver, spleen, pancreas and adrenal glands. Cysts are found throughout the pancreas varying in size from a few millimetres to 10 centimetres. These cysts are benign and usually give rise to symptoms when the common bile duct is obstructed. Microcystic adenoma is represented by a grape-like cluster of multiple cysts separated by thick-walled stroma. The cysts are lined by cuboidal epithelium, rich in glycogen but containing no mucus. These tumours are benign and not premalignant, giving rise to symptoms by mass effect when large. Mucinous cystadenoma is premalignant and not associated with von Hippel–Lindau disease. Microcystic adenoma may appear solid at ultrasound because of the multiple interfaces caused by the cysts of varying sizes, mostly small. Other pancreatic tumours reported with von Hippel–Lindau disease include adenoma, haemangioblastoma, and adenocarcinoma of the pancreas and ampulla of Vater. Islet cell tumours appear unrelated to pancreatic cystic disease in von Hippel–Lindau disease. There is a frequent association with pheochromocytoma. A number of endocrinopathies have been reported with pancreatic cell tumours in von Hippel–Lindau disease. These tumours are solid initially but as they grow central necrosis may occur. They may contain calcification. Because of their small size at presentation they may not be visualised on ultrasound. However intraoperative sonography is extremely useful in identifying and staging these tumours.

Dysontogenic pancreatic cysts

These are hamartomatous cysts, often associated with renal cysts, cerebellar angioma and encephalocoele. Imaging reveals a large thin-walled cyst with a mulberry configuration.

Pseudoaneurysm

Pseudoaneurysms are usually not truly intrapancreatic but may be confused with a pancreatic cyst. These aneurysms are a complication of pancreatitis in 3.5 to 10 per cent of patients. Doppler ultrasound may show turbulent arterial flow within a pseudoaneurysm, while colour flow Doppler shows bidirectional flow and swirling within the anechoic mass. Doppler ultrasound may permit tentative identification of the artery feeding the pseudoaneurysm.

Retroperitoneal neurofibroma or schwannoma

These tumours may be hyperechoic or hypoechoic cystic lesions with sporadic internal echoes which are a common feature in larger tumours in which cystic degeneration and haemorrhage has occurred. The tumours are retroperitoneal but may mimic pancreatic masses. Obstructed Roux loop after pancreatic cancer or bile duct surgery may present as a cystic mass in the pancreatic bed. Ultrasound demonstrates obstructed Roux loop as well as a patent biliary–enteric anastamosis. Echoes due to gas with or without comet-shaped artefacts are usually demonstrated.

Duodenal diverticula

Duodenal diverticula may mimic pancreatic neoplasms on ultrasound as they may have both complex as well as cystic appearances and may cause obstructive jaundice. With careful scanning it is possible to demonstrate the presence of air within the diverticulum and its continuity with the duodenum. ERCP may be diagnostic.

Cystic neoplasms of the pancreas

Cystic neoplasms of the pancreas are uncommon and represent less than 5 per cent of the pancreatic tumours. Two distinct types have been described.

Mucinous cystic tumours

There is a lot of confusion in the terminology used to describe these tumours and they have been described by several other names including

- intraductal mucin-producing tumours
- mucinous cystadenoma
- mucinous cystadenocarcinoma
- mucin-hypersecretory carcinoma
- 'ductectatic' mucinous cystadenoma
- mucinous ductal ectasia
- mucin-producing tumours.

Nakozawa *et al.* advocated the use of 'mucin-producing tumours' of the pancreas which included mucin-producing tumours (main duct type), ductectatic mucinous cystic tumour (branch duct type) and classic mucinous cystic tumours (peripheral type). These tumours have a malignant potential, are more common in women in the age range 20 to 82 years, with most patients presenting in the fifth to sixth decade. At presentation they are usually greater than 5 cm. The walls of mucinous cysts are composed of thick fibrous stroma containing dystrophic calcification. Sonography reveals a large cystic or complex mass with numerous septae, tumour excrescences and sometimes debris. The tumour size may vary from 2 to 23 cm, they usually have sharply marginated walls but have lobulated borders. The cystic portions show a good through transmission.

Microcystic adenoma (serous cystadenoma)

These tumours have no malignant potential. They tend to be large at presentation with an average diameter of 10 to 12 cm. Pathologically they tend to be lobulated masses with a thick fibrous capsule and contain multiple cysts of varying sizes. The cysts do not communicate with the pancreatic ducts. A central stellate fibrous scar is commonly seen, which may calcify. These tumours occur most frequently in women in the age range 34 to 88 years, however the average age at presentation is 65 years. Rare cases have been reported in children. On sonography these tumours are mostly complex with numerous internal echoes resulting in the appearance of a solid mass. Occasionally the tumour may be composed of a single cyst, differentiation from a mucous tumour is then based on the lack of internal septae and excrescences. The central scar and calcification may be demonstrated on CT.

Papillary cystic neoplasms of the pancreas

Papillary tumours of the pancreas may be solid or cystic. These are rare tumours often mistaken for mucin-secreting tumours or non-functioning adenomas. They present a low-grade malignancy, with females affected nine times more often than men, at an average age of 27 years. They are most often located within the pancreatic tail. They are large well-encapsulated masses with areas of haemorrhage and necrosis. On sonography they appear as a heterogeneous round solid mass with a cystic necrotic centre and dystrophic calcification which may shadow.

Gastric and duodenal leiomyosarcoma or leiomyoma

These tumours represent complex masses with a multicystic component; they may be confused with pancreatic masses, see p. 245.

Pancreatic sarcoma

Pancreatic sarcoma is a rare tumour of mesenchymal supporting structures of the pancreas. It is a relatively sonolucent mass which may be mistaken for a fluid collection or pseudocyst. Sonography may be normal or it may demonstrate a retroperitoneal mass which is relatively sonolucent compared to the surrounding tissues; it may therefore be confused with a cystic pancreatic mass.

Pancreatic lymphoma

Primary pancreatic lymphoma is rare. The clinical presentation is not unlike that of pancreatic carcinoma. Sonography may reveal a homogeneous sonolucent or complex mass. These masses are usually echopoor and mimic cystic lesions. As the prognosis of a pancreatic lymphoma is favourable, differentiation from a carcinoma is crucial.

Correlation of ultrasound, CT and angiography may result in a correct diagnosis, but if doubt exists an ultrasound-guided biopsy may reveal the true nature of the mass.

Pancreatic metastases

A variety of tumours may metastasise to the pancreas. Patients may present with acute pancreatitis, caused by pancreatic duct obstruction. The initial findings in this instance may be those of inflammatory disease of the pancreas complicated by pseudocysts and pancreatic ascites. Most metastases are solid but cystic metastases may occur particularly from cystadenocarcinoma of the ovary and melanoma. Pancreatic metastases cannot normally be differentiated from primary tumours on CT or ultrasound.

Differential diagnosis of pancreatic cystic masses

Pseudocysts or pancreatic fluid collections.
Focal pancreatitis (focal hypoechoic mass may mimic fluid collection).
Dilatation of the pancreatic duct.
Dilatation of the distal common bile duct – choledochocoele or choledochal cysts.
Congenital or hereditary cysts.
Trauma – haematoma.
Hydatid cysts.
Mucinous cystic tumours.
Microcystic adenoma.
Papillary cystic pancreatic tumours.
Cystic metastases.
Lymphoma – this may appear anechoic.
Sarcoma – this may appear anechoic.
Pseudoaneurysms.
Adjacent cystic masses – obstructed roux loop, duodenal diverticulum.
Retroperitoneal neurofibroma or schwannoma – this may be hypoechoic or anechoic.

2.3.12 PANCREATIC TRANSPLANTS

Pancreatic transplant drainage

One of the main technical difficulties facing the pancreatic transplant surgeon has been the fashioning of devices to drain exocrine pancreatic secretions. The method of free peritoneal drainage from a transplanted pancreas has now largely been abandoned. Segmental or whole pancreatic grafts are now drained into the small bowel or bladder. Bladder drainage is the preferred technique. The complication rate is high and clinical presentation non-specific.

Complications of pancreatic transplantation

Rejection 35 per cent.
Pancreatic or peripancreatic abscess 8 to 22 per cent.

Pancreatitis.

Thrombosis leading to graft failure 12 per cent.

Fluid collections – haematomas, lymphocoele, urinomas, pseudocysts, pancreatic ascites, leaks of exocrine anastamosis.

Sonography is the imaging of choice in the follow-up of pancreatic transplantation. Ultrasound should include Doppler evaluation of the graft arterial blood supply and venous drainage. Doppler signals are obtained of the pancreas and the transplant vascular pedicle. Knowledge of the vascular reconstruction is therefore vital for accurate evaluation of the transplanted pancreas.

Normal pancreatic transplant appearance

Sonographic appearance of the transplanted pancreas takes several weeks to normalise if no complications ensue. The normal parenchyma following transplantation reflects homogeneous medium level echoes similar to those of muscles. Appearances of the early transplant do not correlate well with endocrine function.

Parenchymal abnormalities

In the immediate postoperative period the graft may be anechoic or hypoechoic, this appearance is non-specific and may be a sign of rejection or pancreatitis but may also be seen normally. In the presence of acute rejection the pancreas is enlarged with patchy foci of decreased echogenicity or small anechoic areas. A sensitivity of 80 per cent is quoted for ultrasound diagnosis of rejection. Inhomogeneous parenchymal echoes and a dilated pancreatic duct are said to represent more specific signs of rejection. An increasingly echogenic pancreas with a reduction in the pancreatic size are related to chronic rejection. Calcification can be identified as bright foci which may shadow. Doppler ultrasound may add further specificity to the diagnosis of pancreatic transplant rejection. Impaired diastolic flow may indicate acute rejection. A parenchymal resistive index of 0.70 per cent or greater has a sensitivity of 76 per cent and specificity of 100 per cent in the diagnosis of acute rejection.

Fluid collections

Peripancreatic, intraparenchymal and pancreatic ascites or pelvic fluid collections are well visualised on ultrasound, although the character of extrapancreatic fluid often cannot be established. Bright echogenic foci within the fluid may be related to gas bubbles secondary to abscess formation.

Vascular complications

Arterial thrombosis and false aneurysms are readily detectable on Doppler ultrasound. Patent vascular supply to the graft is indicated by Doppler signal within the pancreatic parenchyma and vascular pedicle. Inability to detect an arterial or venous signal in the graft vasculature may reflect thrombosis or pancreatic rejection. Allowance should be made for technical difficulties such as gaseous distension and obesity. Doppler signal within a peripancreatic fluid collection suggests a false aneurysm.

2.3.13 SOLID PANCREATIC MASSES

Pancreatic carcinoma

Ductal pancreatic carcinoma is of increasing medical importance in Europe and the United States. Six per cent of all cancer deaths are now known to occur from pancreatic cancer in the US. The incidence of pancreatic cancer is rising. Most cases occur in patients over the age of 60 years, and its incidence is low below the age of 40 years. The risk factors include alcohol abuse, diabetes (increases the risk ×2), smoking (increases the risk ×2), asbestos exposure, hereditary pancreatitis (40 per cent) and chronic calcific pancreatitis (3 to 9 per cent). One to two per cent of acute pancreatitis cases have underlying carcinoma. Sixty per cent are found in the head of the pancreas, 20 per cent in the body or tail of the pancreas (these are often incurable at presentation) and 20 per cent involve the whole pancreas. Histologically 95 per cent of pancreatic carcinomas are adenocarcinoma, which usually originate from ductal elements. Lymphatic spread is to the celiac, superior mesenteric, paracaval, retrocaval and porta hepatis nodes. Vascular invasion is to the liver (55 per cent), lungs and peritoneal cavity. Venous thrombosis may occur especially with the body or tail tumours. Less frequently direct invasion of duodenum, stomach, colon, gallbladder, adrenal gland and kidney may occur. The prognosis is usually poor, 50 per cent of cases are dead within 3 months after the onset of symptoms. Though pancreatic carcinoma is a classic cause of progressive painless jaundice the commonest presenting symptoms are pain and weight loss. If a mass is identified then ultrasound may allow guided biopsy. Without biopsy the false positive rate of diagnosis of pancreatic carcinoma is 25 per cent because of the frequency of inflammatory masses of identical echopattern.

Sonographic signs of pancreatic carcinoma
1. A focal or diffuse mass.
2. The mass is usually greater than 2 cm in diameter at diagnosis.

3. The mass is usually well-defined and smooth in outline.
4. Tumours in the body or tail cause contour anomaly.
5. Tumours in the head may begin as a focal mass but often cause diffuse enlargement.
6. Pancreatic duct dilatation occurs in up to 97 per cent of pancreatic carcinomas.
7. Common bile duct dilatation occurs in 80 to 90 per cent of pancreatic head carcinomas, with small carcinomas common bile duct dilatation may be the only ultrasound abnormality.
8. The presence of calcification or intraductal calculi makes chronic pancreatitis more likely but does not exclude a carcinoma.
9. The majority of masses are hypoechoic but 3 per cent are echogenic. Once inflammatory changes supervene the echopattern becomes heterogenous.
10. Forty-seven per cent of cases are associated with hepatic metastases. These may be echopoor or echogenic.
11. Thickening of tissues around the coeliac axis or mesenteric vessels may be due to invasion of the lymphatics.
12. Masses adjacent to the pancreas may be mistaken for pancreatic masses:
    retroperitoneal varices
    retroperitoneal masses
    lymphatic masses or nodes
    renal tumours
    arterial aneurysms
    focal pancreatitis.

The differential diagnosis of pancreatic masses is difficult because chronic pancreatitis (particularly if the pathological changes are focal) and pancreatic cancer show similar clinical and imaging patterns. This diagnostic difficulty extends to ultrasound including endoscopic ultrasound angiography, CT and MRI. Technical progress in percutaneous aspiration biopsy has resulted in better diagnostic information. The use of 20–22 gauge needles has reduced the frequency of complications. Such biopsy can be performed under CT guidance or ultrasound.

Islet cell tumours

These slowly progressive tumours are of low-grade malignancy with an overall 5-year survival of 44 per cent. Sixty per cent are insulinomas, 18 per cent secrete gastrin and 15 per cent are non-functioning. Other rarer tumours include glucagonoma, enteroglucagonoma, somatostatinoma and vipoma (vasoactive intestinal polypeptide). Islet cell tumours may be associated with multiple endocrine neoplasia syndromes Type 1 (MEN 1). Functioning and non-functioning tumours are small. In the Zollinger–Ellison syndrome only 42 per cent of tumours are visible sonographically whilst only 30 per cent of non-functioning islet cell tumours can be identified by ultrasound. On the whole transabdominal ultrasonography is capable of detecting 60 per cent of solitary islet cell tumours. In cases of non-functioning tumours angiography is usually more rewarding. The typical sonographic appearances of an islet cell tumour are a well-circumscribed mass that is hypoechoic in relation to surrounding pancreatic tissue. In younger patients the tumour may be isoechoic or hyperechoic as the normal pancreas is less echogenic in the younger patient.

2.3.14 PANCREATIC SARCOMA

See p. 197.

2.3.15 PANCREATIC LYMPHOMA

One to two per cent of patients with intra-abdominal non-Hodgkin's lymphoma has pancreatic involvement; nearly all have massive retroperitoneal nodes. Isolated pancreatic lymphoma is rare and identical to adenocarcinoma. A mass of lymph nodes around the pancreas may blend in with the pancreas whether these nodes are from a lymphoma or metastases.

2.3.16 PANCREATIC METASTASES

The pancreas is not a particularly common site for metastases but tumour may affect the pancreas by direct spread from adjacent organs and also via the blood stream and lymphatics. Direct spread occurs particularly from the stomach, colon and kidney. Metastases from distant primary sites occur with several tumours including melanoma, lung, ovary, prostate, hepatoma, thyroid, testes and sarcoma. Melanoma metastases usually infiltrate the pancreas without focal mass formation. The remainder gives rise to hypoechoic masses indistinguishable from primary tumour.

2.3.17 AMPULLARY CARCINOMA

This is an epithelial tumour of the ampulla of Vater, and may represent a benign villous adenoma or an invasive carcinoma. There is an association with an adenomatous polyposis syndrome colon carcinoma. Patients may present with jaundice, gastrointestinal bleeding or pain. The tumour is staged as

- T_1 when confined to the ampulla
- T_2 when the duodenal wall is invaded
- T_3 when there is less than 2 cm pancreatic invasion
- T_4 when there is more than 2 cm pancreatic invasion.

The tumour is visualised on endoscopy in 63 per cent of cases, seen as a submucosal mass in 25 per cent, but not visualised at all in 9 per cent. These tumours are often small at presentation and not often seen on ultrasound. When seen they usually present as small hypoechoic masses within the lower end of the common bile duct with or without adjacent pancreatic infiltration. The common bile duct or intrahepatic ducts are invariably dilated at presentation. The pancreatic duct may also show dilatation. Endoscopic ultrasound is more reliable at ampullary tumour detection. Differential diagnoses include periampullary duodenal adenoma, choledochocoele, pancreatic rest, leiomyoma, carcinoid, impacted calculus and Brunner gland tumour.

2.3.18 INTRAOPERATIVE ULTRASONOGRAPHY

Intraoperative ultrasound identifies tumours as small as 3 mm and has a much higher sensitivity. If intraoperative ultrasound of the pancreas is negative in a patient with a known endocrine syndrome, the stomach and duodenum should be examined for potential extrapancreatic sites of tumour. Endoscopic ultrasound is another sensitive technique for searching for islet cell tumours. Approximately 80 per cent of small endocrine tumours not detected by preoperative conventional CT and ultrasound are visualised by intraoperative ultrasound. Small tumours in the wall of the duodenum have also been visualised with this technique.

2.3.19 INTRADUCTAL ULTRASONOGRAPHY

A 30 MHz probe mounted on a 4.3-F intraductal catheter may be used via an ERCP. Small pancreatic tumours can be identified using this technique, but experience is limited at the time of writing.

2.3.20 MYELOMA AND PLASMACYTOMA

Myeloma and plasmacytoma may cause a hypoechoic solid mass resembling a lymphoma or carcinoma and may cause obstructive jaundice.

2.3.21 FOCAL FATTY SPARING

As in the liver pancreatic fatty infiltration may be focal. Parts of the organ are spared, particularly the head and uncinate process, in the initial stages of fatty change. This gives rise to an impression of a hypoechoic mass lesion within the head or uncinate process, while the rest of the pancreas shows increased echogenicity. As with the liver the fatty sparing may be geographical in shape, for example triangular.

2.3.22 RETROPERITONEAL PSEUDO-TUMOURS IN CHILDREN AND YOUNG ADULTS

Inflammatory pseudo-tumours may clinically and radiologically mimic malignant neoplasms particularly lymphoma and sarcoma.

2.3.23 PANCREATIC IMAGING: ULTRASOUND CHECKLIST

1. The size of the pancreas is relatively large in the newborn and decreases with age, becoming thinner in the elderly, the application of pure measurements as a criteria of disease may therefore be misleading. As with any other organ actual measurement is a guide only.
2. Record echogenicity, this again is variable particularly with age. Changes in echogenicity should be read in the clinical context.
3. Record any focal masses or abnormality in focal echogenicity.
4. Record calcification.
5. Measure pancreatic duct size if appropriate.
6. Look for abnormal fluid collections in and around the pancreas.
7. Record dilatation of the biliary tree.
8. Look for evidence of gallstones.
9. Look for evidence of liver masses or metastases.
10. Look for evidence of liver cirrhosis or portal hypertension.

2.4 SPLEEN

2.4.1 ANATOMICAL RELATIONSHIPS

The spleen is an intraperitoneal lymphoid organ lying in the left upper quadrant of the abdomen beneath the left hemidiaphragm. Posterolaterally the spleen is related to the 9th to 11th ribs. Interiorly the visceral surface is concave and is related to the stomach, left kidney and adrenal and the splenic flexure of the colon. The spleen is contained in a fibrous capsule and is invested in visceral peritoneum which is adherent to its surface except at the hilum. Peritoneal reflections form ligaments which connect the spleen to the diaphragm, stomach and kidney. In 2 per cent of the population these ligaments are lax allowing increased splenic mobility (wandering spleen).

The splenic artery and vein both pass through the splenic hilum, the artery dividing into approximately six branches. The splenic vein runs behind the superior aspect of the pancreas whilst the artery is slightly higher running just above the superior aspect of the pancreas. The splenic vein is less than 1 cm in diameter in 87 per cent of patients. Increasing size is associated with portal hypertension particularly when the vein is large (greater than 1.3 cm). The size of the spleen relative to total body size is greatest in children and falls with age. Average splenic weight in the first year of life is only 17 g increasing to 200 to 300 g in young adults. The spleen then gradually reduces in size weighing around 120 g at 70 to 80 years. In the young adult the spleen measures approximately $3 \times 8 \times 13$ cm but size is very variable and may change in a short space of time in response to infection and other stress. The spleen generally has a 'half-a-moon' configuration being concave inferomedially but it may have a lobulated border or may show an apparent cleft which should not be mistaken for a laceration.

2.4.2 SONOGRAPHIC APPEARANCES OF THE SPLEEN

The spleen is normally slightly more echogenic than the liver and significantly more echogenic than the kidney. Splenic echogenicity increases with age but not to the same extent as the pancreas. The appearance of the splenic parenchyma is not usually affected by the transducer angle or the angle of incidence of the ultrasound beam, but visualisation of the splenic capsule is variable and is dependent on the angle of incidence of the ultrasound beam. The left lobe of the liver extends across the abdomen in neonates and young children and may be in contact with the spleen. This relationship may be seen in adults with hepatomegaly or splenomegaly. In these cases a well-defined margin can usually be seen between the liver and spleen but when they are of a similar echogenicity it may be necessary to scan medially to show portal tracts within the lateral aspect of the left lobe of the liver thus confirming its identity. When a small amount of ascites is present within the abdomen fluid between the spleen and left lobe of the liver is easily mistaken for a splenic laceration. In these cases a wedge of tissue is seen anteromedial to the spleen. It is essential to follow this wedge of tissue medially in order to demonstrate portal tracts within it.

2.4.3 SPLENIC SIZE

Splenic size is most frequently assessed by measuring the craniocaudal length (normally 14 cm). Whilst this is a fairly crude means of evaluating splenic size other methods are prone to error. Measuring the spleen in three dimensions may also prove difficult because of its position under the left hemidiaphragm and ribs. Regardless of the method used to assess splenic size it should be remembered that the size of the spleen is variable and changes quite rapidly in response to infection and other illness. The degree of atrophy, which occurs with age, is variable. Minor changes in splenic size in the absence of haematological evidence of hyper- or hyposplenism are thus of little consequence.

Splenic measurements

Normal splenic measurements are

- length   12 cm (up to 14 cm)
- width   7 to 8 cm
- anteroposterior diameter   3 to 4 cm
- in children splenic length is approximately $5.7 + (0.31 \times$ age in years) cm
- splenic index   length × width × thickness
- splenic volume   220 cm^3 ± 75 cm^3 (variable shape limits the accuracy of measurement).

2.4.4 ACCESSORY SPLENIC TISSUE

Accessory splenic tissue or splenuncles are common, being present in up to 30 per cent of the population, at post mortem. They usually lie on the visceral surface of the spleen close to the splenic hilum. Splenuncles are frequently seen when the spleen is enlarged and after splenectomy but are not usually seen when the splenic size is normal. When visible the accessory splenic tissue is seen as a very well-defined round to ovoid mass with uniform echogenicity identical to that of the adjacent spleen, often with a fine echogenic capsule. Ten per cent of people have multiple nodules of accessory splenic tissue and though the majority of nodules lie around the splenic hilum they have been found in the pelvis. Accessory splenic nodules are usually easy to recognise but can mimic pancreatic tail masses. The diagnosis of accessory splenic tissue can be confirmed by showing branches of the splenic vessels entering the nodules. Nodules of splenic tissue have been reported in the perirenal area, pancreas, liver and testes. These splenic rests may mimic lymphoma and lymphadenopathy. Diagnosis of accessory splenic tissue can be confirmed by Tc-99m sulphur colloid or splenic-specific Tc-99m denatured red blood cells.

2.4.5 SPLENOSIS

Splenosis is the autotransplantation of splenic tissue caused by trauma or surgery. Deposits of splenic tissue have been found on the serosal surface of the bowel, on the mesentery, on the parietal peritoneum and on the diaphragm. When enlarged these masses may mimic neoplasia.

2.4.6 LACK OF VISUALISATION OF THE SPLEEN

Small spleen

A large obese patient.
A barrel chest – the spleen is under the diaphragm / over inflated lungs.

Anatomical distortion – scoliosis, diaphragmatic hernia, etc.

Asplenia, polysplenia or previous splenectomy.

Small spleen – radiation, infarction, traumatic fragmentation, etc.

Hereditary or congenital hypoplasia

Infarction – sickle cell disease

Polysplenia syndrome

Post-radiotherapy.

Atrophy.

Trauma.

Splenectomy – The spleen is a very vascular organ and laceration may cause torrential haemorrhage. Laceration may occur with minimal trauma particularly if the spleen is diseased, for example by infectious mononucleosis. Splenectomy should be avoided if at all possible, as there is significant risk of overwhelming infection post-splenectomy (after splenectomy the risk of death from sepsis such as pneumonia and meningitis is 60 × normal). Despite this, splenectomy may be necessary to prevent fatal haemorrhage and the sonographer should recognise the signs of progressive splenic haemorrhage from early subcapsular haematoma or laceration to the build up of peritoneal fluid due to persistent bleeding. After splenectomy fluid collections may occur in the left upper quadrant or bowel loops may fill the splenic bed mimicking postoperative abscess.

2.4.7 VARIATIONS IN SPLENIC SIZE

Asplenia

Congenital absence of the spleen is rare. Congenital absence of the spleen is associated with an increased risk of overwhelming sepsis, this also occurs after splenectomy. The usual association is with symmetric development of normal asymmetric organs or pair of organs and multiple cardiovascular anomalies is the rule.

Hyposplenism

Functional hyposplenia and small or atrophic spleen is not synonymous. Functional hyposplenia (hyposplenism) can occur with a normal sized spleen and even splenomegaly, where the splenic tissue has been replaced by granulomas, amyloid, myeloma deposits or the splenic phagocytes have been paralysed by large doses of corticosteroids or cytotoxic drugs. Actual atrophy is less common than evidence of hypofunction.

Functional hyposplenia refers primarily to loss of phagocyte function of the spleen. It is defined by lack of uptake of heat-damaged erythrocytes, labelled with 99m-Tc sulphur colloid or other radionuclides and evidence of impaired remodelling of erythrocytes. The circulating erythrocytes reflect the loss of splenic filtration function, which can be detected by a peripheral blood smear.

Causes of hyposplenism

Anatomic causes.
Asplenia.
Hyposplenism.
Splenectomy.
Splenic vein thrombosis.
Splenic artery or coeliac axis thrombosis.
Sarcoidosis.
Amyloidosis.
Myeloma.
Haemangiosarcoma.
Iatrogenic causes.
Corticosteroids.
Cytotoxic drugs.
Thorotrast exposure.
Radiotherapy.
Immunoglobulin G.
Haematological causes.
Sickle cell disease.
Primary thrombocytopenic purpura.
Fanconi anaemia.
Lymphoma.
Autoimmune disease.
Systemic lupus erythematosis.
Mixed connective tissue disorder.
Rheumatoid arthritis.
Sjogren's syndrome.
Graft-versus-host reaction.
Chronic active hepatitis.
Thyroiditis or thyrotoxicosis.
Miscellaneous causes.
Coeliac disease.
Ulcerative colitis.
Crohn's disease.
Dermatitis herpetiformis.
Intestinal lymphangiectasis.
Tropical sprue.
Fulminant bacteraemia.

Hypersplenism

Hypersplenism is uncommon only occurring in a small percentage of patients with splenomegaly. It is characterised by

1. splenic enlargement
2. increased sequestration of blood cells reducing one or more of the blood cellular elements, particularly the platelets
3. correction of the haematological disturbance by splenectomy.

Ultrasound cannot predict which patients with splenomegaly will suffer from hypersplenism.

Splenomegaly

The size and shape of the spleen are very variable, some being long and thin while others are short and broad. This variation, together with the natural tendency of splenic size to vary during infective episodes, makes minor changes in size very subjective. Despite this splenomegaly is usually evident sonographically before it can be demonstrated clinically. The enlarged spleen may extend inferiorly over the left kidney improving renal visualisation. When very large the spleen may extend into the left iliac fossa. Any spleen over 13 cm long should be considered enlarged particularly if it also shows an increase in the anteroposterior diameter.

Causes of splenomegaly

Infection - non-specific reactive splenomegaly, for example viraemia, SBE (subacute bacterial endocarditis), infectious mononucleosis, tuberculosis, typhoid fever, cytomegalovirus infection, malaria, leishmaniasis, hepatitis, toxoplasmosis, schistosomiasis, histoplasmosis, syphilis, trypanosomiasis, hydatid disease.

Congestive disorders – right heart failure, cirrhosis or portal hypertension, splenic vein thrombosis.

Lymphoproliferative or haematogenous disorders – lymphomas, histiocytosis, myeloma, polycythaemia rubra vera, myelofibrosis, acute and chronic leukaemia, haemolysis, thrombocytopenic purpura, extramedullary haemopoiesis.

Collagen vascular disease – systemic lupus erythematosis, rheumatoid arthritis, Felty's syndrome.

Storage disease and infiltration – Gaucher's disease, Niemann–Pick disease, mucopolysacharidosis, haemodialysis, amyloidosis, sarcoidosis (in up to 60 per cent), haemochromatosis, diabetes mellitus.

Neoplastic disorders – haematological malignancy (leukaemia, lymphoma), sarcoma, haemangioma, chondroma, osteoma, fibroma, metastases (uncommon usually late in disease).

Congenital and acquired cysts and masses – post-traumatic masses.

Splenic vein thrombosis – splenic vein thrombosis is usually secondary to venous congestion or adjacent inflammation such as portal hypertension, pancreatitis and pancreatic neoplasm. When long standing splenic vein thrombosis can result in varices with massive splenomegaly.

Splenomegaly with a normal echopattern

Portal hypertension – although the spleen may be hypoechoic or show a splenic interface sign.

Hepatocellular disease.

Early stages of sickle cell disease – in the later stages multiple infarcts lead to atrophy.

Hereditary spherocytosis.

Leukaemia.

Chronic anaemia.

Still's disease.

Felty's syndrome.

Wilson's disease.

Reticulum cell sarcoma.

Tumour infiltration.

Splenomegaly with a hypoechoic pattern

Reaction to sepsis.

Hepatocellular disease or portal hypertension.

Hodgkin's disease.

Myeloma.

Non-gaseous granulomatous infection.

Leukaemia..

2.4.8 SPLENIC CYSTS

Cysts within the spleen are relatively uncommon compared to hepatic and renal cysts. They may be true congenital cysts with epithelial lining but at least 80 per cent are acquired secondary to trauma, infection or infarction. Congenital cysts may have the same appearance as simple cysts elsewhere in the body. They are well-defined anechoic spaces, which may show no demonstrable wall or capsule. There is distal acoustic enhancement and unless haemorrhage or infection has complicated the cyst there are no internal echoes. Haematomas may form cysts as they liquefy. Often the patient cannot recall the episode of trauma responsible. Acquired cysts including those caused by infection, haematomas and infarcts usually have a fibrous capsule which may not be visible on ultrasound. Hydatid cysts are the most important infective cysts in the spleen. Their appearance is that of hydatid disease of the liver. Both hydatid cysts and haematomas can calcify giving rise to dense cyst wall echogenicity and distal shadowing. Post-inflammatory cysts usually have well-defined margins with internal septations and a fairly well-defined wall. Diagnosis may be confirmed by cyst aspiration but this should not be attempted if there is a risk of hydatid disease.

Differential diagnosis of splenic cysts

Congenital cysts or primary cysts are subdivided by histological types

Endothelial lined – haemangioma, lymphangioma.
Epithelial lined – dermoid, epidermoid, transitional cell.

2.4.9 SPLENIC HAEMANGIOMA

Benign haemangiomas are the commonest primary splenic tumour being found in up to 14 per cent of individuals at autopsy. They are usually single and relatively small in size although they have been recorded up to 17 cm in size. They are generally of little significance and are found within the vascular splenic parenchyma. They are not easy to see on CT or ultrasound. When large they may result in hypersplenism causing anaemia, thrombocytopenia and coagulation disorders. The vast majority are small capillary lesions isoechoic with the spleen. Larger lesions may show mixed echogenic areas and cystic spaces whilst very large lesions may show anechoic cystic spaces. The cystic spaces usually show no flow on Doppler assessment whilst the adjacent parenchyma shows flow.

2.4.10 SPLENIC LYMPHANGIOMA

Lymphangioma of the spleen is a rare condition usually associated with osseous and hepatic involvement. Part or all of the spleen is replaced by multiple endothelial-lined cystic spaces that vary in diameter from a few millimetres to several centimetres. Echogenicity of the mass depends upon cyst size and cyst contents, for example amorphous eosinophilic debris, cholesterol crystals, calcium, haemosiderin and pigment-laden macrophages. When cystic they usually appear multiloculate.

2.4.11 EPIDERMOID CYST

These are congenital in origin. They are usually solitary well-defined cysts which initially may have the appearance of a simple cyst. However, with time they may become large and complex or show calcification. The average age at diagnosis is 18 years, the cysts often being as large as 10 cm at diagnosis. Cysts over 15 cm have been recorded. They may show septations, 20 per cent being multiple or multilocular.

2.4.12 SPLENIC PSEUDOCYSTS

These cysts resemble the congenital variety of splenic cysts on sonography and other imaging. These cysts can only be differentiated on histology as they are not epithelial or endothelial lined. The majority of splenic cysts (80 per cent) are of this variety. They are invariably secondary to previous trauma as a result of splenic haematoma or laceration, however the history of trauma may not be forthcoming. They have also been reported after splenic infarction, especially in sickle cell disease. These cysts as well as the epithelial-lined cysts may expand and become symptomatic. Splenic pseudocysts, as well as epithelial-lined cysts are characteristically unilocular, solitary non-calcified and surrounded by a smooth well-defined wall.

2.4.13 PANCREATIC PSEUDOCYSTS INVADING THE SPLEEN

This is a rare occurrence when a pancreatic pseudocyst at the hilum of the spleen invades the spleen. This is a serious complication of pancreatitis and usually requires urgent surgical treatment.

2.4.14 SPLENIC ABSCESS

Despite the vascular nature of the spleen and frequency of septicaemia, splenic abscesses are uncommon. Seventy-five per cent are due to haematological spread from SBE, intravenous drug abuse and immune compromise. Fifteen per cent follow trauma whilst 10 per cent are related to infected infarcts. The rest are related to direct inoculation by trauma, percutaneous procedure or secondary infection of an epidermoid or a pseudocyst. Rarely direct spread may occur from the colon or subphrenic space. Abscesses are seen with increasing frequency in patients with immune compromise because of chemotherapy or HIV. In these cases abscesses are frequently multiple and atypical organisms such as fungi may be involved. A splenic abscess is seen as an anechoic or hypoechoic focus, which is usually ill defined but can be well defined with a recognisable wall. There may be internal echoes or even gas bubbles giving rise to highly echogenic foci. The clinical history and sonographic findings usually suggest the diagnosis of splenic abscess, if necessary confirmed by needle aspiration. The main differential diagnosis is splenic haematoma or haemorrhagic infarct. The diagnosis is important as splenic abscess has a high mortality of up to 60 per cent.

NB although abscesses are usually ill defined and round or oval they may be wedge shaped and may mimic infarcts and metastases.

2.4.15 SPLENIC HAEMATOMA

The majority of splenic haematomas are post-traumatic but some are due to spontaneous bleeding from bleeding diathesis or anticoagulant therapy. The spleen is the intraperitoneal organ most frequently injured by blunt abdominal trauma.

Ultrasonography is valuable both for the demonstration of splenic haematomas and lacerations and also for the examination of other organs such as the liver and kidneys which may also be damaged. Small volumes of intraperitoneal fluid may also be demonstrated and in the context of abdominal trauma (and the absence of other disease) this may be assumed to be blood.

Blunt trauma sufficient to cause significant splenic injury will frequently result in other abdominal injuries. Forty per cent of patients with splenic injury will have an injury to the lower left ribs. Ten per cent have a left renal injury and 2 per cent have a left hemidiaphragm injury. Conversely 25 per cent of patients with significant left renal trauma also have a splenic injury and 20 per cent with lower left rib fracture have a splenic injury.

Splenic haematomas are initially seen as an anechoic collection which may become echogenic as the blood clots. Haematomas can be echogenic from the outset if the blood clots and layers as the haematoma forms. Liquefaction may give a complex or cystic appearance. Subcapsular collections are crescent shaped or lenticular and conform closely to splenic shape. Subcapsular haematomas may result in delayed splenic rupture over 48 hours after the episode of trauma, causing severe sudden haemorrhage in patients who have previously been stable.

2.4.16 SPLENIC LACERATION

Splenic lacerations are reliably demonstrated provided the spleen can be adequately visualised. This is often difficult after trauma as the patient is usually acutely tender over the area of interest. Lacerations are seen as anechoic or echo-poor defects in the splenic margin and parenchyma. This is because of blood within the laceration. As the blood clots the laceration becomes echogenic. Extensive lacerations may cross both capsular margins resulting in a complete splenic fracture.

Both CT and ultrasound have a major role in the evaluation of splenic trauma. Which modality is used as first choice will depend upon local preference and clinical circumstances. CT has the advantage that it may also be used to evaluate cranial and thoracic trauma. Ultrasound has the advantage that it is mobile and can be taken to the patient and can be repeated regularly over a short period of time. This is useful as the spleen is a very vascular structure and may show a very significant reduction in size during periods of hypotension. Changes in perfusion may affect post-contrast CT appearances of the spleen and sonography provides a useful means of assessing the spleen if CT appearances are confusing or equivocal. When evaluating a spleen after trauma always consider the possibility that any hypoechoic or echogenic areas that are seen may antedate the trauma and are not necessarily due to haematoma or laceration. An abnormal spleen is more susceptible to trauma and rupture than a normal spleen thus a proportion of patients who present with post-traumatic splenic haemorrhage will have underlying abnormalities.

Whenever possible splenic trauma is treated conservatively. When surgery is unavoidable there is usually little chance of repair thus surgery usually results in splenectomy. In children the risk of death from overwhelming infection in the years following splenectomy is 1.2 per cent whilst in adults the risk of death from sepsis is 0.3 per cent. Care is thus taken to preserve the spleen if at all possible. Follow up of splenic injury may require repeated abdominal imaging in which case ultrasound is preferable to CT.

Ultrasound signs of splenic trauma

Visible laceration.
Splenic fracture (laceration across the entire width of spleen).
Heterogeneous parenchyma (contusion or haematoma).
Perisplenic fluid.
Double splenic margin.
Irregular margin.
Peritoneal fluid.
Ipsilateral pleural fluid.
Splenic enlargement – hypotension causes a reduction in splenic size. If the patient is hypotensive following trauma then as the blood pressure returns to normal the spleen will enlarge returning to normal size. A pathologically enlarged spleen after trauma will usually have an abnormal texture and should be distinguished from a normal spleen.

Differential diagnosis of splenic laceration

Congenital cleft.
Adjacent liver edge.

NB some anatomical texts incorrectly state that the left lobe of the liver does not reach the spleen. This is in fact the normal anatomical relationship in children and fluid between the spleen and left lobe of the liver is easily mistaken for a splenic laceration.

2.4.17 HYDATID CYST

Splenic hydatid cysts are almost solely caused by *Echinococcus granulosus*. In endemic areas the spleen is involved in 5 per cent of cases and it is about twice as common as other benign cysts. The cysts tend to have a fairly well-defined wall and are usually multiloculate. However they may be unilocular which may resemble a simple cyst, caution is therefore required in endemic areas. Splenic hydatid cysts may calcify.

2.4.18 VASCULAR SARCOMAS

Ascites and hepatosplenomegaly usually accompany vascular sarcomas. The cystic nature of these sarcomas varies with the degree of vascularity and the degree of cystic degeneration in the solid component of the tumour.

2.4.19 SPLENIC ARTERY ANEURYSM

These aneurysms when lying close to the splenic hilum may mimic splenic cysts, however with careful attention to detail and with the use of colour Doppler the nature of these 'cysts' will become obvious.

2.4.20 VARICES

Splenic hilum varices from splenic vein thrombosis or portal hypertension appear as serpiginous cystic spaces. Careful scanning should reveal other signs of portal hypertension or splenic vein thrombosis. There is often splenomegaly. Doppler sonography is diagnostic.

2.4.21 SURROUNDING FLUID COLLECTIONS

A left pararenal cyst, a left adrenal cyst and loculated fluid collections in the left upper quadrant usually should not cause any confusion.

2.4.22 CYSTIC OR NECROTIC SPLENIC TUMOURS

These changes are particularly prevalent in metastases rather than primary tumours, see p. 211.

2.4.23 SPONTANEOUS SPLENIC RUPTURE

Spontaneous rupture of the spleen is uncommon but is a well-recognised and life-threatening complication of many splenic diseases.

2.4.24 SPLENIC TUMOURS AND MASSES

Mesothelial cysts.

Splenic abscesses.

Splenic infarct.

Metastases – especially angiosarcoma, haemangioendothelioma and metastatic carcinoma.

Infiltrative processes – Hodgkin's lymphoma, non-Hodgkin's lymphoma, acute lymphatic leukaemia.

Iatrogenic causes – colonoscopy, electroconvulsive therapy, porta hepatis occlusion during surgery, induction chemotherapy in acute leukaemia.

Infections – typhoid fever, malaria, *Legionella* spp., infectious mononucleosis, rubella, cytomegalovirus, tuberculosis, *Streptococcus pneumoniae*, *Haemophilus influenzae*, *Salmonella* spp., Staphylococcus spp., typhus, *Campylobacter* spp.

Raised intra-abdominal pressure – vomiting, pregnancy, sudden extreme exertion.

Haematological disorders – idiopathic thrombocytopenic purpura, haemophilia, anticoagulant or thrombolytic therapy, congenital afibrinogenaemia.

Miscellaneous conditions – vasculitis, pancreatitis (acute and chronic), hepatitis or cirrhosis.

Fluid-filled left upper quadrant masses

Fluid-filled gastric fundus.

Left renal cyst.

Cystic or necrotic renal tumour.

Left hydronephrosis.

Left adrenal cyst.

Cystic or necrotic adrenal tumour.

Splenic cyst.

Necrotic splenic tumour.

Splenic abscess.

Giant splenic artery aneurysm.

Splenic haematoma or laceration.

Pancreatic pseudocyst.

Pancreatic cystadenoma or cystadenocarcinoma.

Cystic left lobe of the liver.

Necrotic mass or abscess in the left lobe of the liver.

Loculated ascites or abscess, for example subphrenic.

Perisplenic fluid.

Pseudo-perisplenic fluid – uniform hypoechoic tissue, for example lymphoma.

Hydatid cyst – spleen, left lobe of liver, pancreas or retroperitoneum.

Enteric duplication cyst.

Dilated loops of bowel, especially with ileus.

Varices.
Plexiform neurofibroma.
Leiomyoma or leiomyosarcoma of the stomach.

Solid splenic masses

Metastases, for example primary sites – melanoma, ovary, pancreas, endometrium, breast, colon, prostate, testis and chondrosarcoma.
Infarct.
Haemangioma.
Lymphangioma.
Leukaemia.
Hamartoma.
Sarcoma – fibrosarcoma, leiomyosarcoma, angiosarcoma.
Fibrous histiocytoma.
Sarcoid.
Inflammatory pseudo-tumour.
Extramedullary haemopoiesis.
Gaucher's disease.
Fibroma.
Myxoma.
Chondroma.
Haemangioendothelioma.
Infected or haemorrhagic cyst.
Tuberculoma.
Intrasplenic lymph node.
Thrombosed aneurysm.
Malignant splenic neoplasia.

Primary splenic tumours are rare but lymphoma or metastases may involve the spleen. Benign tumours include fibrous, solid and cystic hamartomas, lymphangioma and haemangiomas. Malignant tumours include lymphoma and sarcomas particularly leiomyosarcoma, fibrosarcoma, haemangio-sarcoma, etc. The spleen is commonly involved by lymphoma but in 30 per cent of Hodgkin's patients who have splenomegaly the splenic enlargement is reactive and not due to splenic tumour. Splenomegaly is a more reliable indicator of disease in the spleen in non-Hodgkin's lymphoma. Splenic involvement by lymphoma may cause splenomegaly with or without focal defects, tumour masses may be large or small and there may be associated lymphadenopathy at the splenic hilum. Unfortunately the great variation in splenic size from person to person makes the diagnosis of minor splenic involvement unreliable though ultrasonography is more reliable than pal-pation for the assessment of splenic size.

Signs of splenic lymphoma

Lymphoma deposits are often hypoechoic and may mimic an abscess, infarct or cysts, particularly complicated cysts.

Diffuse splenomegaly without focal defect.

Large nodules up to 20 cm in diameter.

Small miliary nodules.

Lymphadenopathy at the splenic hilum.

50 per cent of cases show focal lesions.

Metastases within the spleen

Although the spleen is very vascular it is an uncommon site for metastases. Metastases within the spleen are usually clinically silent; thus the presence of splenic metastases in advanced cancer is probably under diagnosed clinically. In late stage neoplasia metastases may be found in the spleen in up to 50 per cent of cases of melanoma, 12 to 21 per cent of cases of breast carcinoma and 9 to 18 per cent of cases of bronchogenic carcinoma. Less common sources of metastases within the spleen is carcinoma of the colon, kidney, prostate, ovary, pancreas, stomach, endometrium, testes and chondrosarcoma. Metastases may be microscopic (30 per cent) causing splenomegaly with a normal echopattern.

Splenic angiosarcoma

Angiosarcoma is usually an aggressive malignancy with a poor prognosis (only 20 per cent survive 6 months from diagnosis). It may be present as a solitary splenic mass or as multiple nodules. These may show bizarre and prominent vascular flow or contrast enhancement patterns on CT and colour flow Doppler ultrasound. This reflects the formation of an extensive pathological circulation. These tumours frequently spread to the liver (70 per cent) and up to 30 per cent cause spontaneous splenic rupture due to rapid tumour growth. This may result in catastrophic splenic haemorrhage.

Benign splenic tumours

Benign splenic tumours are rare. Various histological types have been described including haemangioma, lymphangioma, fibroma, chondroma, osteoma, hamartoma and myxoma. While haemangioma, lymphangioma and hamartoma can be either solid or cystic the rest are usually solid. There are no characteristic features on imaging that will differentiate these tumours.

2.4.25 SPLENIC INFARCTION

Splenic infarction is uncommon but is by no means rare. It is usually the result of a systemic disease process such as leukaemia, sickle cell disease, subacute bacterial endocarditis, systemic lupus erythematosus, etc. Focal splenic infarction may affect the overlying visceral peritoneum resulting in acute left upper quadrant pain particularly on respiration and movement. The pain is thus easily mistaken for pleurisy and pulmonary embolism, acute pain and tenderness may make ultrasonography difficult. Initially the spleen may appear normal but significant infarcts become visible as hypoechoic wedge-shaped defects. These can be diffuse and ill defined but are usually peripherally situated, the broadest part of the defect bordering the splenic margin. The defect becomes echogenic and later atrophies leaving a small echogenic scar. Haemorrhage into the infarct will change its appearance making it anechoic, hypoechoic or complex depending upon the stage of resolution of the haemorrhage. Infarcts may be single or multiple and when multiple may lead to autosplenectomy with a small spleen with multiple echogenic nodules representing old infarcts. Uncommonly these may calcify. Splenic infarcts are multiple in 50 per cent of cases and may be massive in 25 per cent of cases. Solitary infarcts may mimic irregular cysts, abscesses or haemangiomas.

Causes of splenic infarction

Sickle cell anaemia.
Leukaemia.
Subacute bacterial endocarditis.
Septic emboli.
Systemic lupus erythematosus.
Pancreatitis.
Trauma.
Left upper quadrant surgery.
Vasculitis – polyarteritis nodosa.
Myelofibrosis.
Polycythaemia rubra vera.
Mitral valve disease.
Acute myocardial infarction – emboli.
Hepatic arterial catheter placement, hepatic chemoembolisation.
Local spread – gastric carcinoma.
Myeloid leukaemia – subendothelial infiltration.
Granulomatous splenic infections – the most commonly encountered granulomatous splenic infections are tuberculosis and histoplasmosis. Infection is usually secondary to haematogenous spread from disease elsewhere. Symptoms are usually

caused by generalised disease and not local splenic involvement. Granulomatous foci may occur in the spleen with sarcoidosis and are usually asymptomatic. Evidence of granulomatous disease in the spleen is often only detected many years after the illness, which may be subclinical. Acute military tuberculosis may give rise to a generally bright splenic echopattern but this appearance is non-specific and may also occur in other inflammatory states and malignancy, particularly multiple metastasis. Healed granulomas calcify giving rise to multiple echogenic foci, which may be visible on plain radiograph.

2.4.26 TORSION OF WANDERING SPLEEN

Although the ligamentous attachments of the spleen are lax in 0.2 per cent of the population, significant splenic mobility is rare and is usually a cause of symptoms. However, ligamentous laxity can allow torsion of the spleen, particularly in women of childbearing age. Once torsion occurs the patient suffers acute left upper quadrant pain with signs of acute abdomen. Sonography will show an abnormal homogeneous splenic mass which may be ectopic lying in the midabdomen, in which case a normal spleen will not be seen in the left upper quadrant.

2.4.27 MULTIFOCAL HYPOECHOIC SPLENIC MASSES

Lymphoma.
Splenic lymphangiomatosis.
Infarction – lesions are of different ages and therefore of varying appearance.
Septic emboli – multiple small abscesses.
Metastases.
Splenic cysts – pseudocysts, epidermoid and hydatid cysts.
Abscesses.

2.4.28 ECHOGENIC SPLENIC MASSES

Infarct.
Haematoma.
Metastases – melanoma.
Calcified granulomas – tuberculosis, histoplasmosis.
Calcification in a cyst wall – hydatid cyst.
Phlebolith.
Lymphoma or leukaemia (more frequently hypoechoic).
Kaposi's sarcoma.
Micro-abscesses especially with gas but also the following with or without calcification:

Pneumocystis carinii causing innumerable tiny reflective foci. Ultrasound is more sensitive than CT in detecting extrapulmonary disseminated pneumocystis in the early stages.

Candida albicans – besides highly reflective foci other patterns have been described which include (1) wheel within a wheel i.e. three concentric rings alternating hypo- and hyper- and central hypoechogenicity, (2) bull's-eye appearance, (3) hypoechogenic foci.

Aspergillus spp.

Cytomegalovirus.

Mycobacterium avium intracellular.

*Due to microcalcification.

All micro-abscesses can give rise to sonographic snowstorm in the liver, spleen, kidney, bowel, lung and pleura.

Schistosoma mansoni.

Extramedullary haemopoisis – *sickle cell anaemia, *hereditary spherocytosis, *Neimann–Pick disease, *myelofibrosis.

Nodules and multiple channels in portal hypertension.

Gamma-Gandy nodules.

Haemangioma – focal well-defined solitary or multiple masses predominantly hyper-echoic, they may occasionally calcify.

2.4.29 CAUSES OF SPLENIC CALCIFICATION

Calcification is frequently seen in the spleen particularly in the elderly. Old granulomas and old infective scars are the most frequently seen lesions thus they are generally of no relevance at the time of scanning.

Differential diagnoses

Cyst wall calcification.

Micronodular calcification in granulomas – tuberculosis, histoplasmosis, brucellosis, sarcoidosis, toxoplasmosis, *Pneumocystis carinii,* fungal abscesses.

Phleboliths or arteriovenous fistula.

Haematoma.

Post-infarction.

Splenic artery calcification.

Dermoid.

Epidermoid.

Splenic artery aneurysm at the splenic hilum.

Lymphangioma.

Haemangioma.

Haemosiderosis.

Subcapsular infarct or haematoma.
Thorotrast spleen.

2.4.30 SPLENIC IMAGING: ULTRASOUND CHECKLIST

1. Look for the presence of the spleen (splenectomy, congenital absence).
2. Check the size of the spleen.
3. Are there splenecules?
4. Check the outline of the diaphragm, subdiaphragmatic and subcapsular collections.
5. Look for focal lesions: calcification, echogenic, echopoor or cystic.
6. Are there extrasplenic abnormalities: liver enlargement, evidence of cirrhosis, ascites, lymphadenopathy (lymphoma), gallbladder calculi in haemolytic anaemia, etc.?

2.5 FURTHER READING

Abu-Yousef MM, Milam SG, Farner RM: Pulsatile portal vein flow: a sign of tricuspid regurgitation on duplex Doppler sonography. Am J Roentgenol *155*:785–788, 1990.

Ali M, Khan AN: Sonography of hepatobiliary ascariasis. J Clin Ultrasound *24*:236–241, 1996.

Altuntas B, Erden A, Karakurt C *et al.*: Severe portal hypertension due to congenital hepatoportal arteriovenous fistula associated with intrahepatic portal vein aneurysm. J Clin Ultrasound *26*:357–360, 1998.

Angelico M, De Santis A, Capocaccia L: Biliary sludge: a critical update. J Clin Gastroenterol *12*:656–662, 1990.

Barzilai M, Lerner A, Branski D: Increased reflectivity of the pancreas in rare hereditary pancreatic insufficiency syndromes. Clin Radiol *51*:575–576, 1996.

Bellamy PR, Hicks A: Assessment of gallbladder function by ultrasound: implication for dissolution therapy. Clin Radiol *39*:511–512, 1988.

Benya EC, Bulas DI: Splenic injuries in children after blunt abdominal trauma. Semin Ultrasound CT MR *17*:170, 1996.

Benya EC, Sivit CJ, Quinones RR: Abdominal complications after bone marrow transplantation in children: sonographic and CT findings. Am J Roentgenol *161*:1023–1027, 1993.

Bismuth H: Surgical anatomy and anatomical surgery of the liver. World J Surg *6*:3–9, 1982.

Bolinger B, Lorentzen T: Torsion of a wandering spleen: ultrasonographic findings. J Clin Ultrasound *18*:510–511, 1990.

Brazilai M, Vadasz Z: Hypoechoic periportal encasement in Chediak-Higashi syndrome. Am J Roentgenol *166*:726–727, 1996.

Bretagne JF, Horsebach D, Darnault P *et al.*: Pseudoaneurysms and bleeding pseudocyst in chronic pancreatitis. Radiological findings and contribution to diagnosis in 8 cases. Gastrointest Radiol *15*:9–16, 1990.

Brouland JP, Boudiaf M *et al.*: Color velocity imaging and power Doppler sonography of the gallbladder wall: a new look at sonographic diagnosis of acute cholecystitis. Am J Roentgenol *171*:183-188, 1998.

Buetow PC, Usar MC, Buck JL *et al.*: Biliary cystadenoma and cystadenocarcinoma: clinical imaging – pathologic correlation with emphasis on the importance of ovarian struma. Radiology *196*:805-810, 1995.

Buscarini E, Buscarini L, Civardi G *et al.*: Hepatic vascular malformations in hereditary hemorrhagic telangiectasis:imaging findings. Am J Roentgenol *163*:1105-1110,1994.

Cameron EW, Beale TJ, Pearson RH: Case report: torsion of the gallbladder on ultrasound: differentiation from acalculus cholecystitis. Clin Radiol *47*:285-286, 1993.

Carpenter HA: Bacterial and parasitic cholangitis (review). Mayo Clin Proc *73*:473-478, 1998.

Cava RK, Rose SC, Miller FJ: Gallbladder volvulus as a complication of percutaneous manipulation. J Vasc Interv Radiol *1*:117, 1990.

Chen JJ, Lin HH, Chiu CT, Lin PY: Gallbladder perforation with intrahepatic abscess formation. J Clin Ultrasound *18*:43-45, 1990.

Chernoff DM: Pancreatic pseudocyst and obstructive jaundice associated with a transcaval penetration by a bird's nest vena cava filter. Am J Roentgenol *171*:179-180, 1998.

Chiu KW, Changchien CS, Chuah SK: Gallbladder compression sign: an indicator of small isoechoic hepatic tumours. J Clin Ultrasound *24*:17-20, 1996.

Choi BI, Han JK, Kim YI *et al.*: Combined hepatocellular carcinoma and cholangiocarcinoma of the liver: sonography, CT, angiography and iodized-oil CT with pathologic correlation. Abdom Imaging *19*:43-46, 1994.

Chong WK, Malisch TW, Mazer MJ: Sonography of transjugular intrahepatic portosystemic shunts. Semin Ultrasound CT MR *16*:69-80, 1995.

Choyke PL, Glenn GM, Walther MM *et al.*: Von Hippel–Lindau disease genetic, clinical and imaging features. Radiology *194*:629, 1995.

Chung-Jyi Tsai: Unusual ultrasonographic appearance of a solitary retroperitoneal neurofibroma. Br J Radiol *67*:210-211, 1994.

Coelho JC, Wallbach A, Kasting G, Moreira RR: Ultrasonic diagnosis of primary sarcoma of the gallbladder. J Clin Ultrasound *12*:168-170, 1984.

Colli A, Cocciolo M, Riva C *et al.*: Abnormalities of Doppler waveforms of the hepatic veins in patients with chronic liver disease: correlation with histological findings. Am J Roentgenol *162*:833-837, 1994.

Collins CD, Kedar RP, Cosgrove DO: Case report: myeloma of the breast – appearance on ultrasound and colour Doppler. Br J Radiol *67*:399-400, 1994.

Cooper M, Bass P, Tung K: Multiple myeloma: a cause of obstructive jaundice. Clin Radiol *56*:874-875, 1995.

Couinaud C: Le foie: etudes anatomiques et chirugicales. Paris, Masson, 9-12, 1957.

Crowley JJ, McAlester WH: Congenital pancreatic pseudocyst rare cause of abdominal mass in a neonate: report of two cases. Pediatr Radiol *26*:210, 1996.

Curtis JM, Pellegrini V, Tappin JA: Case report: multiple myeloma – a rare presentation. Clin Radiol *50*:63-64, 1995.

Dachman AH, Ros PR, Goodman ZD *et al.*: Nodular regenerative hyperplasia of the liver: clinical and radiologic observations. Am J Roentgenol *148*:717-722, 1987.

Dalla Palma L: Diagnostic imaging and interventional therapy of hepatocellular carcinoma. Br J Radiol *71*:808-818, 1998.

de Campo M, de Campo JF: Ultrasound of primary hepatic tumours in childhood. Pediatr Radiol *19*:19-24, 1988.

De Silva F, Boudghene F, Lecomte I *et al.*: Sonography in AIDS related cholangitis: prevalence and cause of an echogenic nodule in the distal end of the common bile duct. Am J Roentgenol *160*:1205–1207, 1993.

DeMaioribus CA, Lally KP, Sim K *et al.*: Mesenchymal hamartoma of the liver. A 5-year review. Arch Surg *125*:596–600, 1990.

Deng-Yu Lin, Cheng-Shyong Wu, Sen-Yung Hsieh: 'String sign' of portal vein as a precursor of portal vein thrombosis: color Doppler ultrasonographic study of one case. J Clin Ultrasound *25*:77–81, 1997.

Denys A, Helenon O, Lajortune M *et al.*: Thickening of the wall of the bile duct due to intramural collaterals in three patients with portal vein thrombosis. Am J Roentgenol *171*:455–456, 1998.

Di Maggio EM, Roberto Dore MS, Preda L *et al.*: First case diagnosed with CT. Am J Roentgenol *167*:56–57, 1996.

Dodds WJ, Erickson SJ, Taylor AJ *et al.*: Caudate lobe of the liver: anatomy, embryology and pathology. Am J Roentgenol *154*:87–93, 1990.

Dodds WJ, Grah WJ, Darweesh RMA *et al.*: Sonographic measurement of gallbladder volume. Am J Roentgenol *145*:1009–1011, 1985.

Doehring E, Reider F, Dittrich M, Coddi Z: Ultrasonographic findings in livers of patients with lepromatous leprosy. J Clin Ultrasound *14*:179–183, 1986.

Donnelly LF, Bisset GS 3rd: Pediatric hepatic imaging. Radiol Clin North Am *36*:413–427, 1998.

Durr-e-Sabih, Sabih Z, Khan AN: 'Congealed waterlilly' sign a new sonographic sign of liver hydatid cyst. J Clin Ultrasound *24*:297–303, 1996.

Edmondson HA, Steiner PE: Benign epithelial tumors and tumor-like lesions of the liver. In Okuda K, Peters RL (eds): Hepatocellular carcinoma. New York, Wiley, 309, 1976.

Everson GT, Braverman DZ, Johnson ML, Kern FJR: A critical evaluation of real time ultrasonography for the study of the gallbladder volume and contraction. Gastroenterology *83*:773–776, 1980.

Feldstein VA, LaBerge JM: Hepatic vein flow reversal of duplex sonography: a sign of transjugular intrahepatic portosystemic shunt dysfunction. Am J Roentgenol *162*:839–841, 1994.

Finlay DE, Mitchell SL, Letourneau JG, Longley DG: Leukemic infiltration of the gallbladder wall mimicking acute cholecystitis. Am J Roentgenol *160*:63–64, 1993.

Foulner D: Case report: granular cell tumour of the biliary tree – the sonographic appearance. Clin Radiol *49*:503–504, 1994.

Fujimoto M, Moriyasu F, Nishikawa K *et al.*: Color Doppler sonography of hepatic tumours with galactose-based contrast agent: correlation with angiographic findings. Am J Roentgenol *163*:1099–1104, 1994.

Fujita N, Mochizuki F, Lees S *et al.*: Carcinoid tumor of the bile duct: case report. Gastrointest Radiol *14*:151–154, 1989.

Furst G, Malms J, Heyer T *et al.*: Transjugular intrahepatic portosystemic shunts: improved evaluation with echo-enhanced color Doppler sonography, power Doppler sonography and spectral duplex sonography. Am J Roentgenol *170*:1047–1054, 1998.

Furui S, Itai Y, Ohtomo K *et al.*: Hepatic epithelioid hemangioendothelioma: report of five cases. Radiology *171*:63–68, 1989.

Furukawa H, Kosuge T: Epidermoid cyst in an intra-pancreatic accessory spleen: CT and pathologic findings. Am J Roentgenol *171*:271, 1998.

Gaia E, Babini G, Dughera L *et al.*: Intrasplenic penetration of a pancreatic pseudocyst: early detection. J Clin Ultrasound *20*:608, 1992.

Gembola RB, Flynn DE, Radecki PD *et al.*: Sonographic diagnosis of traumatic gallbladder avulsion. J Ultrasound Med *5*:299–301, 1993.

Giorgio A, Francica G, De Stefano G *et al.*: Sonographic recognition of intra-parenchymal regenerating nodules using high-frequency transducers in patients with cirrhosis. J Ultrasound Med *10*:355-359, 1991.

Goerg C, Schwerk WB: Color Doppler imaging of focal splenic masses: Eur J Radiol *18*:214, 1994.

Golzerian J, Braude P, Bank WO *et al.*: Color Doppler demonstration of pseudo-aneuryms, complicating pancreatic pseudocysts. Br J Radiol *67*:91-93, 1994.

Gore RM, Mathieu DG, White EM *et al.*: Passive hepatic congestion: cross sectional imaging features. Am J Roentgenol *162*:71-75, 1994.

Gorg C, Weide R, Schwerk WB: Malignant splenic lymphoma: sonographic patterns, diagnosis and follow up. Clin Radiol *52*:535, 1997.

Gorgul A, Kahan B, Dogan I, Unal S: Disappearance of the pseudo-cholangiocarcinoma sign after TIPS. Am J Gastroenterol *91*:150-154, 1996.

Goritsas CP, Repanti M, Papadaki E *et al.*: Intrahepatic bile duct injury and nodular regenerative hyperplasia of the liver in a patient with polyarteritis nodosa. J Hepatol *26*:727-730, 1997.

Gorman B, Reading CC: Imaging of gastrointestinal neuroendocrine tumours. Semin Ultrasound CT MR *16*(4):331-341, 1995.

Grant EG: Doppler imaging of the liver. Ultrasound Quarterly *10*:117-154, 1992.

Hamadani SD, Baron RL: Ectopic liver simulating a mass in the gallbladder wall: imaging findings. Am J Roentgenol *162*:647-648, 1994.

Hann LE, Greatrex KV, Bach AM: Cholangiocarcinoma at the hepatic hilus: sonographic findings. Am J Roentgenol *168*:985-989, 1997.

Harty MP, Hebra A, Ruchelli ED, Schnaufer L: Ciliated hepatic foregut cyst causing portal hypertension in an adolescent. Am J Roentgenol *170*:688-690, 1998.

Hasan AKH, Negrette JJ: Case report: duodenal diverticula and jaundice. Clin Radiol *44*:128-129, 1991.

Hasan AKH, Negrette JJ: Duodenal diverticula and jaundice, ultrasound can be mis-leading. Clin Radiol *44*:128-129, 1991.

Hernanz-Schulman M, Ambrosino MM, Freeman PC, Quin CB: Common bile duct in children: sonographic dimensions. Radiology *195*:193-195, 1995.

Hirooka Y, Naitoh Y, Goto H *et al.*: Differential diagnosis of gallbladder masses using colour Doppler ultrasonography. J Gastroenterol Hepatol *11*:840-846, 1996.

Holland CL, Olliff JF: Ultrasound diagnosis of obstructed Roux loop after cancer of the pancreas of the bile duct. Br J Radiol *67*:309-312, 1994.

Hopper KD, Fisher ME, Kasales CJ *et al.*: Gastrointestinal case of the day. Am J Roentgenol *162*:1448-1451, 1994.

Houston JP, Collins MC, Cameron I *et al.*: Xanthogranulomatous cholecystitis. Br J Surg *81*:1030-1032, 1994.

Itai Y: Different terms for the same disease: intraductal mucin-producing tumour versus mucinous tumour of the pancreas. Radiology 200:285, 1996

Ito Y, Kojiro M, Nakashima T, Mori T: Pathomorphologic characteristics of 102 cases of thorotrast-related hepatocellular carcinoma, cholangiocarcinoma and hepatic angiosarcoma. Cancer *62*:1153-1162, 1988.

Jain R, Sawhney S, Bhargava D, Berry M: Gallbladder tuberculosis: sonographic appear-ance. J Clin Ultrasound *23*:327-329, 1995.

Kanterman RY, Darcy MD, Middleton WD *et al.*: Doppler sonography findings associ-ated with transjugular intrahepatic portosystemic shunt malfunction. Am J Roentgenol *168*:467-472, 1997.

Keane MAR, Finlayson C, Joseph AEA: Histological basis for the 'sonographic snow-storm' in opportunistic infection of liver and spleen. Clin Radiol *50*:220, 1995.

Kedar RP, Cosgrove DO: Echo-poor periportal cuffing: ultrasound appearance of significance. J Clin Ultrasound *21*:464–467, 1993.

Kedar RP, Cosgrove DO: Retroperitoneal varices mimicking a mass, diagnoses by colour Doppler. Br J Radiol *67*:661–662, 1994.

Kedar RP, Merchant SA, Malde HH, Patel VH: Multiple reflective channels in the spleen: a sonographic sign of portal hypertension. Abdom Imaging *19*:453–458, 1994.

Kelly IMG, Lees WR, Russell RCG: Tumefactive biliary sludge: a sonographic pseudotumour. Appearances in the common bile duct. Clin Radiol *47*:251–254, 1993.

Kessler E, Turani H, Kayse S *et al.*: Inflammatory pseudotumour of the liver. Liver *8*:17–23, 1988.

Khan AN, Wilson I, Sherlock DJ, Dekretser D: Sonographic features of mucinous biliary papillomatosis: case report and review of imaging findings. J Clin Ultrasound *26*:151–154, 1998.

Kirejczyk WM, Crowe HM, Mackay IM *et al.*: Disappearing 'gallstones': biliary pseudolithiasis complicating ceftriaxone therapy. Am J Roentgenol *159*:329–330, 1992.

Koito K, Namieno T, Morita K: Differential diagnosis of small hepatocellular carcinoma and adenomatous hyperplasia with power Doppler sonography. Am J Roentgenol *170*:157–161, 1998.

Kong MS, Wong HF: Multiseptate gallbladder: an unusual sonographic pattern in acute hepatitis. J Clin Ultrasound *24*:86–89, 1996.

Koslin B, Mulligan SA, Berland LL: Duplex assessment of the portal venous system. Semin Ultrasound CT MR *13*:22–33, 1992.

Kruskal JB, Kane RA: Correlative imaging of malignant liver tumours. Semin Ultrasound CT MR *13*:336–354, 1992.

Kubota K, Bandai Y, Araki Y *et al.*: Giant hyperplastic polyp of the gallbladder. J Clin Ultrasound *24*:203–206, 1996.

Kuo CH, Changchien CS: Sonographic features of retroperitoneal neurolimoma. J Clin Ultrasound *21*:309–312, 1993.

Laing FC, Frates MC, Vickie A *et al.*: Hemobilia: sonographic appearance in the gallbladder and biliary tree with emphasis on intra-cholecystic blood. J Ultrasound Med *16*:537–543, 1997.

Lebovics E, Dworkin BM, Heier SK, Rosenthal WS: The hepatobiliary manifestations of immunodeficiency virus infection. Am J Gastroenterol *83*:1–7, 1988.

Lee P, Mather S, Owens C *et al.*: Hepatic ultrasound findings in the glycogen storage diseases. Br J Radiol *67*:1062–1066, 1994.

Letourneau JG, Hunter DW, Payne WD, Day DL: Imaging and intervention for biliary complications after liver transplantation. Am J Roentgenol *154*:729–733, 1990.

Lev-Toaff AS, Bach AM, Wechsler RJ *et al.*: The radiologic and pathologic spectrum of biliary hamartomas. Am J Roentgenol *165*:309–313, 1995.

Lim JH: Radiological findings of clonorchiasis. Am J Roentgenol *155*:1001–1008, 1990.

Lim JH, Ko YT, Lee DH, Hong KS: Oriental cholangiohepatitis: sonographic findings in 48 cases. Am J Roentgenol *155*:511–514, 1990.

Linstedt-Hilden M, Brambs HJ: Two different manifestations of botryoid sarcoma (embryonal rhabdomyosarcoma) of the biliary tree. Bildgebung *40*:40–43, 1994.

Longo JM, Bilboo JI, De Villa VH *et al.*: Gallbladder perforation and bile leakage diagnosis by colour Doppler sonography and percutaneous treatment. Br J Radiol *66*:1052–1054, 1993.

Low RA, Kuni CC, Letourneau JG: Pancreatic transplant imaging: an overview. Am J Roentgenol *155*:13–21, 1990.

Lyttkens K, Prytz H, Forsberg L *et al.*: Ultrasound, hepatic lymph nodes and primary biliary cirrhosis. J Hepatol *15*:136–139, 1992.

Lyttkens K, Prytz H, Forsberg L, Hagerstrand I: Hepatic lymph nodes as follow-up factor in primary biliary cirrhosis. an ultrasound study. Scand J Gastroenterol 30:1036–1040, 1995.

Mahr MA: Bile-plug syndrome. Pediatr Radiol 19:61–64, 1988.

Marks WM, Filly RA, Callen PW: Ultrasonic evaluation of normal pancreatic echogenicity and relationship to fat deposition. Radiol 137:475–479, 1980.

Maymind M, Mergelas JE, Seibert DG et al.: Primary non-Hodgkin's lymphoma of the common bile duct (review). Am J Gastroenterol 92:1543–1546, 1997.

McGarth FP, Lee SH, Gibney RG, Burhanne HJ: Hepatic subcapsular hematoma: an unusual complication of biliary lithotripsy. Am J Roentgenol 154:1015–1016, 1990.

Mendez Montero JV, Arrazola Garcia J, Lopez Lufuente J et al.: Fat-fluid level in hepatic hydatid cyst: a new sign of rupture into the biliary tree? Am J Roentgenol 167:91–94, 1996.

Michielsen PP, Pelckmans PA, Van Maercke YM et al.: Hepatoportal sclerosis demonstrated by abdominal ultrasonography. J Clin Ultrasound 19:513–515, 1991.

Millener P, Grant EG, Rose S et al.: Color Doppler imaging findings in patients with Budd–Chiari syndrome: correlation with venographic findings. Am J Roentgenol 161:307–312, 1993.

Miller FH, Gore RM, Nemcek AA, Fitzgerald SW: Pancreaticobiliary manifestations of AIDS. Am J Roentgenol 166:1269–1274, 1996.

Miller WJ, Dodd GD 3rd, Federle MP, Baron RL: Epithelioid hemangioendothelioma of the liver: imaging findings with pathologic correlation. Am J Roentgenol 160:53–57, 1993.

Muller MF, Meyenberger C, Bertschinger P et al.: Pancreatic tumours: evaluation with endoscopic ultrasound, CT and MR imaging. Radiology 190:745–751, 1994.

Murray JG, Patel MD, Lee S et al.: Microabscesses of the liver and spleen in AIDS. Radiology 197:723, 1995.

Nakozawa S, Yamao K, Yamada M et al.: Study of the classification of mucin-producing cystic tumour of the pancreas. Jpn J Gastroenterol 85:924–932, 1988.

Nelson RC, Shorbourne GM, Spencer HB, Chesmer J: Splenic venous flow exceeding portal venous flow at Doppler sonography: relationship to portosystemic varices. Am J Roentgenol 161:563–567, 1993.

Neshiwat LF, Friedland ML, Schorr-Lesnick B et al.: Hepatic angiosarcoma (review). American Journal of Medicine 93:219–222, 1992.

Neste MG, Francis IR, Bude RO: Hepatic metastases from granulosa cell tumour of the ovary: CT and sonographic findings. Am J Roentgenol 166:1122–1124, 1996.

Newmark H 3rd, Kliewer K, Curtis A et al.: Primary leiomyosarcoma of gallbladder seen on computed tomography and ultrasound. Am J Gastroenterol 81:202–204, 1986.

Nghiem HV, Bogost GA, Ryan JA et al.: Cavernous hemangiomas of the liver: enlargement over time. Am J Roentgenol 169:137–140, 1997.

Nisenbaum HL, Rowling SE: Ultrasound of focal hepatic lesions. Semin Roentgenol 4:324–346, 1995.

Numata K, Tanaka K, Kiba T et al.: Use of hepatic tumour index in color Doppler sonography for differentiating large hepatic tumours. Am J Roentgenol 168:991–995, 1997.

Okada A, Fukuzawa M, Oue T et al.: Thirty-eight years experience of malignant hepatic tumors in infants and childhood. Eur J Pediatr Surg 8:17–22, 1998.

Pandolfo I, Zimbaro G, Bartiromo G et al.: Ultrasonographic and cholecystographic findings in a case of fascioliasis of the gallbladder. J Clin Ultrasound 19:505–507, 1991.

Parvey HR, Raval B, Sandler CM: Portal vein thrombosis: imaging findings. Am J Roentgenol *162*:77–81, 1994.

Peristic VN, Howard ER, Milhailovic T *et al.*: Cholestasis caused by biliary botryoid sarcoma. Eur J Pediatr Surg *1*:242–243, 1991.

Pokharna DS, Sharma SK: Ultrasonic measurements of portal vasculature in diagnosing portal hypertension: a controversial subject reviewed. J Ultrasound Med *9*:45–48, 1990.

Powel FC, Spooner KM, Shawker TH: Symptomatic interleukin 2 induced cholecystopathy in patients with HIV infection. Am J Roentgenol *163*:117–121, 1994.

Price J, Leung JWC: Ultrasound diagnosis of *Ascaris lumbricoides* in the pancreatic duct: the 'four-line' sign. Br J Radiol *61*:411–413, 1988.

Principe A, Lugaresi ML, Lords RC *et al.*: Bile duct hamartomas: diagnostic problems and treatment. Hepatogastroenterology *44*:994–997, 1997.

Radin DR, Craig JR, Colletti PM *et al.*: Hepatic epithelioid hemangioendothelioma. Radiology *169*:145–148, 1988.

Radin R, Kanel GL: Peliosis hepatis in a patient with human immunodeficiency virus infection. Am J Roentgenol *156*:91–92, 1991.

Ralls PW, Johnson MB, Radin DR *et al.*: Hereditary hemorrhagic telengiectasia: findings in the liver with color Doppler sonography. Am J Roentgenol *159*:59–61, 1992.

Ralls PW, Mack LA: Spectral and color Doppler sonography. Semin Ultrasound CT MR *13*:355–366, 1992.

Ralls PW: Color Doppler sonography of the hepatic and portal venous system. Am J Roentgenol *155*:517–525, 1990.

Ralls PW: Focal inflammatory disease of the liver. Radiol Clin North Am *36*:377–389, 1998.

Ralls PW, Mack LA: Spectral and color Doppler sonography. Semin Ultrasound CT MR *13*:355–366, 1992.

Ramage JK, Donaghy A, Farrant JM *et al.*: Serum tumour markers for the diagnosis of cholangiocarcinoma in primary sclerosing cholangitis. Gastroenterology *108*:865–869, 1995.

Robledo R, Muro A, Prieto ML: Extrahepatic bile duct carcinoma: ultrasound characteristics and accuracy in demonstration of tumors. Radiology *198*:869–873, 1996.

Roca M, Sellier N, Mensire A *et al.*: Acute acalculus cholecystitis in salmonella infection. Pediatr Radiol *18*:421–423, 1988.

Rusin JA, Sivit CJ, Rakusan TA, Chandra RS: AIDS-related cholangitis in children: sonographic findings. Am J Roentgenol *159*:626–627, 1992.

Sameda H, Moriyasu F, Hamato N *et al.*: Changes in hepatic arterial hemodynamics induced by hepatocellular carcinoma, detected with Doppler sonography. J Clinical Ultrasound *25*:359–365, 1997.

Saul SH, Titelbaum DS, Gansler TS *et al.*: The fibrolamellar variant of hepatocellular carcinoma. Its association with focal nodular hyperplasia. Cancer *60*:3049–3055, 1987.

Saverymuttu SH, Grammatopoulos A, Meanock CI *et al.*: Gallbladder wall thickening (congestive cholecystopathy) in chronic liver disease: a sign of portal hypertension. Br J Radiol *63*:922–925, 1990.

Scerpella EG, Villareal A, Casanova PF, Moreno JN: Primary lymphoma of the liver in AIDS: report of one new case and review of the literature. J Clin Gastroenterol *22*:51–53, 1996.

Schinki-Nicki DA, Muller MF: Lymphoepithelial cyst of the pancreas. Br J Radiol *67*:601, 1996.

Schlesinger AE, Null DM: Enlarged common hepatic duct secondary to morphine in a neonate. Pediatr Radiol *18*:235-236, 1988.

Selby DM, Stocker JT, Ishak KG: Angiosarcoma of the liver in childhood: a clinico-pathologic and follow-up study of 10 cases (review). Pediatr Pathol *12*:485-498, 1992.

Seo JB, Chung JW, Park JH *et al.*: Benign obstruction of the hepatic inferior vena cava, complicated by hepatocellular carcinoma, combined interventional management. Am J Roentgenol *170*:655-659, 1998.

Shawker TH: Intraoperative ultrasound: a decade later. Ultrasound Quarterly *9*:35-39, 1991.

Shirkhoda A, Freeman J, Armin AR *et al.*: Imaging features of splenic epidermoid cyst with pathologic correlation. Abdom Imaging *20*:449, 1995.

Simeone JF, Mueller PR, Ferric JT *et al.*: Sonography of the bile ducts after a fatty meal: an aid in detection of obstruction. Radiology *143*:211-215, 1982.

Simmons MZ: Pitfalls in ultrasound of the gallbladder and biliary tract. Ultrasound Quarterly *14*:2-24, 1998.

Simmons MZ, Miller JA, Levine CD *et al.*: Myelomatous involvement of the liver: unusual ultrasound appearance. J Clin Ultrasound *25*:145-148, 1997.

Siniluoto TMJ, Tikkakoski T, Lahde ST *et al.*: Ultrasound or CT in splenic disease? Acta Radiol *35*:597, 1994.

Smith D, Downey D, Spouge A, Soney S: Sonographic demonstration of Couinaud's liver segments. J Ultrasound Med *17*:375-381, 1998.

Smith MD, Robbins PD, Cullingford GL, Levitt MD: Cholangiocarcinoma and familial adenomatous polyposis (review) Aust N Z J Surg; *63*:324-327, 1993.

Solomon MJ, Stephen MS, Gallinger S, White GH: Does intraoperative hepatic ultra-sonography change surgical decision making during liver resection? Am J Surg *168*:307-310, 1994.

Summerfield JA, Elias E, Hungerford GD *et al.*: The biliary system in primary biliary cirrhosis. A study by endoscopic retrograde cholangiopancreatography. Gastro-enterology *70*:240-243, 1976.

Suqiyama M, Atomi Y, Kuroda A *et al.*: Large cholesterol polyps of the gallbladder. Diagnosis by means of ultrasound and endoscopic ultrasound. Radiology *196*:493-497, 1995.

Talarico HP, Rubens D: Gallbladder wall thickening in acute pyelonephritis. J Clin Ultrasound *18*:653-657, 1990.

Tameda Y, Kosaka Y, Shiraki K *et al.*: Multiple microhamartomas of the biliary tract system (Von Meyenberg complexes) with multiple liver cysts – diagnostic imaging and laparoscopic findings. Digestive Endoscopy *5*:161-168, 1993.

Tan A, Shen JF, Hecht AH: Sonogram of multiple bile duct hamartomas. J Clin Ultra-sound *17*:667-669, 1989.

Tanaka S, Kitamura T, Fujita M *et al.*: Color Doppler flow imaging of liver tumours. Am J Roentgenol *154*:509-510, 1990.

Tartar VM, Balfe DM: Lymphoma in the wall of the bile ducts: radiologic imaging. Gastrointest Radiol *15*:53-57, 1990.

Thuluvath PJ, Rai R, Venbrux AC, Yeo CJ: Cholangiocarcinoma: a review. Gastro-enterologist *5*:306-315, 1997.

Torres WE, Baumgartner BR, Casarella WJ: Abnormalities of the gallbladder after extracorporeal shock-wave lithotripsy: imaging findings. Am J Roentgenol *159*:325-327, 1992.

Traynor O, Castaing D, Bismuth H: Preoperative ultrasonography in the surgery of hepatic tumours. Br J Surg *75*:197-202, 1988.

Ueno N, Tomiyama T, Tano S, Kimura K: Diagnosis of gallbladder carcinoma with color Doppler ultrasonography. Am J Gastroenterol *91*:1647–1649, 1996.

Uggowitzer M, Kugler C, Machan L *et al.*: Power Doppler imaging and evaluation of the resistive index in focal nodular hyperplasia of the liver. Abdom Imaging *22*:268–273, 1997.

Urrutia M, Mergo PJ, Ros LH *et al.*: Cystic masses of the spleen: radiologic-pathologic. Radiographics *16*:107, 1996.

Vassiliades VG, Bree RL, Korobkin M: Focal and diffuse benign hepatic disease: correlative imaging. Semin Ultrasound CT MR *13*:313–335, 1992.

van Sonnenberg E, Casola G, Cubberlty DA *et al.*: Oriental cholangiohepatitis: diagnostic imaging and interventional management. Am J Roentgenol *146*:327–331, 1986.

Wachsberg RH: Sonography of liver transplants. Ultrasound Quarterly *14*:76–94, 1998.

Wachsberg RH, Kyung HK, Sundaram K: Sonographic versus endoscopic retrograde cholangiographic measurements of the bile duct revisited: importance of transverse diameter. Am J Roentgenol *170*:669–674, 1998.

Wadsworth DT, Newman B, Abrahamson SJ *et al.*: Splenic lymphangiomatosis. Radiology *202*:173, 1997.

Wanless IR, Mawdsley C, Adams R: On the pathogenesis of focal nodular hyperplasia of the liver. Hepatology *5*:1194–2000, 1985.

Wedmann B, Schmidt G, Wegener M *et al.*: Sonographic evaluation of gallbladder kinetics: in vitro and in vivo comparison of different methods to assess gallbladder emptying. J Clin Ultrasound *9*:341–349, 1991.

Weltman DI, Zeman AK: Acute diseases of the gallbladder and biliary ducts. Radiol Clin North Am *32*:933–950, 1994.

West MS, Garra BS, Horis SC *et al.*: Gallbladder varices: imaging findings in patients with portal hypertension. Radiology *179*:179–182, 1991.

Worthy SA, Elliot ST, Bennett MK: Low-reflectivity periportal collar on hepatic ultrasound. Am J Roentgenol *67*:1050–1051, 1994.

Wu CS, Yao WJ, Hsiao CH: Effervescent gallbladder: sonographic findings in emphysematous cholecystitis. J Clin Ultrasound *26*:272–275, 1998.

Yang CC, Chen JH, Yang KC: Gallbladder perforation with cholecysto-enteral fistula. J Clin Ultrasound *24*:536–539, 1996.

Yass NA, Stain S, Ralls PW: Recurrent pyogenic cholangitis. Ultrasound Quarterly *14*:41–47, 1998.

Yeung EYC, McCarthy P, Gompertz RH *et al.*: The ultrasonographic appearances of hilar cholangiocarcinoma (Klatskin tumours). Br J Radiol *61*:991–995, 1988.

Zwiebel WJ: Sonographic diagnosis of hepatic vascular disorders. Semin Ultrasound CT MR *16*:34–38, 1995.

3
Gastrointestinal tract

3.1 INTRODUCTION

Visualisation of the upper abdomen and the bowel in particular is frequently compromised by the presence of gas within the bowel. To a certain extent this can be overcome by performing ultrasound examinations in the morning when bowel gas is at a minimum. Water can be used to distend the stomach and provide an acoustic window but many people swallow air when drinking and this can cause further artefacts. Methylcellulose, simethicone and simethicone-coated cellulose have been used as oral contrast agents to aid viewing of the stomach and retroperitoneum by providing an acoustic window. The use of an antifoaming agent has the advantage that swallowed air causes less problems than when water alone is taken. However these substances have not yet gained wide acceptance as their use complicates what is usually a quick and straightforward examination.

3.1.1 THE BOWEL

During abdominal sonography the bowel wall is seen as a hypoechoic muscle layer lined by hyperechoic mucosa. When scanning with a high resolution or endoluminal probe it may be possible to differentiate five layers within the bowel wall

- mucosa: echogenic
- muscularis mucosa: hypoechoic
- submucosa: echogenic
- muscularis propria: hypoechoic
- serosa: echogenic.

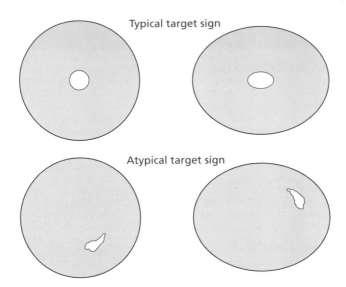

Figure 3.1 The typical and atypical target sign.

Bowel wall thickening may be measured preferably when the bowel is distended. The anterior wall should be measured as the thickness of the posterior wall may be exaggerated by the luminal contents. Care should be taken to exclude bowel contraction during measurement as this may also lead to artefactual bowel wall thickening.

Most bowel pathology causes thickening of the bowel wall. When examining the bowel, it usually presents as a 'target sign' where a hypoechoic wall surrounds the echogenic mucosa, intraluminal mucus, air and other bowel contents. This 'target' may be round or oval (the pseudo-kidney sign). The hypoechoic bowel wall under normal physiological conditions measures less than 4 mm. With a few exceptions mentioned later this 4 mm rule can be applied to the whole of the bowel (Figure 3.1). Under pathological conditions the bowel wall thickens symmetrically in target fashion or asymmetrically when the echogenic lumen is displaced to one side on a true cross section – the 'atypical target' sign. Most bowel pathology whether inflammatory or neoplastic can be inferred from these signs. As with most imaging these signs are non-specific and only a differential diagnosis can be offered.

Technique and artefact

Upper bowel

Drinking fluids cuts down the amount of air swallowed.

Lower bowel

No preparation is necessary if scanned early in the morning when less air is in the abdomen.

Stomach

This may mimic a mass, especially in infants following a feed (milk curd), examine the gastroduodenal junction. Some clinicians facilitate visualisation of the stomach by administering 1000 mL water or tea by straw in combination with intravenous glucagon or Buscopan® to relax the stomach. With this technique 82 per cent of stomach lesions are found. When the stomach is normal 95 per cent of scans are normal.

Duodenum

The duodenum frequently covers the pancreatic head and may mimic a mass but with administration of oral fluids it may be possible to show the duodenal configuration and gastroduodenal junction.

Small bowel

The small bowel has a tubular long axis and round short axis when distended with fluid, valvulae conniventis may be seen.

Appendix

Use graded compression to examine the appendix.

Colon

This is not usually examined by ultrasound but ultrasound can show colonic masses, and intestinal obstruction by showing fluid-filled distended bowel loops. The colon can be examined by means of a water enema/isotonic saline 1500 ml, whilst buscopan can be used to arrest peristalsis.

Gas in bowel

This is echogenic with mottled distal shadowing due to scattered sound, mucus does not shadow but is echogenic.

Bowel wall should measure up to 5 mm or up to 3 mm if the bowel is distended.

3.2 OESOPHAGUS

The distal 3-cm portion of the oesophagus lies within the abdomen having passed through the diaphragm at the level of the 19th thoracic vertebral body. It can usually be identified lying behind the left lobe of the liver on the left side of the caudate lobe anterior to the aorta. It is seen as a tube or ring with hypoechoic walls representing the oesophageal wall muscle with a central echogenic band representing the mucosa. The lumen is not usually visualised unless the patient is drinking or there is gastro-oesophageal reflux. The gastro-oesophageal junction is seen in over 93 per cent of normal subjects and usually presents the pseudo-kidney sign. The length of abdominal oesophagus in adults is 38.7 ± 5.3 mm (range 30 mm to 48 mm). The mean thickness of the oesophageal wall in normal adults is 3.8 ± 1.2 mm.

Ultrasonography is not always the initial investigation of choice for oesophageal pathology but even so it should be visualised during routine upper abdominal ultrasonography, particularly in patients with liver disease and possible varices.

3.2.1 OESOPHAGEAL VARICES

These are seen as multiple anechoic tubes around the distal oesophagus. They are usually associated with portal hypertension, thus full evaluation of the liver spleen and the portal splenic and umbilical veins should be undertaken. Varices may also be found at the umbilicus because of recanalisation of the umbilical vein.

Demonstration of oesophageal varices is important as there is 40 per cent mortality at each episode of variceal bleeding. Ninety per cent of patients who bleed from oesophageal varices will have a second episode of haemorrhage within 1 year. Two-thirds of patients with varices have cirrhosis, often due to alcohol abuse in the western world. These patients have an incidence of peptic ulcer disease so bleeding should not always be assumed to be variceal.

3.2.2 ACHALASIA OF CARDIA

Achalasia is a condition characterised by incomplete relaxation of the lower oesophageal sphincter, increased sphincter tone and progressive loss of oesophageal peristalsis. Initially the oesophagus is of normal calibre but drainage is delayed resulting in stasis after eating. Progressive oesophageal dilatation follows and a dilated fluid-filled oesophagus may be evident particularly if the epigastrium is scanned with the patient semi-erect. Identical appearances may be seen in Chaga's disease, a trypanosomal infection that destroys ganglia within the oesophageal wall. If the diagnosis is considered then oesophageal manometry should be undertaken to confirm or exclude sphincter dysfunction. Unfortunately many cases are not diagnosed until the late stages of disease when the oesophagus is already dilated.

Sonography may reveal a dilated fluid-filled lower oesophagus that tapers into a funnel shape at the gastro-oesophageal junction. Following a drink there is persistent water retention at the gastro-oesophageal vestibule, symmetrical parietal thickening and/or delayed or intermittent opening of the cardiac orifice after drinking. High-resolution endoluminal sonography has revealed that all muscle layers are significantly thickened at the lower oesophageal sphincter in patients with achalasia when compared with normal controls. The thickness of the muscle layer has been correlated to the severity of the disease and therefore the procedure may be useful for grading the severity grade and for deciding on the therapy. Echoendoscopy can also be useful in differentiating idiopathic megaoesophagus from secondary megaoesophagus by visualising a perioesophageal infiltration. Care should be taken when measuring oesophageal wall thickening in a patient with an irregular shaped tortuous oesophagus which may result in a tangential image and production of artefacts simulating submucosal lesions.

The differential diagnosis of achalasia cardia include peptic oesophagitis and oesophageal obstruction from lower oesophageal tumours.

3.2.3 HIATUS HERNIA

Hiatus hernia represents herniation of the stomach into the thorax via the oesophageal hiatus. Ninety nine per cent are sliding hernias where the gastro-oesophageal junction remains within the thorax. There is an increasing incidence with age. There is an association with reflux oesophagitis, duodenal ulcers, diverticulosis and biliary calculi.

About 1 per cent of hiatus hernias are of the rolling or paraoesophageal variety where part of the stomach is displaced into the thorax along with the oesophagus but the gastro-oesophageal junction remains within the abdomen. Occasionally an irreducible hiatus hernia is seen where the stomach lies entirely within the thorax. This type of hernia is usually associated with a defect in the central tendon of the diaphragm in combination with non-compromising volvulus in the transverse axis of the stomach, retrocardially. The cardia in the majority of patients is also placed within the thorax although rarely this may be placed below the diaphragm.

Sonography

In normal subjects the gastro-oesophageal junction can be visualised in nearly all patients with a cross-sectional diameter of 7.1 to 10.0 mm at the diaphragmatic hiatus level. The gastro-oesophageal junction is not visualised in a hiatus hernia and the bowel diameter measured at the diaphragmatic hiatus is 16.0 to 21.0 mm. Each of the aforementioned signs has a predictive value of 100 per cent. The negative predictive value of the bowel diameter is 90 per cent and that of non-visualisation of the gastro-oesophageal junction is 94.7 per cent.

Signs of sliding hiatus hernia in infants and young children

Intra-abdominal oesophagus measuring less than 2 cm.
Rounding of the gastro-oesophageal angle.
The presence of a beak at the gastro-oesophageal junction.

The predictive value of these criteria is quite good however they cannot be applied if the gastric fundus, distal oesophagus and gastro-oesophageal junction no longer lie within the abdominal cavity.

3.2.4 GASTRO-OESOPHAGEAL REFLUX

Gastro-oesophageal reflux is relatively common and is seen so frequently in the newborn that it is regarded as physiological at this age. Reflex usually occurs because of loss of the normal gastro-oesophageal sphincter mechanism that may be secondary to shortening of the intra-abdominal oesophageal segment.

Sonography

Gastro-oesophageal reflux may be diagnosed sonographically with a 95 per cent sensitivity but reflux is an intermittent phenomenon and therefore prolonged scan times may be required which are not always practical. To detect reflux it is also necessary to position the patient so that there is fluid lying over the gastro-oesophageal junction. The examination may start with the patient lying in the supine position but it may be necessary to raise the left side or even place the patient in a head-down position to allow reflux to occur. Fluid refluxing into the lumen of the oesophagus is seen sonographically as an anechoic column. With slight reflux the column is small, transient and easily missed. In more severe reflux cases the column of fluid is long and may persist for some time. The fluid often contains small echogenic air bubbles caused by turbulent flow. With care the accuracy of sonography in the diagnosis of gastro-oesophageal reflux is similar to the accuracy of barium meal examination, though these two examinations are less accurate than portal hypertension probe studies. One of the disadvantages of using ultrasound for reflux is that it allows poor assessment of the severity of reflux and is not very sensitive at detecting oesophagitis. However associated hiatus hernia can be detected reliably.

3.2.5 PERSISTENT VOMITING IN INFANTS

Ultrasound of the abdomen is an accurate and rapid screening method to differentiate the causes of persistent vomiting in infants. It can reliably differentiate between oesophageal and duodenal causes. A test feed is usually given followed by sonography concentrating on the duodenum to document or exclude pyloric stenosis. Once pyloric stenosis has been excluded attention is paid to the gastro-oesophageal junction to detect reflux and/or hiatus hernia.

3.2.6 OESOPHAGEAL DUPLICATION CYSTS

Oesophageal duplication cyst represents 10 to 20 per cent of all the gastrointestinal duplications and make up about 2 per cent of all the oesophageal masses. Nearly half of these cysts will contain gastric mucosa and therefore have the potential to become symptomatic. There is an association with vertebral anomalies, oesophageal atresia and small bowel duplication cysts. Sixty per cent of these anomalies are in association with the lower oesophagus and are often located in the paraspinal region.

Sonography

Sonography may reveal hypoechoic fluid-filled cysts of varying shape with an echogenic inner mucosal lining. These usually present in neonates or young children where other anomalies such as neuroenteric cysts may also be seen as cystic or complex fairly well-defined structures just above the diaphragm.

3.2.7 OESOPHAGEAL TUMOURS

The oesophagus is a common site of malignancy, particularly in the elderly, which often gives rise to a visible mass within or around the oesophageal wall. Tumour spread usually occurs longitudinally along the oesophageal wall and there may be extensive tumour spread without a sonographically detectable mass lesion.

Carcinoma of the oesophagus is a common condition accounting for 10 per cent of gastrointestinal malignancies. The majority are squamous cell tumours although 5 to 10 per cent are adenocarcinomas. Alcohol, tobacco, Barrett oesophagus, asbestosis, tylosis, coeliac disease, Plummer-Vinson syndrome, achalasia, caustic stricture and radiation are known risk factors.

Benign oesophageal strictures and ulceration are associated with a thirty-fold increase in the risk of malignancy. The other tumour types include carcinosarcoma, leiomyosarcoma, rhabdomyosarcoma, malignant lymphoma and fibrosarcoma. Benign tumours also occur including leiomyoma, fibroma, lipoma, stromal cell tumour, neurofibroma and lymphangioma. The clinical presentation is usually with dysphagia, weight loss, retrosternal pain and regurgitation. The tumour may be polypoid, ulcerative or infiltrative.

Staging oesophageal cancer

The TNM system
T1   tumour invading submucosa or lamina propria.
T2   invasion of muscularis propria.
T3   invasion of adventitia.
T4   invasion of adjacent structures.
Stage I = T1, N0, M0.
Stage II A = T2–3, N0, M0.
Stage II B = T1/2, N1, M0.
Stage III = T3, N1, M0 or T4, N0/1, M0.
Stage IV = T1–4, N0/1, M1.

CT staging
● I   intraluminal mass, no wall thickening, no mediastinal metastases.
● II   wall thickening, no adjacent invasion.
● III thick wall with extension into other tissue, nodes, etc.
● IV   further extension or metastases.

Sonography

As patients usually present with dysphagia, oesophageal tumours are often diagnosed by endoscopy and barium studies. Sonography will occasionally demonstrate an unexplained distal oesophageal mass but its great use is in evaluating the liver, portal and para-aortic nodes and para-oesophageal areas to demonstrate tumour spread. Oesophageal tumour usually spreads longitudinally along the oesophageal wall thus there may be extensive tumour spread without sonographically detectable mass lesions.

Endoscopic ultrasound

The clinical use of endoscopic ultrasound at the present moment is an established technique for TNM staging of oesophageal and gastric cancer. Submucous tumours can be clearly demonstrated and definitely distinguished from extrinsic masses.

Although endoscopic ultrasound does not usually allow differentiation of malignant from benign lesions, it can give a clue as to the nature of the submucous tumour such as a cyst, lipoma or a leiomyoma. Endoscopic ultrasound is ideally suited to TNM staging as it depends on the depth of invasion of cancer and its involvement of various layers of the oesophageal wall. The five layers of the oesophageal wall are well seen on endoscopic ultrasound enabling such staging. However the ability to stage nodal involvement is limited by the fact that endoscopic ultrasound can detect lymph nodes within 3 cm of the primary tumour. When endoscopic ultrasound is combined with abdominal sonography, liver and upper abdominal lymph node metastases can be detected and peritoneal metastases inferred in the presence of ascites. On endoscopic ultrasound an oesophageal tumour is usually seen as an area of wall thickening which is usually hypoechoic but which may present a more complex echopattern. With cancer penetration the wall differentiation is lost and the smooth outer border of the oesophagus is no longer seen. Tumour invasion into the echogenic paraoesophageal fat can be easily detected. In comparative studies endoscopic ultrasound has been shown to be superior to CT in TNM staging of oesophageal cancer. The most recent studies have reported a T-stage accuracy of 82 to 86 per cent and an N-stage accuracy of 70 to 90 per cent. Endoscopic ultrasound is also helpful in the follow-up of patients with operative resection of cancer and with non-Hodgkin's lymphoma follow-up during radiotherapy or chemotherapy.

3.2.8 CAUSES OF A THICKENED INTRA-ABDOMINAL OESOPHAGEAL WALL

The normal thickness of the intra-abdominal oesophageal wall is 3.8 ± 1.2 mm.

Carcinoma – usually more than 10 mm thick.
Acute inflammation or corrosive injury (7.8 ± 2.1)
Lymphoma.
Oesophagitis or oesophageal ulceration.
Oesophageal Crohn's disease.
Oesophageal amyloid.
Right-sided heart failure.
Oesophageal varices.

3.3 STOMACH

Conventional transabdominal scanning of the stomach walls shows two layers. The inner echogenic layer represents the mucosa whilst the outer hypoechoic layer represents the gastric muscle. Intraoperative or endoscopic ultrasound with a high frequency probe shows five layers.

1. The innermost layer on the luminal aspect is hyperechoic, this usually represents an acoustic interface between the probe or balloon and mucosa.
2. A hypoechoic layer, the muscularis mucosa.
3. A hyperechoic layer, the interface between submucosa and muscularis propria.
4. A hypoechoic layer, the muscularis mucosa.
5. A hyperechoic subserosa and serosa interface echo.

When the patient is supine fluid collects in the gastric fundus which is posterior in position. This is seen as an anechoic collection medial to the spleen and upper pole of the left kidney. In babies' food, such as milk, curds may appear solid and echogenic and may be mistaken for a mass. Echogenic foci are usually present within gastric fluid because of the presence of debris and air bubbles. The gastric wall is usually clearly defined and the fluid-filled stomach may be mistaken for a cystic structure. The pylorus lies anteriorly as it crosses the spine and has a ring or 'bull's-eye' appearance in sagittal section. At this point it is anterior to the pancreas and superior mesenteric vein.

Gastric wall thickness is usually less than 4 mm. A wall thickness of 5 mm or over is highly suspicious of disease though transient thickening is seen when the stomach is collapsed or during peristalsis.

3.3.1 CAUSES OF A THICKENED GASTRIC WALL

Artificial (peristalsis).
Peptic ulceration.
Tumours – benign and malignant (primary or secondary).
Gastritis – including viral and eosinophilic.
Lymphoma.
Portal hypertension gastropathy.
Varioliform gastritis.
Focal foveolar hypertrophy.
Ménétrier's disease.
Hypertrophic pyloric stenosis.
Lymphoid hyperplasia.
Henoch–Schönlein purpura.
Chronic granulomatous disease of childhood.
Haematoma – particularly post-endoscopy.
Crohn's disease.
Chemical agents and toxins – ingestion of acid, alkali, iron, etc.
Gastric amyloidosis.
Interstitial emphysema.

Ectopic pancreas.
Gastric sarcoidosis.
Gastric tuberculosis.

3.3.2 PEPTIC ULCERATION

The majority of gastric and duodenal ulcers are far too small to be visualised by transabdominal ultrasound. However, oedema cellular infiltration cause gastric wall thickening which may be seen as echogenic or hypoechoic areas of gastric wall thickening. Distension of the stomach with fluid aids visualisation of larger ulcer craters. However when a large ulcer is seen it is more likely to be neoplastic than peptic in origin. Ultrasound cannot usually differentiate between malignant and peptic gastric ulcers unless there is an extrinsic mass or lymphadenopathy to suggest malignancy. Endoscopy and biopsy are therefore necessary. On endoscopic ultrasound gastric carcinoma may present as polypoid, flat ulcerated hyperechoic and inhomogeneous lesions with irregular margins disrupting the normal layered architecture. Carcinomas that infiltrate the deeper layers may be seen on endoscopic ultrasound with a reported accuracy of 67 to 92 per cent in local TNM staging.

When duodenal ulcers are seen they may have a central hyperechoic focus due to the presence of fibrinoid debris with an adjacent hypoechoic halo representing oedematous thickening of the duodenal wall.

Complications of peptic ulcer are relatively common and include haemorrhage, obstruction and perforation. Twenty-six per cent will penetrate the bowel wall and involve adjacent organs including the pancreas, biliary tract, liver, lesser sac and the greater omentum. Whenever you see an abscess or fluid collection always look for a tract leading to adjacent bowel or evidence of air within the collection.

Approximately a third of patients with peptic ulcer disease are hypersecretors producing excess gastric acid. The highest basal gastric acid output is in the morning and ultrasound can be used to provide a rough estimate of resting gastric fluid volume. This is assessed by placing the patient in the right lateral decubitus position. The maximum cross-section area (cm^2) of the pylorus is roughly proportional to the gastric fluid volume. Excess fluid is present in hyper-secretors and also gastric outlet obstruction. The maximum cross-sectional area of the distal stomach or pylorus can also be used to assess gastric emptying after a test feed. The area is measured against time giving a graphic display of the gastric volume after feeding and hence the rate of emptying.

Gastric ulcers in infants may be the result of stress, hyperacidity or food allergies especially milk. Ultrasonically the thickened mucosa (more than 4 mm in thickness) may be uniform or lumpy associated with delayed gastric emptying.

Sonographic features of gastric ulceration

Scan the gastric walls with the patient's stomach distended.

Wall thickening.
Loss of the five-layered structure of the gastric wall.
Crater may not be evident.
Wall can be thinned.
Crater can be disc shaped.
Crater can go through the wall.
Loss of definition of external structures.

3.3.3 GASTRIC TUMOURS

Ultrasonography is an unreliable means of demonstrating bowel masses and is thus not regarded as the investigation of choice in cases of suspected bowel pathology. However recent work has shown that conventional ultrasound is a simple, rapid and useful method to detect tumours of the gastrointestinal tract particularly when the stomach is fluid filled. Sensitivity has been touted at 77.8 per cent, specificity of 99.1 per cent positive predictive value of 94.9 per cent and negative predictive value of 95.5 per cent. The stomach is identified in 99 per cent of patients. Often ultrasound demonstrates totally unsuspected bowel masses on scans performed for unrelated reasons, particularly those which tend to present late clinically.

Primary gastric neoplasms are rare in childhood, the commonest being teratomas. These are seen as anechoic or hypoechoic masses which may show evidence of calcification. These usually occur in the first year of life and are more common in boys than girls. Hamartomas of the gastric wall produce marked wall thickening and protrude into the gastric lumen in a polypoid fashion. They may be mistaken for food residues. Benign gastric tumours comprise three distinct entities

1. submucous tumours are rare, most often conjunctive but may also be heterotopic or congenital, these include leiomyoma, schwannoma, neurofibroma, aberrant pancreas, fibroma, lipoma, haemangioma, glomus tumours and gastric wall cysts – because of their subepithelial location samples taken during endoscopic examination are rarely contributory
2. polyps, they are of epithelial origin, are common, most often small and best seen on endoscopic ultrasound
3. carcinoids.

On endoscopic ultrasound benign tumours result in thickening of the wall without disruption of the layered structure. Adenocarcinoma of the stomach is rare in children but is common in the elderly. It causes thickening of the gastric wall with mixed but generally hypoechoic echopattern. Anechoic areas occur because of focal necrosis. Gastric lymphoma and lymphosarcoma give rise to relatively anechoic masses and similar changes occur with leiomyoma and leiomyosarcoma, though these tumours may also give rise to complex or multicystic masses. Haematomas of the gastric wall also give rise to anechoic or hypoechoic masses and these are a not uncommon cause of small masses in the stomach particularly after endoscopy. They usually occur in the body of the stomach and are rare in the pylorus. Sonographic appearance of intramural gastric masses is thus often quite non-specific, although endoscopic ultrasound can differentiate between benign and malignant lesions.

Gastric carcinoma

This is the third most common gastrointestinal malignancy. The incidence of carcinoma of the stomach has fallen over the last decade although there has been an increasing incidence of cardia tumours as compared to antrum tumours. The risk factors include dietary factors such as nitrites, nitrates, low vegetable and fruit diet, pickled vegetables and low acid output states such as chronic gastritis, partial gastrectomy, gastrojejunostomy, bile reflux and pernicious anaemia. Ninety-five per cent are adenocarcinomas. Morphologically carcinoma of the stomach may present as an intraluminal polyp, ulcerative lesion or infiltrative scirrhous lesion.

Staging gastric carcinoma

T1   cancer confined to the mucosa or submucosa.
T2   muscular layer or serosa involved.
T3   cancer penetrating through the serosa.
T4a   invasion of extragastric contiguous tissue.
T4b   adjacent organs invaded.
N1   lymph node invasion within 3 cm of the primary lesion along gastric curvatures.
N2   lymph node invasion at a distance greater than 3 cm from the primary lesion along branches of the coeliac axis.
N3   involvement of the aortic, pancreatic, duodenal and mesenteric group of lymph nodes.
M1   distant metastases.

Sonography

The sonographic features of gastric carcinoma on transabdominal scanning are the presence of an intraluminal mass, focal or diffuse wall thickening and/or an exophytic mass. A target or atypical target sign may be present. An atypical target sign corresponds more frequently to adenocarcinoma while a typical target sign due to more uniform diffuse involvement is more common with lymphomas. The presence of ascites in association with a stomach mass is strongly suggestive of peritoneal metastases. Some tumours present a high echogenic dot with an acoustic shadow, which has been interpreted as an ulcer in the centre of the tumour. On endoscopic ultrasound gastric cancers may appear polypoid, flat, ulcerated, hyperechoic and inhomogeneous lesions with irregular margins disrupting the normal layered anatomy of the stomach.

Technique of endoscopic ultrasound The procedure is performed under conscious sedation using a fibreoptic endoscope equipped with 7.5 to 12 MHz probes. The probes are of rotating types that can achieve a 360 degree image. A depth of 3 cm is achieved with a 12 MHz probe and 7 cm with a 7.5 MHz probe. Thus distant organ metastases beyond 7 cm from the field of vision cannot be detected. Endoscopic ultrasound is the only modality that allows preoperative staging according to the TNM classification and differentiation between early and advanced cancer. However, endoscopic ultrasound is rather disappointing for lymph node assessment at 50 to 80 per cent sensitivity but compares favourably with CT. Lymph nodes that appear well defined and hypoechoic with an echopattern similar to the primary lesion are more likely to be cancerous rather than inflammatory. Distant lymph node metastases require abdominal ultrasound, CT or MRI.

Sonography of pancreatic invasion with gastric carcinoma
Gastric carcinoma not infrequently invades the lymph nodes, liver, pancreas, duodenum, spleen, colon and the peritoneal cavity. Accurate staging is essential to plan therapy. It is a common observation when performing abdominal sonography that intraperitoneal and extraperitoneal organs move differently on respiration. Pancreatic invasion is difficult to detect on CT and the reported accuracy has been poor. The sliding sign on sonography has been found to be useful in assessing and localising a right upper abdominal mass by the fact that retroperitoneal organs move differently on respiration. This sign has recently been applied to pancreatic invasion by gastric carcinoma. When a gastric mass had no sliding motion against the pancreas or partial motion against the background of disrupted fat planes between the stomach and pancreas, the sliding sign was considered negative and was taken as evidence of pancreatic invasion. This sign has yielded a sensitivity of 80 per cent, 96 per cent specificity and 90 per cent accuracy for pancreatic invasion.

Anastamotic recurrence of gastric carcinoma
Endoscopic ultrasound is a reliable method in identifying cancer recurrence with a sensitivity of 95 per cent and specificity of 80 per cent. In normal anastamosis a three-layered structure with a maximum thickness of 6 mm is seen with a normal five-layered stomach wall above and below. Recurrence

leads to modularity and hypoechoic thickness at the site of anastamosis with thickness over 7 mm. Regional lymphadenopathy may be recognised.

Lipoma

Lipoma is a rare benign tumour of the stomach that usually arises from the submucosal layer of the stomach. The majority are asymptomatic but may present with haemorrhage due to superficial ulceration. Sonographically they are well-defined hyperechoic tumours originating from the submucous layer. Endoscopic ultrasound gives better resolution, the tumours are seen confined to the submucous layer, they are diffusely homogeneous and hyperechoic. Small tumours can be detected on endoscopic ultrasound. Computed tomography would confirm these tumours to be sharply defined intramural masses of fat density.

Leiomyoma

This is the most common benign extramucosal tumour of the stomach. With an average size of 4.5 cm they are submucosal hypoechoic masses with smooth margins. Growth may be confined to the wall of the stomach, but they may grow either into the lumen of the stomach forming a pedunculated mass or in an exophytic subserosal direction. It results in a focal gastric mass often with overlying mucosal ulceration. Histology is identical to that of uterine leiomyoma. Dystrophic calcification can occur (mucinous adenocarcinoma of stomach also show foci of calcification), endoscopic ultrasound shows the tumour to arise from the muscularis propria (fourth layer) but occasionally from the muscularis mucosa (second layer). The normal layered wall structure is maintained.

Leiomyosarcoma

Sixty per cent of leiomyosarcomas involve the stomach. They are usually large focal mass lesions up to 10 cm in diameter. Although they have been described in children as young as 10 years old, the majority occur in the fifth and sixth decades of life with a slight male preponderance. Although this is a mural lesion its size results in gastric displacement and an exophytic position. Central necrosis is common and calcification can occur. They are generally globular or irregular in shape and sometimes acquire huge proportions outstripping their blood supply and undergoing central necrosis, hence the cystic ultrasound appearance. In females they may reach the pelvis mimicking ovarian masses. The demonstration of a convex lower border to the mass excludes an ovarian or pelvic mass. Sonographic appearance is variable. In tumours that have undergone necrosis without liquefaction the appearance is that of an echopoor mass without enhancement. With liquefactive necrosis cystic spaces that enhance are seen. The appearance of a solid mass, anteriorly placed with no relation to a solid viscus, the presence of cystic spaces in relation to a gas-filled viscus is highly suggestive of a leiomyosarcoma. Better still when an atypical target sign is seen in the epigastrium in association with a large multicystic or complex mass the appearances may be even more suggestive. Malignant transformation may occur in a leiomyoma. On endoscopic ultrasound the tumour is often hypodense as a result of liquefaction necrosis or has irregular outer margins associated with destruction of the normal wall layers. Malignant change is possible in a benign-looking lesion and hence the value of biopsy.

Leiomyoblastoma

This is a rare gastric neoplasm that cannot be differentiated sonographically from leiomyoma or leiomyosarcoma. These tumours may be intramural or present as pedunculated exophytic masses. These tumours are usually fairly well defined and have both hypoechoic solid as well as cystic components.

Gastric carcinoid

Whilst being the most common primary tumour of the small bowel its occurrence in the stomach is rare. On transabdominal sonography these tumours cannot usually be differentiated from other gastric neoplasms. They may present as hypoechoic atypical target lesions or as a hypoechoic intramural mass. Endoscopic ultrasound is an effective method of looking at these tumours. The smallest sized tumour detectable on endoscopic ultrasound is 2 mm in diameter. They are well-defined tumours that are hypoechoic, homogeneous and primarily oval to round. The tumours are mainly located in the third layer. The second layer usually covers the tumour whilst the third layer forms the base of the tumour. With malignant transformation the layered wall of the stomach is disrupted. Endoscopic ultrasound is useful in determining local metastases and in detection of local lymph node metastases.

Gastric lymphangioma

Lymphangioma of the stomach is a rare tumour, it is a thin-walled cyst lined by a flattened endothelium. The tumour has a submucous location. There is no association between lymphangioma and lymphatic obstruction. The age range affected has been reported as 8 days to 79 years. Vague abdominal symptoms are usually present. On abdominal sonography the appearance is that of a fairly well-defined cystic mass within the gastric wall. Endoscopic ultrasound shows a characteristic submucosal cystic lesion with internal septations. Septations in these tumours are difficult to see on abdominal CT or ultrasound.

Kaposi's sarcoma

Kaposi's sarcoma is an AIDS-associated malignant neoplasm originating from the endothelial cells of vascular channels. The gastrointestinal tract is involved in 40 per cent of patients. Any part of the gastrointestinal tract may be involved but involvement is usually in association with lymph node, skin or liver. Gastrointestinal involvement in isolation occurs in less than 5 per cent of cases. Nodular thickened mucosal folds, polypoid masses and diffuse infiltration manifest gastrointestinal involvement. Lymph node involvement is common. Sonographically the masses are hypoechoic and poorly defined, an atypical target sign may occur and regional lymphadenopathy may be detected.

Gastric lymphoma

Lymphoma accounts for 1 to 5 per cent of gastric tumours. It most frequently results in generalised thickening of the gastric wall but occasionally focal involvement may occur. The gastric wall is usually greater than 1 cm thick and can be as much as 5 cm thick. The mucosa is usually intact but can be ulcerated. When using the stomach fluid-filled technique, lymphomatous infiltration may be seen as extensive wall thickening of varied echogenicity while the inner wall may be normal or thrown into infiltrated polypoid folds. Circumferential involvement may be associated with bulky focal masses and nodular exophytic involvement. A target or atypical target sign may occur. The echogenicity of lymphoma infiltration tends to be echopoor. Occasionally giant gastric folds with a central star-like configuration of echogenicity may be visible on ultrasound. Seventy-two per cent of lymphomas of the stomach present with a target-like pattern of the gastric antrum with uniform hypoechoic wall thickening.

Gastric metastases

The stomach is an uncommon site for metastatic disease deposits occurring in only 2 per cent of patients with primary malignancy elsewhere. Tumours more commonly invade the stomach directly. Primary tumours giving rise to gastric metastases include lymphoma, leukaemia, melanoma, carcinomas from bronchus, breast, colon, prostate, thyroid, ovary, pancreas, uterus and testicular malignancy. Metastatic deposits lie within the gastric wall usually within the submucosa. They are usually lobular but may form plaques or are occasionally infiltrative with a linitis plastica appearance. Uncommonly aggressive tumours are infiltrative. Sonography will usually shows a focal mural mass which may or may not have a target appearance. Visualisation is aided by distension of the stomach with fluid.

3.3.4 PORTAL HYPERTENSION GASTROPATHY

Portal hypertension is associated with a variety of signs, for example splenomegaly, ascites, varices, other portosystemic shunts and a dilated portal vein. Portal hypertension causes significant thickening of the stomach wall probably as a result of congestive gastropathy although hypoproteinaemia from liver disease may also play a role. In the majority of patients the increased thickness is generalised and mostly confined to the inner region of mixed echogenicity.

In control groups the mean thickness of the antrum is 13.8 mm (SD 3.02, range 8–20 mm) and the mean thickness of the body is 14.05 mm (SD 2.70, range 11–19 mm). In patients with cirrhosis the mean thickness of the antrum was 22.15 mm (SD 5.63, range 13–31 mm) and the mean thickness of the body is 22.2 mm (SD 5.73 mm, range 13–31 mm).

3.3.5 FOCAL FOVEOLAR HYPERPLASIA

Focal foveolar hyperplasia is the commonest cause of gastric polyps in adults but is rare in infants. These polyps are thought to occur because of hyper-regeneration of gastric mucosa after injury and may be associated with partial gastrectomy, bile reflux, inflammation and Ménétrier's giant rugal hypertrophy. These polyps are usually asymptomatic but have been implicated in gastric outlet obstruction in infants. A polypoidal mass may be evident lying within the mucosa surrounded by normal gastric muscle. The mass has similar echogenicity to gastric mucosa. The appearance may be identical to peptic ulceration, inflammation and Ménétrier's disease. It may cause gastric obstruction in infants as a result of a polypoid mucosal mass. The lobulated mass may be seen on ultrasound with an echogenicity similar to a normal gastric mucosa and submucosa. Large gastric folds may be seen impinging upon the gastric lumen. Endoscopic ultrasound shows a normal layered structure of the stomach without disruption.

3.3.6 MÉNÉTRIER'S DISEASE

Ménétrier's disease or transient protein-losing gastropathy is characterised by giant rugal hypertrophy. It is a rare abnormality of the gastric wall. It may affect both adults and children though paediatric cases are particularly rare and do not behave in the same manner as the adult form. The disease in adults, which occurs predominantly in middle-aged men, is usually chronic and associated with a 10 per cent risk of complicating carcinoma. In children it tends to have a shorter more benign course with allergies and viral infections being implicated. The disease is characterised by the presence of hypertrophic gastritis (giant rugal hypertrophy) and protein-losing enteropathy. The clinical symptoms include oedema occasionally associated with ascites, pleural effusions, anorexia, abdominal pain, vomiting and diarrhoea.

Sonography

In a fasting state the stomach displays polypoid mucosal thickening especially in the body and fundus of the stomach. The entire wall of the stomach is thickened and hypoechoic. The rugae are best seen with a fluid-filled stomach but may flatten after fluid ingestion. There are hypoechoic areas behind the rugae because of gland hypertrophy and therefore this condition looks different from a neoplasm of the stomach. As the condition gets better the ultrasound appearance improves On endoscopic ultrasound the first and second layers of the stomach wall are usually thickened but generally the layered structure is maintained unless the gastropathy is complicated by a gastric carcinoma.

3.3.7 DIFFERENTIAL DIAGNOSIS OF THICKENED RUGAE SEEN ON SONOGRAPHY

Benign causes – gastritis, Ménétrier's disease, portal hypertension gastropathy, gastric varices, multiple polyps, for example Peutz–Jeghers syndrome, Zollinger–Ellison syndrome, lymphangiectasia, gastric amyloidosis.
Malignant causes – gastric carcinoma, linitis plastica, lymphoma.

3.3.8 GASTRIC VARICES

In portal hypertension gastric varices are seen in 2 to 78 per cent of patients, the commonest location is at the gastro-oesophageal junction and along the lesser curve, occasionally they may be located in the antrum of the stomach. On abdominal sonography the appearance is that of thickened gastric wall in association with cirrhosis or other ultrasound features of portal hypertension. On a fluid-filled stomach polypoid projection into the stomach lumen may be apparent. Endoscopic ultrasound shows characteristic anechoic tubular structures with smooth margins.

3.3.9 GASTRIC PANCREATIC RESTS

Ectopic pancreatic rests have an incidence of 2 to 10 per cent at autopsy series. Males have twice the incidence. Eighty per cent are said to occur in the stomach whilst the others are distributed in the small bowel and Meckel's diverticulum. This is one of the causes of focal gastric thickening on sonography but as the rests are submucosal endoscopic ultrasound is the best method of looking at these. They are seen as well-circumscribed submucosal lesions of varying echogenicity with central cystic or tubular structures corresponding to a duct system. They tend to arise from the innermost three sonographic layers.

3.3.10 HENOCH–SCHÖNLEIN PURPURA

Henoch–Schönlein purpura is the most common allergic vasculitis in children but may occur in adults. Bleeding may occur in various organs including the gastrointestinal tract. Sonography is the examination of choice in Henoch–Schönlein purpura to assess stomach/bowel involvement and detection of complications. Sonography reliably shows mural thickening, bowel haematomas, ileus, ascites and intussusception. Sonography distinguishes between a tight intussusception and a loose intussusception, the former is unlikely to respond to conservative treatment while the latter can safely be managed conservatively. The presence of air or fluid between the layers of the intussusception indicates looseness. Sonography is also useful in demonstrating other complications of Henock–Schönlein purpura such as pleural effusions, bladder wall haemorrhage and scrotal oedema. Colour flow Doppler shows blood flow signals in the diseased small bowel wall. The analysis of the Doppler waveform showed the arterial blood flow signals with a resistive index value of 0.642 to 0.6669.

3.3.11 CHRONIC GRANULOMATOUS DISEASE

Chronic granulomatous disease of childhood is an X-linked recessive disorder, which results in a defect in the bacterial activity of polymorphonuclear leukocytes. The phagocytes are able to engulf bacteria but are not able to kill them; this leads to an increased susceptibility to bacterial infection particularly with *Staphylococcus* spp. Chronic infection leads to granulomatous tissue formation particularly in the lungs, liver and gastric antrum. These granulomata may eventually calcify and may become visible on plain radiographs. Involvement of the pyloric antrum causes wall thickening and luminal narrowing. This wall thickening is usually circumferential and give rise to the target sign. Affected children are usually older than those with hypertrophic pyloric stenosis and have slower onset of symptoms.

Antibiotic treatment is often successful at relieving the symptoms of gastric outlet obstruction without the need for surgery. The sonographic features are relatively non-specific and, depending upon the patient's age, may mimic peptic ulceration, Crohn's disease, carcinoma, the effect of radiotherapy, etc.

3.3.12 GASTRIC AMYLOIDOSIS

Gastrointestinal involvement is more common with primary than secondary amyloidosis. Although gastrointestinal amyloidosis is often asymptomatic widespread dysfunction may occur. With stomach involvement postprandial epigastric pain and heartburn may occur. The oesophagus is involved in 11 per cent, the stomach in 37 per cent and small bowel in 74 per cent of cases. The stomach may be infiltrated diffusely resulting in a rigid stomach resembling linitis plastica. The gastric rugae may be thickened associated with diminished peristalsis and a degree of gastric outlet obstruction. Localised infiltration may occur usually confined to the gastric antrum associated with hypertrophied rugae and superficial ulceration. A well-defined low echogenicity submucous amyloidoma is a rare occurrence. The differential diagnosis is from other causes of stomach wall thickening and hypertrophied rugae.

3.3.13 BOWEL WALL HAEMATOMAS

Small intramural haematomas are common in the oesophagus and stomach particularly after endoscopy. These rarely cause symptoms and are not visualised on abdominal sonography. Large haematomas may be recognised as anechoic masses. Large symptomatic haematomas of the oesophagus and stomach are rare and are often associated with trauma (including endoscopy and non-accidental injury), bleeding diathesis, for example haemophilia, anticoagulant therapy, etc. or other underlying pathology such as leukaemia, lymphoma, Henoch–Schönlein purpura or thrombocytopenic purpura. A pyloric haematoma has been recorded as a cause of gastric outlet obstruction in a baby. The haematoma was seen as an anechoic ring around the normal hypoechoic muscle thus differentiating the haematoma from hypertrophic pyloric stenosis.

3.3.14 GASTRIC GRANULOMATOUS DISEASE

Crohn's disease, sarcoidosis and tuberculosis may rarely affect the stomach and cause focal or diffuse wall thickening. The diagnostic clues may be in the patient's history, otherwise differentiation from other causes of bowel thickening may not be possible without a biopsy.

3.3.15 THE WATER MELON STOMACH

The water melon stomach or gastric antral vascular ectasia is seen endo-scopically as thickened, red vascular folds radiating from the pylorus to the gastric antrum. On endoscopic ultrasound focal thickening of the inner layers of the gastric wall are noted and may reflect the diagnosis of gastric antral vascular ectasia.

3.3.16 ENTERIC DUPLICATION CYSTS

Enteric duplication cysts are caused by errors of canalisation of the ali-mentary canal during embryonic development which may result in two forms of morphologic aberrations

1. duplication of the lumen
2. development of closed cysts in relation to bowel wall.

They have a common muscular wall with the gastrointestinal tract but have a separate mucosal lining (ectopic mucosa). Enteric cysts are rare in adults and more often found in children. They account for 15 per cent of paedi-atric abdominal masses and 9 per cent are associated with gastrointestinal atresia. The incidence is

- 17 to 20 per cent in the oesophagus
- 4 per cent in the stomach
- 4 to 5 per cent in the duodenum
- 30 to 33 per cent in the ileum
- 13 to 30 per cent in the colon
- 4 per cent at the ileocaecal junction
- 4 per cent in the rectum, and
- 7–15 per cent are multiple.

On cross-sectional imaging they appear as spherical, saccular cysts in 82 per cent of patients, in the rest they appear tubular, sausage-shaped cysts.

The stomach is an uncommon site for duplication cysts. They are twice as common in females and usually involve the greater curve of the stomach.

Sonography

All enteric cysts have an inner echogenic mucosal layer and an outer hypo-echoic layer. The two layers can often be seen circumferentially in any one image. The inner echogenic layer may be fuzzy and is 1 to 2 mm thick which is the same thickness as the muscle layer of the cyst. This combina-tion is highly suggestive of duplication cysts. Other cystic structures do not show the double layer as completely. Uncommonly in the case of the stomach they may communicate with a gastric lumen causing a complex appearance.

Differential diagnosis of enteric cysts

Omental cysts.
Mesenteric cysts.
Choledochal cysts.
Liver cysts.
Pancreatic cysts or pseudocysts.
Renal cyst.
Ovarian cysts.
Abscesses.
Splenic cysts.
Meckel's diverticulum.
Lymphangioma.
Lymphoma.
Intramural tumours.

3.3.17 GASTRIC PNEUMATOSIS

Interstitial gas within the gastric wall is uncommon but can occur after gastrostomy tube placement, which is an increasingly common procedure with emphysema or bronchitis. Occasionally it occurs because of infection with gas-forming organisms. This may be associated with previous gastritis, alcohol abuse or corrosive ingestion and has a high mortality. It may be a complication of biliary stenting, gastric manipulation, gastric outlet obstruction, overzealous gastric distension during gastroscopy, aerophagia ischaemia and trauma including non-accidental injury and gastric bezoar.

Gas in the gastric wall may be difficult to appreciate as the stomach is often obscured by the contained gas. When visible it is seen as echogenic lines with distal reverberation artefact.

3.3.18 GASTRIC BEZOAR

A bezoar is an insoluble mass within the gastric lumen. The mass may be formed from hair (trichobezoar) particularly in young women or from vegetable or fruit fibre (phytobezoar) or from concretions of inorganic material. Recently bezoar formation has been reported with sucralfate, a complex aluminium hydroxide and sulphated sucrose used in the treatment of peptic ulcer. The drug is also used to prevent stress ulceration and gastrointestinal haemorrhage on intensive care units. Newborn infants who receive sucralfate 36% may have problems with bezoar formation and present with gastric occlusive syndrome. A gastric bezoar reduces gastric capacity and causes nausea, pain and weight loss. In middle-aged and elderly patients these symptoms often mimic carcinoma. Ultrasonography demonstrates a complex mass within the gastric lumen. The mass usually has echogenic areas, it is mobile within the stomach and will often cause shadowing.

3.3.19 GASTRIC DILATATION

A large fluid-filled stomach may extend inferiorly into the lower abdomen and may be mistaken for a distal bowel loop. The presence of air within a dilated stomach may further complicate matters as it may obscure the upper abdomen. Causes of gastric dilatation include biochemical imbalance, diabetes mellitus, drugs (such as prostaglandins and non-steroidal anti-inflammatory drugs), pyloric or duodenal stricture, tumour, amyloid, chronic granulomatous disease, Bouveret's syndrome (gastric outlet obstruction caused by a gallstone impacted in the duodenal bulb). Sonography may reveal a large fluid-filled upper abdominal structure with fine echoes caused by air bubbles or food debris. With gastric outlet obstruction the cause may be identified, for example lymphoma, amyloid, tumour, gallstone, bezoar, etc.

3.3.20 GASTRIC EMPTYING

The variable shape of the stomach makes the assessment of gastric volume measurement inaccurate. However, a reasonably accurate assessment of gastric emptying can be made by sonography. The half time ($t_{1/2}$) of gastric emptying calculated by sonography correlates fairly well with the estimation of gastric emptying by scintigraphy. The degree of gastric filling is assessed by measuring a transverse section of the stomach and the diameter. The diameter or circumference of the stomach may be plotted against time to give a measure of gastric emptying. The mean of the product of parasagittal and transverse diameters (the gastric filling index) has also been used.

3.3.21 HYPERTROPHIC PYLORIC STENOSIS

Hypertrophic pyloric stenosis is a condition characterised by pyloric muscle hypertrophy resulting in gastric outlet obstruction. It is a relatively common condition affecting 1 in 150 boys and 1 in 775 girls. The exact aetiology is uncertain but there appear to be hereditary factors, though interestingly it is more common in the children of affected females than affected males. It especially affects the first-born son. There is a high concordance in twins. It has also been suggested that trauma caused by the presence of a nasogastric tube in a neonate may also increase the risk of hypertrophic pyloric stenosis. The pylorus has been shown to be normal at birth and it is thought that the pyloric muscle hypertrophy may occur in response to trauma caused by the passage of milk curds. Spasm induced by this trauma leads to muscle hypertrophy but also increases the pyloric narrowing. Therefore hypertrophic pyloric stenosis is not an 'all-or-nothing' phenomenon but a condition which evolves over a period of time, usually a few days. The majority of cases present in the 2- to 8-week age group with a history of increasing vomiting that becomes projectile. Gastric peristalsis may be visible and a pyloric muscle mass is usually palpable after a test feed. Five per cent of cases are associated with jaundice which clears after surgery.

In 83 per cent of cases the findings are sufficiently characteristic to proceed to surgery without any form of imaging. In the remaining 17 per cent ultrasonography is the investigation of choice to confirm or exclude the diagnosis. Ultrasonography has replaced barium meal examination which has an error rate of up to 10 per cent in the diagnosis of hypertrophic pyloric stenosis, this error rate is because of lack of specificity of barium meal findings which cannot differentiate pylorospasm from true hypertrophic pyloric stenosis and may also miss early cases. Ultrasonography is also safer and less time consuming than barium meal examination. On ultrasonography the normal pylorus is seen as a ring of hypoechoic muscle with an inner ring of echogenic mucosa. In hypertrophic pyloric stenosis there is marked thickening of the pyloric muscle relative to the rest of stomach mucosa and this compresses the mucosa into a single echogenic band. The lumen is only seen in 10 per cent of cases of hypertrophic pyloric stenosis and then it is only seen on prolonged scanning when it is visible for a short period of the time during the passage of a short 'jet' of fluid. Even when visible the lumen never dilates to its normal calibre. The gallbladder is a good landmark of pyloric location. If the pylorus is still not identified the whole of the upper abdomen should be examined as the pylorus may be displaced to the right lateral abdominal wall or it may be directed posteriorly instead of transversely. If a nasogastric tube has not drained the stomach then it will usually be full, even 4 hours after the last feed or after vomiting. An empty stomach in the absence of vomiting or nasogastric drainage makes hypertrophic pyloric stenosis unlikely.

Once located the pylorus is evaluated and the muscle compared with that of the body of the stomach. In hypertrophic pyloric stenosis the pylorus assumes a 'doughnut' appearance because of the marked muscle thickening. In some cases the normally hypoechoic muscle may appear anechoic. The mucosa is compressed into a single echogenic band. Pyloric measurements may be useful aids to diagnosis but when the experienced sonographer sees classic hypertrophic pyloric stenosis configuration the diagnosis has been made. Lack of visualisation of pyloric muscle mass does not exclude the diagnosis but rather a search should be made for the pylorus and its normality confirmed by demonstration of the normal muscle thickness and full dilatation during the passage of fluid. If these rules are followed there should be no false positive results, though false negatives may occur in early cases where pyloric muscle hypertrophy is not fully developed. In cases of doubt the examination is simply repeated on the following day. False positive results may occur if the sonographer relies solely upon measurement of the pyloric dimensions for diagnosis, as the pyloric diameter may be above the normal range when it is transiently dilated during gastric emptying. In these cases the pyloric configuration is not that of hypertrophic pyloric stenosis and there is no evidence of muscle mass. The great variation in children's dimensions, even in the neonatal period, may cause difficulties when tables of normal values are used in diagnosis.

Pyloric muscle dimensions

Thickness measured from the base of the echogenic mucosa to the outer edge of the muscle (Figure 3.2)

- normal 1.8 ± 0.4
- hypertrophic pyloric stenosis 4.8 ± 0.8

Total pyloric diameter

- normal ≤10 mm
- hypertrophic pyloric stenosis ≥15 mm.

Pyloric length

- normal 9.1 mm (5–16)
- hypertrophic pyloric stenosis 22.1 mm (16–28)

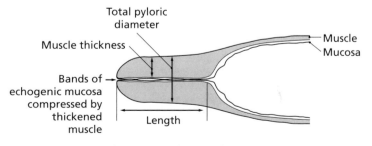

Figure 3.2 Pyloric canal measurements.

Pyloric volume

pyloric volume $> 1.4\,cm^3$ ($= 1/4 \times \pi$ (diameter)$^2 \times$ length
$1.4\,cm^3 = 1/4\,\pi \times$ (max. diameter)$^2 \times$ length
Pyloric length $+ 3.64 \times$ thickness $> 25\,mm$

Generally if the muscle thickness is greater than 4 mm or total pyloric diameter is greater than 15 mm then a confident diagnosis of hypertrophic pyloric stenosis can be made, providing a pyloric mass is clearly present. Muscle thickness is the most reliable feature, other parameters show overlap between normal and abnormal. In the early stages of hypertrophic pyloric stenosis pyloric muscle thickness has not reached a critical stage at which gastric outlet obstruction occurs and hence the lack of cases with measurements in the intermediate range between normal and abnormal. Muscle thickness increases with age of patient and with duration of symptoms. Length of pylorus is the single most reliable measurement but there is considerable overlap between normal and abnormal, therefore the whole appearance must be reviewed rather than a single parameter. Other signs described with hypertrophic pyloric stenosis are the cervix sign – an elongated narrowed pylorus which looks like a cervix – and the double track sign of compressed tracks of fluid. Pyloric haematomas are very rare and are seen as anechoic collections around or adjacent to the muscle. Chronic granulomatous disease of childhood does not usually cause gastric obstruction at such an early age and focal foveolar hypertrophy causes irregular wall thickening with an irregular inner surface without mucosal compression into a single band. If doubt remains after evaluation of the pylorus then the infant should be given fluid either orally or by a nasogastric tube and the pylorus evaluated during the passage of this fluid.

3.3.22 CAUSES OF ANTROPYLORIC NARROWING IN YOUNG CHILDREN

Pylorospasm.
Hypertrophic pyloric stenosis – complete or incomplete.
Pyloric stenosis – atypical short segment.
Chronic granulomatous disease.
Focal foveolar hypertrophy.
Focal pyloric haematoma.
Gastric duplication cyst.
Tumours (these are very rare in infants) – leiomyoma, leiomyosarcoma, leiomyoblastoma, lipoma, liposarcoma, neurofibroma, etc.
Aberrant pancreatic tissue.
Hamartoma.
Congenital stenosis – atresia.

Chemical gastritis.
Regional enteritis.

3.3.23 PYLOROSPASM (ANTRAL DYSKINESIA)

Pylorospasm is relatively common in infancy and may cause symptoms similar to hypertrophic pyloric stenosis but without a palpable pyloric mass. It may be related to vagal over-stimulation and hyperacidity. Increased pyloric tone also occurs in association with neurological disorders and these cases are easily mistaken for hypertrophic pyloric stenosis on barium meal examination. Sonographically the pylorus shows normal muscle thickness but it appears narrowed with ineffective transmission of peristalsis and delayed gastric emptying. Muscle thickness is usually between 1.5 to 3 mm with variable canal narrowing associated with increased peristalsis, delayed emptying and an elongated pylorus. The condition resolves over a period of days.

3.3.24 PSEUDO-HYPERTROPHIC PYLORIC STENOSIS

The pyloric muscle may appear thickened during muscle contraction particularly in the presence of pylorospasm. This transient phenomenon may be exaggerated if the sections through the pylorus are oblique. Imaging the pylorus in several dimensions over a period of time will reveal the transient nature of the finding.

3.3.25 FOCAL FOVEOLAR HYPERPLASIA

See p. 248.

3.3.26 CHRONIC GRANULOMATOUS DISEASE

See pp. 250–251.

3.3.27 ANTROPYLORIC MEMBRANES

The presence of membranes across the bowel is a form of focal atresia which is thought to be caused by intrauterine stress such as anoxia or focal ischaemia. As the bowel heals scarring causes focal narrowing. Bowel obstruction is usually incomplete because of the presence of a small opening in the membrane. The membrane may be seen as a constant band surrounded by fluid. If the membrane lies in the distal pylorus it is easily mistaken for the division between the pylorus and duodenum.

3.3.28 PYLORIC HAEMATOMAS

Small intramural haematomas are common in the oesophagus and stomach particularly after endoscopy. These rarely cause symptoms and are not usually visualised sonographically. Larger haematomas may be recognised as anechoic intramural masses. Large symptomatic haematomas are rare and are often associated with haemorrhagic disease or other underlying pathology. A pyloric haematoma has been recorded causing gastric outlet obstruction in a baby. It was seen as an anechoic ring around normal pyloric muscle and was thus differentiated from hypertrophic pyloric stenosis.

3.3.29 RETROGASTRIC MASSES

Differential diagnosis of a retrogastric mass

Pancreatic (most common):
Pancreatitis or pseudocyst.
Tumour – adenocarcinoma, cystadenoma, cystadenocarcinoma, etc.
Gastric wall masses – leiomyoma or leiomyosarcoma, carcinoma, lymphoma, etc.
Retroperitoneal masses – lymphadenopathy, renal mass or tumour, adrenal cyst or tumour, haematoma, abscess, retroperitoneal tumour, aortic aneurysm, omental hernia, enlarged caudate lobe of the liver, loculated ascites, obesity, choledochal cyst.

Endoscopic ultrasound of retrogastric masses

Endoscopic ultrasound allows characterisation and diagnosis of a mass displacing or compressing the stomach by the adjacent viscera such as the spleen, liver, kidney, gallbladder, aorta, lymph nodes and pancreas. The use of high-resolution probes makes it possible to evaluate pancreatic tumours such as islet cell adenomas. Local invasion of pancreatic carcinoma to the lymph nodes, portal veins, arteries (encasement) can be identified. Cysts and tumours arising from adjacent organs may compress all five gastric layers.

3.4 DUODENUM

The first and second parts of the duodenum are frequently filled with air giving rise to areas of marked echogenicity and distal shadowing and reverberation echoes. If the patient drinks fluids then lies in the right-side-down position, visualisation of the duodenal lumen is facilitated. When distended by fluid the second part of the duodenum defines the lateral aspect of the head of the pancreas. The first and second parts of the duodenum frequently bulge into the medial side of the distended gallbladder.

3.4.1 NEONATAL DUODENAL DISTENSION AND OBSTRUCTION

The overall sensitivity and specificity of fluid-aided sonographic evaluation of the causes of duodenal obstruction in the neonatal period are 100 per cent and 99 per cent respectively.

Duodenal atresia – double bubble appearance of distended stomach and duodenal cap.

Duodenal stenosis.

Transient duodenal obstruction of the newborn – this may be a form of superior mesenteric artery syndrome with compression of the fourth part of the duodenum.

Preduodenal portal vein.

Oesophageal atresia – without a tracheo-oesophageal fistula this may be associated with a fluid-filled duodenal loop.

Midgut volvulus.

Annular pancreas.

Duodenal or proximal jejunal haematoma.

Proximal small bowel obstruction.

Duodenal bands – Ladd's bands may compress and obstruct the third and fourth parts of the duodenum. They are usually associated with malrotation which predisposes to midgut volvulus. An upper gastrointestinal barium series is the most reliable means of confirming the diagnosis that requires urgent surgery.

Paraduodenal hernia – a rare condition in which the duodenum is herniated internally through the mesenteric origin.

3.4.2 MALROTATION AND MIDGUT VOLVULUS

Malrotation of the bowel occurs when the distal limb of the developing midgut fails to rotate on returning to the abdomen. The normal midgut undergoes a total rotation of 270 degrees to achieve its final configuration. Malrotation is a spectrum of congenital abnormalities ranging from reverse rotation to non-rotation of the bowel, to lesser degrees of rotation in which the bowel has failed to rotate the full 270 degrees. Mild cases are not uncommon and simply result in a high-placed caecum. More severe cases are uncommon but potentially fatal, as malrotation is often associated with a short small bowel mesentery origin which predisposes to volvulus. Midgut volvulus is an acute surgical emergency most often occurring in the neo-natal period. A volvulus causes acute bowel ischaemia which, without urgent surgery, leads to bowel infarction with fatal consequences. The neonate presents with an acute onset of bile-stained vomiting. In 20 per cent of patients midgut volvulus is associated with duodenal atresia, duo-denal diaphragm, duodenal stenosis and annular pancreas. The plain radio-graph may show signs of intestinal obstruction, but a diagnosis of volvulus can only be entertained in the presence of duodenal distension. A normal radiograph does not exclude the presence of midgut volvulus in an infant. Sonographically malrotation with volvulus may be identified by alteration in the normal relationship of the superior mesenteric artery and vein. The vein normally lies on the right of the artery but this relationship may be reversed. Ultrasound assessment of the relative positions of the superior mesenteric artery and vein is an important consideration in the evaluation of infants with suspected duodenal obstruction. Patients in whom ultra-sound shows transposition of these vessels should have further investiga-tions to detect malrotation. In lesser degrees of malrotation alterations in vascular anatomy may not be so clear and thus in any suspected case a barium examination should be performed as delayed diagnosis may be fatal. In 81 per cent of patients with malrotation the superior mesenteric vein is located to the left of the superior mesenteric artery, in 11 per cent the supe-rior mesenteric vein is directly anterior to the superior mesenteric artery while in 7 per cent the arteries have a normal relationship. Sonographic visualisation of the superior mesenteric vein and superior mesenteric artery is possible in 84 per cent of infants. However inversion of the superior mesenteric vein and superior mesenteric artery on the transverse abdomi-nal scans is highly suggestive but not specific for malrotation. It has been described with abdominal masses causing displacement of mesenteric vessels and with situs inversus. It is therefore not a sensitive test for mal-rotation. A to-and-fro hyperperistaltic motion has been observed in the obstructed duodenal loop with midgut volvulus. The fluid-filled proximal duodenum may be seen ending in a twist or 'arrowhead configuration'. The fluid-filled duodenum does not appear to cross the spine. Another sign called the 'whirlpool sign', where the superior mesenteric vein is seen winding round the superior mesenteric artery, has been described as a sign of midgut volvulus. Colour Doppler studies are ideally suited to recognis-ing this sign, with colour depiction of mesenteric vessels moving clockwise with caudal movement of the transducer. However this sign has been demonstrated recently in a small number of patients with malrotation without volvulus. An additional ultrasonic sign described with midgut mal-rotation is the finding of dilated thick-walled bowel loops mainly to the right of the spine associated with free peritoneal fluid.

3.4.3 INTRAMURAL DUODENAL HAEMATOMA

The duodenum is retroperitoneal throughout most of its course and is thus relatively prone to injury. Intramural duodenal haematoma is rare but most common in children as a result of blunt abdominal trauma. The common causes include road traffic accidents, bicycle handle-bar injuries, play or athletic injuries and invasive endoscopic procedures, also non-traumatic causes like bleeding disorders and Henoch–Schönlein purpura. Children are at higher risk than adults for duodenal injuries because of their weaker abdominal musculature. Diagnosis of duodenal haematoma is often difficult because of delayed presentation, poor history and by the fact that its clinical presentation may mimic other abdominal pathology. Trauma may be mild and often forgotten. The trauma may be non-accidental in 10 per cent of children. Visceral injury is uncommon in non-accidental trauma, but when it occurs it carries a mortality of 50 per cent. Pancreatitis is associated in 21 to 40 per cent of abdominal injuries. Duodenal haematomas are seen as anechoic intramural collections which are usually eccentric. They may remain anechoic or become echogenic. The haematomas may develop internal septations as part of a more complex looking cystic mass. Large haematomas may cause bowel obstruction but usually resolve over a few weeks. A hypoechoic mass may be seen in the pancreas as a result of associated acute traumatic pancreatitis.

3.4.4 DUODENAL ATRESIA

Duodenal atresia is the most common cause of congenital duodenal obstruction, it has an incidence of 1 : 10 000 with no gender predilection. There is an association with Down's syndrome (25 per cent), congenital heart disease, vertebral anomalies, urinary tract and other gastrointestinal abnormalities. Presentation is usually within hours after birth with bilious vomiting. There is a mortality of 36 per cent in neonates. Sonography may reveal a 'double-bubble sign' because of distension of the stomach and the first part of the duodenum associated with hyperperistalsis of the stomach. A 'double-bubble sign' associated with polyhydramnios may be demonstrated on the antenatal ultrasound scans.

3.4.5 DUODENAL DUPLICATION CYSTS

The duodenum is an uncommon site for duplication cysts (4 to 5 per cent). Sonographically they may be spherical or tubular cystic structures in close proximity to the duodenum. They are often located within the 'C' of the duodenum. In common with other enteric duplication cysts they may demonstrate the 'muscular rim sign', that is the echogenic inner mucosal lining with a hypoechoic outer muscle wall.

3.4.6 DUODENAL VARICES

These are usually a result of portal hypertension and are often associated with fundal and oesophageal varices. They are seen sonographically as a 'cluster of grape-like anechoic structures' or a 'bag of worms' in association with other signs of portal hypertension.

3.4.7 DUODENAL TUMOURS

Duodenal tumours, both benign and malignant, are rare, the commonest malignant tumour is an adenocarcinoma (73 per cent) while leiomyosarcomas, carcinoids and lymphomas make up the rest of the malignant tumours. Benign duodenal tumours include leiomyomas, lipomas, adenomatous polyps, Brunner gland adenoma and angiomatous tumours, whilst hamartomas and neurofibromas are exceptionally rare. The tumours may cause gastric outlet obstruction. Sonographically they may appear as a typical or atypical target sign in association with a fluid-filled stomach with residual food or debris within the stomach. It is not usually possible to differentiate malignant from benign tumours on abdominal ultrasonography unless liver or lymph node metastases are seen. However endoscopic ultrasound has the potential of differentiating the two, as malignancy will disrupt the layered gastrointestinal structure.

3.4.8 DIFFERENTIAL DIAGNOSIS OF A THICKENED DUODENAL WALL

Haematoma.
Pancreatitis or adjacent inflammation.
Post-bulbar duodenal ulcer.
Adjacent varices.
Osler–Rendu–Weber syndrome.
Retroperitoneal haemangioma.
Duodenal duplication.
Inflammatory bowel disease or Crohn's disease.
Retroperitoneal abscess – in children periduodenal abscess or haematoma should raise the possibility of non-accidental injury. In adults abscesses are usually caused by duodenal ulceration or perforation.
Duodenal tumours – benign and malignant.
Ectopic pancreas.
Ectopic gastric mucosa.
Tuberculosis.
Strongyloidiasis.
Sprue.

3.5 JEJUNUM AND ILEUM

Small bowel visualisation is improved when it is fluid filled. This may occur in normal individuals particularly after the ingestion of meals or large volumes of fluids. Sonography shows fluid-filled tubes lined by echogenic mucosa which are thrown into folds or valvulae. These may give the inner wall a ribbed appearance. The normal small bowel wall thickness is 3 to 5 mm. Normal loops are compliant and are easily deformed during examination. They may alter configuration during waves of peristalsis. Ileus leads to loss of peristalsis and distension of bowel loops by fluid and air. Progressive distension makes the bowel more tubular with loss of the sharp angles through which loops may normally turn.

3.5.1 SMALL BOWEL OBSTRUCTION

Features of small bowel obstruction

Bowel loop distension.
Loops have a rounded contour and show little deformity due to adjacent bowel loops.
Loss of definition and loss of prominence of valvulae conniventes.
Variable peristalsis – the distended bowel becomes paralysed and bowel close to the
    site of obstruction may be aperistaltic.
Variation in peristalsis may make it difficult to differentiate ileus from obstruction –
    peristalsis is reduced or absent in ileus but peristalsis is frequently reduced or
    absent in bowel immediately proximal to an obstruction.

Neonatal small bowel obstruction

Meconium ileus.
Atresia, stenosis, diaphragm in duodenum, jejunum or ileum.
Midgut volvulus (volvulus neonatorum).
Ladd's bands associated with failure of caecal descent.
Enterogenous cysts.
Milk-curd obstruction.
Meconium ileus and atresia present early with vomiting within hours of birth – vomi-
    ting green rather than yellow bile-stained material suggests obstruction.

Small bowel obstruction beyond the neonatal period

Perforated appendicitis.
Intussusception.
Postoperative adhesions.

Regional enteritis.
Pseudo-obstruction in gastroenteritis.
Peritoneal bands.
Compressing cysts.
Midgut volvulus.
Hernias.
Ascariasis.
Mural haematoma.
Foreign body or bezoar.
Small bowel tumours.

Small bowel obstruction in adults

Tumour.
Hernia.
Adhesions.
Gallstone.
Volvulus.
Intussusception.
Crohn's disease.
Ischaemia or venous thrombosis.
Strictures – ischaemia or radiation.
Mural haematoma.
Ascariasis.
Obstruction secondary to large bowel obstruction.

Paralytic ileus in a neonate

Severe ill health – pneumonia.
Intracranial pathology.
Necrotising enterocolitis.
Hyperbilirubinaemia.

Paralytic ileus in children and adults

Congenital agangliosis.
Postoperative incidence.
Abdominal perforations, inflammations or infections.
Ischaemia.
Sympathetic nervous system – pneumonia, pericarditis, myocardial infarction, visceral pain, intracranial pathology, trauma.
Metabolic causes – diabetes, hypothyroidism, uraemia, hypokalaemia, porphyria, hyperbilirubinaemia.
Drugs – tricyclics, atropine, antidepressants.

Small bowel bezoar

Bezoars may gain entrance into the small bowel from the stomach after endoscopic breakdown of a gastric bezoar, and they may lead to small bowel obstruction. Bezoars are more common with delayed gastric emptying especially following gastric surgery such as vogotomy and diabetes mellitus. Nifedipine (a delayed action preparation) used in the treatment of angina has been associated with small bowel bezoar. Sonographically the bezoar may appear as an echogenic intraluminal mass, if there is air within it or fluid surrounding it the bezoar may shadow.

Intestinal ascariasis

Intestinal ascariasis may present as an acute abdomen with intestinal obstruction or it may mimic or cause an abdominal inflammatory condition such as acute cholecystitis, pancreatitis or appendicitis. On sonography an individual worm may appear as a hypoechoic longitudinal tubular structure with echogenic walls. The tubular central alimentary canal when visualised may appear as an echogenic line when in an empty state or parallel hyperechoic bands when the canal is distended. On a transverse scan the worm appears as a target appearance with echogenic body wall and a central dot representing the worm's alimentary canal. Prolonged scanning may reveal zig-zag movement of the worms. A tangle of worms mixed with faeces and air may present a complex intraluminal bowel mass. These patients usually respond to hypertonic saline enema and seldom require surgery.

Sonography of paralytic ileus

Like mechanical obstruction paralytic ileus is also accompanied by distended fluid-filled bowel. The bowel is aperistaltic or shows pendulating peristalsis, when pressure is applied with the transducer the bowel compresses and appears pliable. Compression with the probe also induces movement of echoes within the bowel luminal fluid. Fluid-filled loops are also seen with gastroenteritis although peristalsis is not abolished.

Sonographic features of fluid-filled bowel

Duodenum   Fluid-filled bowel has a 'keyboard' or 'step-ladder' configuration. Fluid columns may contain debris and may be continuous with the stomach.

Jejunum   The bowel is tubular with a 'keyboard' margin because of valvulae conniventes.

Ileum   Fluid-filled bowel is smoother and more featureless than prominent small bowel.

Colon   Generally the colon is peripherally situated in the abdomen whilst the small bowel is more centrally placed. Ascending and transverse colon show haustral sacculations. The descending colon has a more tubular appearance and the rectum lies deep in the pelvis behind the bladder.

3.5.2 CAUSES OF SMALL BOWEL THICKENING

Oedema – hypoalbuminaemia, portal hypertension, constrictive pericarditis.
Zollinger–Ellison syndrome.
Cystic fibrosis.
Sprue.
Protein-losing enteropathy.
Cancer chemotherapy.
Ischaemia and intramural haemorrhage.
Venous congestion including malrotation and chronic volvulus.
Intestinal lymphangiectasia.
Henoch–Schönlein purpura (this may accentuate the mucosal pattern).
Pelvic inflammatory disease*.
Appendix abscess*.
Trauma*.
Crohn's disease.
Gastroenteritis (including eosinophilic enteritis).
Giardiasis.
Yersinia ileitis.
Campylobacter ileocolitis.
Salmonella ileitis.
Anisakiasis.
Amyloidosis.
Whipple's disease.
Giardiasis or strongyloidiasis.
Behçet's syndrome, the appearance is similar to Crohn's disease.
Radiation.
Lymphoma.
Coeliac disease.
Dermatomyositis.
Abscess*.
Necrotising enterocolitis.
Ameobiasis.
Pseudomembranous colitis.
Adenocarcinoma*.
Tumours including metastases*.

* Changes in these conditions are usually focal.

Pneumatosis intestinalis.
Peritonitis.
Kaposi's sarcoma.

3.5.3 ABNORMAL BOWEL PATTERNS

The jejunum is wider than the ileum and has thicker walls with more circular mucosal folds than the ileum. In the distal ileum the mucosal folds become longitudinal. These appearances are normal findings and should not be mistaken for pathology. The non-distended small bowel loop gives a target appearance with a hypoechoic muscular wall in transverse sections. An echogenic layer representing the mucosa and submucosa lines the muscle. Gas within the bowel lumen frequently prevents visualisation of the distal bowel wall and underlying structures.

1. Thickening of the sonolucent halo (bowel wall). Exact measurement of bowel wall thickness is unreliable owing to the great variation in apparent wall thickness with bowel distension and peristalsis. Slight thickening may be missed but marked thickening is usually obvious.
2. Asymmetric location of the echogenic mucosal band indicating irregular bowel wall thickening. Asymmetric bowel wall thickening or the 'atypical target' appearance is a non-specific appearance but it is indicative of bowel pathology.
3. Lack of change in configuration or peristalsis on prolonged imaging.
4. Irregular bowel contour.

3.5.4 MECKEL'S DIVERTICULUM

Meckel's diverticulum is the remnant of the vitelline-intestinal duct. It lies on the antemesenteric border of the ileum. It is present in 2 per cent of the population being 60 cm from the ileocaecal junction and 5 cm long. A Meckel's diverticulum is usually an incidental finding but they can contain ectopic gastric or pancreatic tissue, which may secrete acid or enzymes resulting in ileal ulceration and bleeding. The orifice of the diverticulum may become occluded. When this occurs the wall becomes inflamed and the diverticulum distends with fluid. Acute inflammation may mimic appendicitis. These diverticula are rarely visible sonographically but have been noted when distended with fluid. Sonographically a Meckel's diverticulum may be identified when complicated, as a fluid-filled over-distended tube connected to the umbilicus. This tubular structure is larger and away from the caecum thus differentiating it from an inflamed appendix. Two target signs of different sizes have been described in a double intussusception of the Meckel's diverticulum into the ileum and the ileum into the colon.

3.5.5 JEJUNAL AND ILEAL DUPLICATION CYSTS

Duplication cysts occur more frequently in the jejunum and ileum than in other segments of the bowel. They usually do not communicate with the bowel lumen and are seen as anechoic structures which may be indistinguishable from mesenteric and peritoneal cysts. The cyst wall is usually hypoechoic with an echogenic lining. They can contain ectopic gastric and pancreatic tissue which may bleed and perforate.

3.5.6 SMALL BOWEL HAEMATOMA

The majority of small bowel haematomas occur in the duodenum because of its fixed retroperitoneal position. Haematomas of the duodenum and proximal jejunum in children are most frequently related to blunt abdominal trauma from non-accidental injury. The clinical presentation is that of duodenal or gastric-outlet obstruction. More distal small bowel haematomas may occur in bleeding diatheses and Henoch–Schönlein purpura. Sonographically small bowel haematomas appear as asymmetrical anechoic masses but they can be echogenic depending upon the age of the haematoma. An atypical target sign may occur. The haematoma may extend into the retroperitoneum; haemorrhagic ascites may also occur.

3.5.7 MECONIUM ILEUS

This is due to distal ileal obstruction caused by inspissated meconium. There is associated cystic fibrosis in 10 to 15 per cent of patients. In USA and Canada virtually all white neonates with meconium ileus have cystic fibrosis. The classic radiographic appearance of meconium ileus is the absence of air–fluid levels and a frothy appearance of the bowel. Meconium peritonitis, perforation, volvulus, bowel gangrene and small bowel atresia complicate 50 per cent of neonates with meconium ileus. Sonography may demonstrate echogenic meconium within the dilated distal bowel lumen. An important differential diagnosis is from ileal atresia, since the management of the former may be medical but the latter requires prompt surgical intervention. Patients with ileal atresia have dilated loops of bowel filled with air and fluid and not thick echogenic material as in meconium ileus. In some patients a diagnosis would have been made on the antenatal ultrasound scan when echogenic bowel, or dilated loops of bowel filled with echogenic material associated with polyhydramnios may be seen. However echogenic bowel *in utero* is non-specific and can be seen in other conditions such as cytomegalovirus infections, chromosomal abnormalities and intrauterine demise. There is a high association of perinatal and neonatal complications when in the second trimester highly echogenic bowel approaching the echogenicity of bone is seen.

3.5.8 GALLSTONE ILEUS

Gallstones may erode directly from the gallbladder or common bile duct into the bowel. Such a stone may impact within the duodenal bulb and cause gastric outlet obstruction – Bouveret's syndrome. More often with gallstones over 2.5 cm in diameter obstruction is caused at the ileocaecal valve causing gallstone ileus. Eighty to ninety per cent of gallstones which erode into the bowel pass spontaneously, and in those cases which come to surgery a preoperative diagnosis is made only in 30 per cent of cases. There is a 15 per cent operative mortality. Sonographically multiple dilated loops of small loops may be seen associated with a contracted gallbladder which may contain air and gallstones. The gallstone causing the obstruction may be directly visualised. Pneumobilia is seen as bright echoes with or without reverberation artefact in 69 per cent of the cases with gallstone ileus.

3.5.9 SALMONELLA ILEITIS

Salmonella ileitis or typhoid fever has a high mortality in the developing world, however even in the Western world mortality is quoted at 2 per cent, which may be because of a delay in diagnosis since the diagnosis may not be entertained in the first instance. Sonographic features include bowel thickening involving the terminal ileum and caecum, associated with mesenteric lymphadenopathy. However the appearances are non-specific and may occur with other bacterial enteritis.

3.5.10 YERSINIA ILEITIS

Yersinia enterocolitis is caused by a Gram negative organism usually affecting the terminal ileum, it is associated with diarrhoea, fever and right upper quadrant pain. There is often thickening of the folds in the terminal ileum, ulceration and lymphoid nodular hyperplasia. Sonography reveals thickened hypoechoic wall between 7 to 10 mm associated with mesenteric lymphadenopathy. The lymph nodes are sharply marginated round to oval, hypoechoic and 7 to 21 mm in diameter (the normal anteroposterior diameter is less than 4 mm). The pathological lymph nodes are also more numerous (normal numbers between three and six). Colour Doppler shows increased vascularity within the mucosa in areas of diffuse concentric wall thickening. Colour Doppler can be seen with several inflammatory bowel processes but is non-specific. However colour Doppler may aid in differentiating primary bowel disease from extrinsic inflammatory conditions such as peritonitis. Unlike inflammatory bowel disease the increased vascularity in thickened bowel from peritonitis is within the periphery of the bowel wall or in adjacent soft tissues.

3.5.11 CAMPYLOBACTER ILEOCOLITIS

Campylobacter jejuni is a common cause of enteritis in the Western world. The symptoms may be mild, mimicking a viral enteritis, or severe enough to resemble an acute surgical abdomen or acute onset ulcerative colitis. Sonographic findings are non-specific and resemble those described for *Yersinia enteritis*. There is mural thickening of the terminal ileum associated with mesenteric lymphadenopathy. The appendix is usually not visualised, thus excluding the diagnosis of acute appendicitis. The ultrasound findings are non-specific but do however tend to exclude conditions that require urgent surgical intervention.

3.5.12 CROHN'S DISEASE

Crohn's disease is the commonest chronic inflammatory disease of the small bowel. Eighty per cent of the cases involve the distal ileum whilst disease is limited to the colon in 10 per cent of cases at presentation. The incidence of Crohn's disease has risen in recent years and 20 per cent of cases are diagnosed in childhood. Ultrasound reliably demonstrates bowel thickening. In Crohn's lesions there is a well-defined echopoor outer rim and a bright inner region, transverse scans may demonstrate a target lesion. The bowel thickening may be focal or found over long segments, characteristic skip lesions may be observed. Bowel masses due to matted loops, rigid bowel segments and abscesses may be observed. In long-standing cases fibrosis results in stiff, thick, echogenic, ill-defined bowel walls. Crohn's disease is associated with fatty liver, hepatic abscesses, gallstones, cholecystitis, sclerosing cholangitis, hepatocellular carcinoma, bile duct carcinoma, renal calculi and renal amyloid. The ultrasonic features of all these conditions have been well described in this volume. Doppler interrogation of the superior mesenteric artery has shown a mean blood flow of 323 ± 103 ml/min (mean $\pm$ SD; range 162–492 ml/min). In patients with active Crohn's disease the flow is 826 ± 407 ml/min (range 242–1455 ml/min). A certain overlap is present. If the threshold value of less than 500 mL/min is used, a sensitivity of 83 per cent and specificity of 87 per cent can be achieved for active Crohn's disease. Activity in the left colon will escape detection because the superior mesenteric artery does not supply it. Colour Doppler in children with Crohn's disease has shown increased vascularity in the mucosa as well as increased transmural vascularity in areas of wall thickening.

3.5.13 SMALL BOWEL ANISAKIASIS

Anisakiasis is a gut parasitic infection caused by ingesting marine products containing *Anisakis marina* larvae. The incidence of the infection is high in Japan where raw fish is consumed. Gastric anisakiasis is readily diagnosed by gastroscopy but small bowel involvement may cause diagnostic problems. Many causes are misdiagnosed as acute abdominal surgical emergencies and diagnosis is made only at laparotomy. Small bowel anisakiasis responds very well to conservative measures and hence early diagnosis is essential. Sonographic features include ascites; small bowel dilatation 2.5 to 3.6 cm (mean 2.9 cm), localised oedema over small bowel segment of 10 to 30 cm length. The oedema is full circumferential and presents as a five-layered structure, with 0.8 to 1.3 cm (mean 1.0 cm) of wall thickening. There is marked thickening of the second hypoechoic layer indicating oedema of Kerckring's folds.

3.5.14 GASTROINTESTINAL RADIATION INJURY

Radiation causes obliterative endarteritis with radiation doses in excess of 4000 rads (40 Grays). Radiation changes usually occur within the field of radiation. Radiation gastritis causes wall thickening, antral narrowing and deformity resembling linitis plastica. Ultrasonography is non-specific and shows a typical or atypical target sign whilst endoscopic ultrasound may demonstrate loss of definition of the layered wall structure. Radiation enteritis may show bowel thickening, strictures and bowel dilatation associated with fixation and immobilisation of bowel loops. There is thickening of the valvulae conniventes with a stacked-coin appearance.

3.5.15 INTUSSUSCEPTION

Children

This is the most common abdominal emergency of early childhood (6 months to 2 years) and is the leading cause of intestinal obstruction. Ninety-five per cent of cases are idiopathic, whilst 5 per cent have a lead point such as Meckel's diverticulum, lymphoma, polyp, duplication cyst, Henoch–Schönlein purpura, etc.

Adults

Eighty per cent are due to a lead point whilst 20 per cent are idiopathic. Most intussusceptions have an acute onset however a small number may have chronic presentation.

Sonography

Sonography may show either a typical or atypical target sign but more specifically there is an appearance of concentric rings comprising alternating echogenic and echopoor rings representing compressed mucosal and serosal surfaces and oedematous bowel wall respectively. Colour Doppler shows blood vessels dragged in between entering and exiting layers of intussusception. Absence of blood flow indicates devitalised bowel segments.

3.5.16 COELIAC DISEASE

Coeliac disease is a gluten sensitive enteropathy characterised by malabsorption as a result of villous atrophy. Diagnosis of coeliac disease is by endoscopic duodenal biopsy which shows partial villous atrophy. Sonography has recently been used in the diagnostic work up. Although ultrasound cannot replace intestinal biopsy, awareness of sonographic abnormalities may lead to earlier diagnosis and prompt introduction of treatment. The various sonographic abnormalities that have been described in children with coeliac disease include

1. diffuse bowel wall thickening in 64 to 94 per cent
2. moderately dilated small bowel (range 2.5 to 3.5 cm, mean 2.9 cm) in 73 per cent
3. ascites in 45 to 76 per cent
4. hyperperistalsis in 73 to 82 per cent
5. moderately enlarged mesenteric lymph nodes (anteroposterior diameter 5 to 10 mm, mean 9 mm)
6. liver steatosis 55 per cent
7. dilated calibre of the superior mesenteric artery (range 8 to 11 mm, mean 9 mm) or portal vein (range 13 to 17 mm, mean 15 mm)
8. pericardial effusions in 47 per cent.

A patient showing diffuse small bowel thickening was observed to show complete resolution of bowel wall thickening associated with clinical, biochemical and histological improvement. There is no identifiable correlation between ultrasound findings of adult coeliac disease and the degree of severity of the mucosal biopsy result. None of the ultrasound signs are specific for coeliac disease but a combination of signs is characteristic and indicates suspicion of this disease in a high percentage of patients.

Differential diagnosis of diffuse bowel wall thickening

Hypoproteinaemia or hypoalbuminaemia.
Intestinal lymphangiectasia.

Coeliac disease.
Venous congestion.
Chronic volvulus.

3.5.17 INTESTINAL LYMPHANGIECTASIA

Intestinal lymphangiectasia is a rare lymphatic disorder in which obstruction of lymph drainage causes lymphatic stasis within the bowel wall and mucosal congestion. Two varieties are known.

1. A congenital form resulting from atresia of the thoracic duct affects children and young adults. These patients present with hypoproteinaemia, chylous pleural effusions, diarrhoea, steatorrhoea and abdominal pain.
2. An acquired variety which may be secondary to mesenteric adenitis, retroperitoneal fibrosis, small bowel lymphoma or pancreatitis.

Cases present with peripheral oedema and pleural effusions or ascites, if the thoracic duct is obstructed pericardial effusions may also occur. The bowel wall and mucosa are thickened and may weep proteinaceous fluid causing malabsorption or protein losing enteropathy. Fluid-filled lacteals may give rise to anechoic spaces but these are rarely seen and the sonographic pattern is usually a non-specific picture of diffuse wall thickening. The mesentery also appears to be thickened. Identical appearances have been described in children with coeliac disease, malrotation, chronic volvulus and venous congestion. Inflammatory bowel disease usually causes focal disease rather than diffuse wall thickening. It is said that the bowel is less rigid in lymphatic congestion than portal venous congestion allowing transmission of peristaltic waves but assessment is subjective.

3.5.18 PNEUMATOSIS INTESTINALIS

This is a condition characterised by the presence of gas within the wall of the bowel. The condition has been attributed to multiple causes, some are life threatening while others are quite benign. The most common life-threatening causes of intramural gas are the result of bowel necrosis due to ischaemia, necrotising enterocolitis, neutropenic colitis and sepsis. These conditions represent surgical emergencies. Pneumatosis is encountered with increasing frequency in immunocompromised (especially AIDS) patients, particularly those treated with radiotherapy, cytotoxic drugs or steroids. Less life-threatening causes include over-distension of the stomach and proximal small bowel. Air may enter the bowel wall because of disruption of the mucosa, as a result erosion trauma including non-accidental trauma and various endoscopic and interventional techniques. Mild forms of mucosal disruption may also occur because of subclinical enteritides. Various pulmonary causes include conditions such as chronic obstructive airway disease, asthma, cystic fibrosis, barotrauma and percutaneous interventional tube placement. Besides imaging findings clinical presentation is all important in arriving at a correct diagnosis and management. There are characteristic changes on plain abdominal radiographs, CT and barium enema. Sonography may show central bright echoes in relation to bowel wall with or without reverberation artefact. These bright echoes remain more or less static while intraluminal air changes with position and peristalsis. With bowel infarction a 'bright ring' appearance may occur caused by intramural gas surrounding the fluid-filled viscus. There is often associated portal venous gas that may lead to the search for intramural bowel gas. Tiny gas bubbles may be seen arising from the dependent portion of the bowel reminiscent of champagne bubbles – the 'effervescent bowel'! The 'aurora sign', long strips of bright echoes separated by acoustic shadows displaying an Antarctic aurora-like image, arising from the bowel may be seen or there may be a continuous undulating reflective line with a posterior acoustic shadow cone.

3.5.19 SMALL BOWEL TUMOURS

Small bowel tumours are uncommon in adults and relatively rare in children. Benign tumours may be polypoid and may form part of a polyposis syndrome, for example Peutz–Jeghers syndrome. Malignant tumours may be primary or secondary to almost any distant tumour. The commonest primary tumour in childhood is lymphosarcoma or Burkitt's lymphoma. In adults metastases are more common particularly in the elderly, for example carcinoma bronchus. Benign small bowel tumours are made up of leiomyoma (45 per cent), adenoma (20 per cent), lipoma (16 per cent), haemangioma (13 per cent), lymphangioma (5 per cent) and neurogenic tumours (1 per cent). The malignant tumours involving the small bowel in descending order of frequency are carcinoid (47 per cent), adenocarcinoma (25 per cent), lymphoma (16 per cent) and vascular tumours (1 per cent). Of the primary tumours 41 per cent are located in the ileum, 36 per cent in the jejunum and 18 per cent in the duodenum. Small bowel tumours are frequently not visualised sonographically. When seen they may have a mass or target appearance. The mass may lie within the bowel lumen or replace the bowel wall. There is usually a thick sonolucent rim though the overall pattern may be heterogeneous. Luminal small bowel tumours may cause intussusception, giving rise to a mass with a layered appearance. Small bowel obstruction may occur causing dilatation of the proximal small bowel with fluid and gas-filled bowel loops.

Leiomyomas or leiomyosarcomas unlike the gastric tumours seldom reach enormous proportions and the majority are less than 5 cm when benign, and over 6 cm when malignant. They may undergo central necrosis but rarely appear cystic on sonography, most tumours appear solid or complex.

Small bowel lymphoma

Lymphomas make up 16 per cent of the small bowel tumours. Lymphoma of the bowel may be primary-localised or diffuse or the bowel may be involved as a part of systemic disease. The median age of onset is around 60 years. Lymphoma is the commonest gastrointestinal tumour in children. The commonest cell type is non-Hodgkin's including Burkitt's and histio- cytic lymphoma. Burkitt's type tends to be a rapidly growing mass. Hodgkin's almost never presents as an isolated gastrointestinal mass but involves the gastrointestinal tract in 50 per cent of late cases. Risk factors for lymphoma includes coeliac disease, Crohn's disease, AIDS, systemic lupus erythematosis and a history of chemotherapy. Sonography may reveal eccentric wall thickening by lymphomatous infiltrate. This is usually an- echoic but haemorrhage and clot may give rise to echogenic areas. There may be aneurysmal dilatation of the bowel lumen and enlargement of adja- cent nodes. Anechoic deposits may mimic duplication cysts. The combina- tion of eccentric bowel wall thickening with aneurysmal dilatation and mesenteric lymphadenopathy produces the so-called 'sandwich sign' which distinguishes lymphoma from Crohn's disease.

3.5.20 ABDOMINAL MANIFESTATIONS OF AIDS

Abdominal complications such as intercurrent infections with cytomegalo- virus, *Mycobacterium avium intracellulare*, pneumocystis, *Cryptosporid- ium* spp. and *Candida* spp., and AIDS-related malignancies are one of the principal sources of morbidity and mortality in this disease. An incidence of over 50 per cent of Kaposi's sarcoma of the gastrointestinal tract has been reported in AIDS-related cutaneous Kaposi's sarcoma, although small bowel involvement in isolation has been reported with Kaposi's sarcoma. Sonog- raphy of the abdomen is of great value in the evaluation of visceral and nodal lesions in AIDS. Opportunistic infections may cause liver, splenic, lymph node, renal and bowel changes. (These are discussed elsewhere in this volume.) Bowel involvement with Kaposi's sarcoma resembles that reported with non-AIDS-related lymphoma, see small bowel lymphoma (above). Chylous ascites has been reported with AIDS-related Kaposi's sarcoma.

3.5.21 ATYPICAL TARGET CONFIGURATION OF THE BOWEL

Bowel usually has a ring-like or target appearance. 'Atypical target' appearance because of asymmetric bowel thickening can be caused by the following conditions.

Tumours – adenocarcinoma, benign bowel wall tumours, lymphoma, carcinoid, leiomyosarcoma, serosal implants.

Inflammations – Crohn's disease, diverticular disease, pancreatitis, appendicitis, tuberculosis.

Others – intussusception, amyloidosis, Whipple's disease, intramural haematoma, duplication cyst, pneumatosis coli or intestinalis, radiation enteritis.

3.6 CAECUM, APPENDIX AND COLON

The large bowel usually contains air and thus is not clearly visualised sonographically in the majority of cases. Despite this, sonography can give valuable information in a variety of circumstances. Normal bowel wall is echopoor, less than 4 mm thick with a smooth boundary. The ventral wall, but not the dorsal wall, is usually visualised because of gaseous distension.

3.6.1 APPENDICITIS

Appendicitis is the second most frequent inflammatory process within the abdomen, gastroenteritis being the most common. It is relatively rare in infancy but is common in children and young adults. Appendicitis occurs when obstruction of the appendix lumen causes a build up of secretions. This stretches the wall causing ischaemia. In the presence of bacterial infection the inflamed appendix may perforate as early as 6 hours after the onset of symptoms and the risk of perforation with resultant peritonitis increases with time. If the right iliac fossa is not obscured by gas and the patient can tolerate the examination ultrasonography may confirm the diagnosis of appendicitis in patients whose symptoms are not sufficiently prominent to warrant urgent surgery. With care 89 per cent of inflamed appendices can be visualised and perforation can be predicted in 80 per cent of cases. Criteria for ultrasound diagnosis are

1. non-compressible aperistaltic sausage appendix with wall thickening, a target appearance and anteroposterior measurement of 7 mm (measurements are made from outer wall to outer wall)
2. demonstration of an appendicolith, which is seen as an echogenic focus within the appendix lumen with shadowing.

Further signs include fluid around the appendix, an inflammatory bowel mass and the formation of abscess. Thirty per cent of patients have demonstrable lymphadenopathy in the adjacent mesentery. Blood flow in the appendix wall or a lower quadrant mass on colour Doppler sonography suggests appendicitis but absence of flow cannot definitively distinguish a normal from an inflamed appendix. Acute appendicitis in children and young adults is accompanied by inflammatory hypervascularity reflected as an increased number of colour signals and higher diastolic Doppler shifts as compared to normal. No Doppler shifts are identified in areas of ischaemia.

In the majority of patients appendicitis remains a clinical diagnosis but sonography is valuable in the assessment of complications such as abscess formation. The majority of abscesses secondary to appendicitis occur in the pelvis or right iliac fossa though pus may spread to the psoas sheath, subhepatic space or the subphrenic space. Intra-abdominal inflammation may also give rise to portal vein thrombosis and liver abscess, both of which may be demonstrated sonographically.

False negative diagnosis of appendicitis

Appendicitis confined to the tip
When appendicitis is suspected it is important to view the entire appendix as early inflammation may be confined to its tip. Thus measurements at the base may be normal giving a false negative diagnosis.

Retrocaecal appendicitis
A retrocaecal appendix may be difficult to visualise because of the presence of gas within the caecum and ascending colon. In right iliac fossa inflammations when the appendix is not visualised it is prudent to obtain sagittal or coronal images of the right iliac fossa via the lateral flank, this often permits visualisation of the appendix in this position.

Gangrenous or perforated appendix
With gangrenous appendicitis the echogenic mucosa is lost because of necrosis and the appendix appears as a jumbled inflammatory mass or abscess. If the appendicolith is lost a confident diagnosis of appendicitis can no longer be made.

Markedly enlarged appendix
A markedly enlarged appendix measuring 1.5 to 2.0 cm may be confused with an inflamed bowel such as that in enteritis or Crohn's disease. In such instances one must always concentrate on the appendix tip which will often provide a clue to the diagnosis.

Gas-filled appendix

Gas within an appendix due to gas forming organisms may cause acoustic shadowing or reverberation artefact obscuring the appendix, however gas within the appendix is often confined to part of the lumen, making diagnosis possible.

False positive diagnosis of acute appendicitis

Meckel's diverticulitis

When inflamed Meckel's diverticulum may be identified as a tubular structure away from the appendix in close association with the umbilicus. This normally should not be confused with an inflamed appendix.

Resolving appendicitis

In a minority of patients acute appendicitis may resolve spontaneously. These patients may have early sonographic features of an inflamed appendix without an appendicolith. These changes seem to resolve on follow up scans weeks later.

Salpingitis or dilated fallopian tube

A dilated right or inflamed right fallopian tube may mimic appendicitis. However the ultrasonic appearance of a fallopian tube mucosa appears different to that of the appendix. The fallopian tube has mucosal folds that are undulating with no echogenic mucosal ring as in the appendix. A transvaginal ultrasound may be instrumental in the diagnosis of hydrosalpinx.

Inspissated faeces mimicking an appendicolith

Inspissated faeces in the caecum or ascending colon may become echogenic and cast a shadow. It is therefore important that one makes sure the shadow is caused by inspissated faeces in the colon and not by an appendicolith in the appendix.

Peri-appendix inflammatory process

Crohn's disease and right-sided diverticulitis can give rise to inflammation or abscess in the right iliac fossa. In these instances the inflammation is in the bowel wall and the appendix appears normal. A peri-appendix abscess can only be diagnosed definitively when an appendicolith is identified.

Psoas muscle fibres mimicking an appendix

The fibro-fatty tissues of the psoas muscle may mimic the echogenic submucosa of the appendix on sagittal scans. Transverse scans should normally clarify this issue.

Symptomatic appendicial wall thickening caused by interleukin-2 therapy

Gallbladder wall thickening mimicking acute cholecystitis and right lower quadrant pain with appendix wall thickening has been reported in HIV-infected patients on interleukin-2 therapy. The appendix wall thickening and symptoms abate following cessation of therapy.

Caecal diverticulitis

This is a rare cause of right lower quadrant pain that clinically mimics acute appendicitis but it is an important entity to diagnose as management is different from an acute appendicitis. Sonographically it should be considered when diverticula (round or oval foci 10 to 22 mm protruding from the caecal wall) are seen with thickened non-compressible caecal wall, and associated with focal tenderness. Outpouching as discrete structures may be seen arising from the caecum, containing echogenic material. There may be segmental irregular wall thickening with air inclusions and luminal narrowing. Hypoechoic rims surrounding hyperechoic diverticula have been reported. An abscess may be demonstrated around the caecum or diverticula. In the absence of demonstrable diverticula such abscesses cannot be assigned to diverticulitis. Patients treated with antibiotics show a decrease in the wall thickening and decrease in the size of the diverticula.

Epiploic appendagitis

This is a rare inflammatory process of one of the numerous epiploic appendages as a result of torsion, venous thrombosis or secondary to an adjacent inflammatory process such as diverticulitis or appendicitis. The process is self limiting and usually resolves spontaneously. Sonographically the inflamed epiploic appendages appear as hyperechoic non-compressible ovoid masses with hypoechoic margins.

Degenerated uterine leiomyoma

This is a degenerating leiomyoma that may mimic an acute appendicitis clinically. Compressive sonography should enable exclusion of an acute appendicitis and identify the leiomyoma as an intrauterine or exophytic mass. The leiomyomas demonstrate a central hypoechoic area but with no Doppler flow indicating necrosis.

Crohn's appendicitis

In approximately a quarter of the patients with Crohn's disease the appendix is involved. An acute inflammation of the appendix may be an initial presentation of Crohn's disease. The involvement of the appendix alone without affecting the terminal ileum or caecum is rare. With Crohn's disease there are usually signs of inflammation and wall thickening in the terminal ileum and/or caecum. If the appendix alone is affected by Crohn's disease it cannot usually be differentiated from non-Crohn's appendicitis by sonography.

Radiation appendicitis

The appendix may be caught in a radiation beam in patients receiving radiation therapy for advanced rectal carcinoma. The appendix has been shown to be abnormal or inflamed at subsequent surgery, although these patients had no symptoms of acute appendicitis. The diagnosis of radiation appendicitis should be considered in patients having an abdominal ultrasound scan following radiation therapy in which the ultrasonic criteria of appendicitis are met though the patients may not have symptoms of an inflamed appendix.

Appendix abscess

Abscesses are not uncommon in appendicitis particularly if surgery was delayed or the appendix ruptured. Abscesses usually lie in the pelvis or right iliac fossa and are seen as irregular anechoic collections. Small collections are easily mistaken for bowel loops and in cases of doubt the examination should be repeated after an interval to allow bowel loops to change configuration. Large collections can be clearly identified as extraluminal and may contain debris.

Mucocoele of the appendix

Progressive cystic dilatation of the appendix resulting from obstruction of the lumen may occur without bacterial infection. In these cases accumulation of mucus may give rise to a cystic right iliac fossa mass. The majority of cases are due to the presence of a faecolith or inflammatory stricture but 10 per cent of cases are due to malignancy (usually mucinous cystadenocarcinoma of the appendix). Other causes include the presence of a foreign body, carcinoid, adhesions and endometriosis. Twenty-five per cent are asymptomatic. Some present with right lower quadrant pain. Rupture of the mucocoele may lead to pseudomyxoma peritoneii.

Sonography

The appearance is that of an oblong well-encapsulated cystic mass extrinsic to solid abdominal organs. The cystic mass is heterogeneous containing mucin that is both fluid and gelatinous and viscous. The degree of internal echogenicity is related to the acoustic interfaces provided by the mucous contents. Excellent through transmission and posterior enhancement is usually present. The mass may be highly echogenic because of the presence of calcification which is a known association.

Mucosal hypertrophy

Adherent debris and tumour nodules may give rise to a nodular luminal surface. However the wall thickness is seldom over 6 mm as in acute appendicitis, moreover the target appearance characteristically seen in appendicitis due to an echogenic submucosal layer sandwiched by an oedematous inner hypoechoic lamina propria or muscularis mucosa and outer hypoechoic muscularis layer will not be seen. Multiseptate mucocoeles have been described on CT and will presumably be demonstrable sonographically. Mobile dependent echoes may occur because of the presence of debris or protein aggregates. A mucocoele may appear heterogeneous without distal enhancement particularly if the iliac wing is directly posterior. An intussusception may complicate a mucocoele and may be detected on sonography.

Pseudomyxoma peritoneii

This may also be demonstrable sonographically, the appearance is similar to ascites but the bowel loops may be depressed by the mucus rather than floating in it and scalloping of the hepatic outline has also been recorded. Septae may also be seen within the mucinous collection.

Myxoglobulosis

This is a rare variant of mucocoele of the appendix where mucous balls appear within mucous fluid. It may appear as an acute appendicitis.

Appendix stump abscess

Recurrence of conventionally treated appendicitis is very rare but it is a known phenomenon in the form of a stump abscess. Sonography is helpful in detecting pericaecal inflammatory changes or the development of an abscess.

3.6.2 INTUSSUSCEPTION

Intussusception is the invagination or herniation of a segment of bowel in a manner analogous to the shortening of a telescope. The majority of cases occur in children and of these 9 per cent involve the passage of ileum into the caecum and colon (ileocaecal). In children 75 per cent of cases occur in boys, frequently the incidence is highest in spring and autumn and lymphoid inflammation is thought to play a part in the origin of the intussusception. The diagnosis is usually suspected clinically as patients develop bowel obstruction with colic and vomiting. The child may in addition pass 'recurrent jelly' stool. Five per cent of childhood cases have an underlying abnormality at the apex of the intussusception such as a polyp, Meckel's diverticulum, hamartoma, Crohn's disease, Henoch–Schönlein purpura or tumour. This incidence of underlying pathology is much higher in adult cases. Sonographically the intussusception is seen as a bowel mass with multiple concentric echogenic rings produced by alternating mucosal and muscular layers. This has been described as a 'doughnut' appearance on transverse scans and 'pseudo-kidney' appearance on longitudinal section. The outer rim is usually relatively sonolucent because of oedema whilst the centre of the mass may show one or more layers of echogenic infolded mucosa. Peritoneal fluid trapped inside the intussusception is associated with irreducibility and ischaemia. Colour Doppler may demonstrate mesenteric vessels between the layers of intussusception, absence of blood flow is indicative of bowel necrosis. The sensitivity of sonography in the diagnosis of intussusception is almost 100 per cent. A similar appearance may be seen with bowel tumours but they usually give a different history. Other reported causes of these appearances are necrotising enterocolitis, volvulus and inflammatory bowel disease. Hydrostatic reduction has been attempted under ultrasound guidance and it has been said that the greater the echogenicity of the central mucosal band the greater would be the difficulty in reduction. It is felt that a narrow central mucosal band reflects greater mucosal compression. Although ultrasonography is a reliable means of diagnosing intussusception, its accuracy is not as great as radiography in monitoring reduction and thus we prefer diagnosis and therapy by traditional methods.

3.6.3 INFLAMMATORY DISEASES OF THE COLON

Excluding infective and toxic states, Crohn's disease and ulcerative colitis are the commonest causes of chronic large bowel inflammation. Sonographic features are non-specific and include bowel wall thickening that may involve both the hypoechoic muscular coat and the echogenic mucosa. There is wall thickening that extends longitudinally, decreased echogenicity and luminal narrowing. Localised perforation may occur that may lead to the formation of an abscess which may be clinically silent if the patient is receiving steroid therapy.

Crohn's and ulcerative colitis

Several criteria have been described for the detection of Crohn's colitis and ulcerative colitis. The water-filled colon technique may be used to get better definition of the large bowel mucosa. With Crohn's colitis the whole bowel wall is thickened, all layers being involved with oedema, fibrosis, inflammation and lymphangiectasis. Sonographically the wall is clearly thickened, hypoechoic and homogeneous initially but may become inhomogeneous because of fat deposition. The layered anatomy of the bowel wall and the haustra are lost. The bowel becomes rigid with diminished compressibility and peristalsis. The diameter of the wall is around 13 mm.

In ulcerative colitis the wall thickness is not as great, averaging 7.8 mm. Early disease is confined to the mucosa, the wall stratification is preserved but haustra are lost. Ultrasound is said to be 100 per cent specific for Crohn's colitis and 97 per cent specific for ulcerative colitis. However sonography is unlikely to replace contrast radiography and endoscopy in the near future but will have an impact in diminishing the numbers of invasive examinations. In Crohn's disease as well as ulcerative colitis presence of Doppler parietal flow throughout the affected thickened segment indicates an acute condition, similarly an abnormally high mean portal velocity of 30 to 48 cm/s (normal 15 ± 7 cm/s) and an abnormally low resistive index of 0.58 to 0.78 (normal 0.908 to 0.026) in the superior mesenteric artery are detected. These Doppler findings are known to revert to normal with successful therapy.

Necrotising enterocolitis

Necrotising enterocolitis is an inflammatory disorder which occurs mainly in preterm infants, although it can affect full-term infants usually in an epidemic form of disease. Aetiology is multifactorial. Hypoxia induces vasospasm and thus intestinal ischaemia. This reduces intestinal mucosal integrity and resistance to bacteria. Initially the ischaemic bowel is paralysed causing gaseous distension. The bowel wall is thickened but gas may penetrate the wall. In severe cases the gas may enter the portal venous system and the bowel may perforate causing peritonitis. Sonographically the large volume of gas present may obscure the bowel. When visible there is exaggeration of the normal target appearance because of bowel wall thickening. High amplitude intramural echoes with distal shadowing may occur caused by the presence of intramural air. Portal venous gas is seen as high amplitude echoes within the peripheral portal vein radicles in the liver. Ultrasonography may show these changes before any abnormality is evident on the plain abdominal radiograph.

Pseudomembranous colitis

This is a severe form of colitis caused by infection with *Clostridium difficile* whose enterotoxin is cytotoxic. The condition is usually associated with antibiotic use, although it has followed chemotherapy, surgery, vascular insufficiency, bowel obstruction and other debilitating illnesses. Presentation is with severe diarrhoea, abdominal pain, pyrexia and metabolic disturbance. Diagnosis is bacteriological or by endoscopy. A pseudomembrane due to accumulation of necrotic epithelium, fibrin and leukocytes characteristically lines the mucosa. Sonographically there is hypoechoic moderate to marked large bowel wall thickening ranging from 6 to 28 mm. The bowel thickening affects the mucosal and submucosal layers. The pseudomembrane may be visible as an irregular hyperechoic luminal layer. Marked gaseous distension of the right colon or caecum may be apparent. Ascites is present in 15 to 25 per cent of patients. Although the ultrasound appearances are non-specific they can suggest the diagnosis in the appropriate clinical setting and lead to the appropriate tests being performed to achieve a definitive diagnosis.

Amoebic colitis

Amoebic colitis is a result of infection of the colon by the protozoan *Entamoeba histolytica*. The disease has wide distribution in the tropics. The trophozoite burrows into the bowel wall, giving rise to flask-shaped submucous ulcers associated with inflammatory thickening of the bowel wall. The right colon or caecum is most commonly involved. With chronic infection a hyperplastic granuloma with bacterial invasion of a pre-existing amoebic abscess may develop. This amoeboma forms a constricting annular intraluminal mass, which may mimic a colonic carcinoma. However it responds well to medical treatment and shows shrinkage within a few weeks. Sonographically the colonic wall is asymmetrically thickened – the atypical target. The wall thickness varies from 8 to 17 mm and appears hypoechoic. A concomitant liver abscess may be identified adding confidence to a diagnosis of amoebic colitis. The appearances are otherwise non-specific but in the right clinical context a diagnosis can be offered or the findings can lead to a more specific test.

Typhlitis (neutropenic colitis)

Typhlitis is necrotising colitis usually involving the caecum. It is an infection of the bowel which develops in patients with profound neutropenia secondary to leukaemia on chemotherapy or other patients in which malignancy is being treated with cytotoxic drugs. The condition has a poor prognosis if untreated. It usually presents with right side abdominal pain, pyrexia and bloody diarrhoea. Sonographically there is thickening of the bowel wall associated with marked echogenic thickening, irregularity and convolutions of the mucosa. The marked mucosal thickening and polypoid appearance of the mucosa make the ultrasound appearances different from any other disease affecting the caecum.

3.6.4 ABDOMINAL COMPLICATIONS OF BONE MARROW TRANSPLANTATION IN CHILDREN

Neutropenic colitis The bowel appears echogenic and appendicial enlargement may be present, see p. 285 for ultrasound appearances.

Pneumatosis intestinalis This is not usually associated with bowel necrosis and often resolves with conservative management, see p. 274 for sonography.

Veno-occlusive disease see p. 124.

Haemorrhagic cystitis There is focal or diffuse thickening of the bladder wall, blood clot or sloughed mucosa may be seen within the bladder lumen.

Graft versus host disease The imaging appearance of the acute and chronic forms of this disease is similar with focal or diffuse thickening of the bowel wall, hepatomegaly and infiltration of mesenteric fat.

Lymphoproliferative disorder after transplantation There is abdominal or pelvic lymphadenopathy, a periportal zone of low attenuation, hepatomegaly, splenomegaly and ascites.

Tumour recurrence This may occur at the site of the primary tumour or at distant sites, recurrence usually occurs within 2 years.

3.6.5 ACUTE DIVERTICULITIS

Diverticular disease occurs in about 50 per cent of adults. In asymptomatic patients colonic diverticula are seldom seen on routine abdominal sonography. However acute inflammation of the bowel wall associated with spasm and increased wall thickness improves visualisation of the diverticula as inflammation of the diverticular wall accentuates the diverticulum. Ninety-five per cent of colonic diverticula involve the sigmoid colon. The sigmoid colon can be distinguished from the small bowel by its location (behind the bladder), lack of valvulae conniventes and the lack of characteristic small bowel peristalsis. Sonographically acute diverticulitis can be diagnosed by

1. bowel thickening greater than 4 mm with a range of 5 to 15 mm and a typical or atypical target
2. direct visualisation of the diverticula, echogenic shadowing foci are seen as colonic outpouchings or as round or oval hypoechoic foci protruding from segmentally thickened bowel wall

3. pericolic fluid collection
4. intramural fluid collections
5. oedema of pericolic fat
6. intraluminal sinus tracts.

Paracolic abscesses and colovesical fistulae may be missed by sonography.

3.6.6 COLOVESICAL FISTULA

Colovesical fistula is commonly caused by diverticular disease but can occur secondary to a neoplasm. The majority of patients present with pneumaturia and the passage of faeculant urine. Sonography may show a mass in continuity with the bowel and adherent to the bladder wall. An echogenic tract may be seen connecting the peristaltic bowel lumen to the bladder. One may be able to see a jet of echogenic material forced from the bowel lumen into the bladder cavity by compressing the lower abdomen with the ultrasound probe. This appearance has to be differentiated from an episodic bilateral jet of urine from the ureteric orifices. The bladder contents may be echogenic because of the presence of air and faeces and reverberation artefact may be seen emanating from the superficial portions of the bladder because of the presence of air.

3.6.7 ISCHAEMIC BOWEL DISEASE

Bowel ischaemia is mainly a disease of old age caused by atheroma of mesenteric vessels. Other causes include embolic disease, vasculitis, fibromuscular hyperplasia, aortic aneurysm, blunt abdominal trauma and disseminated intravascular coagulation, radiation and hypovolaemic or endotoxic shock. With occlusive mesenteric infarction (embolus or thrombosis) there is a 90 per cent mortality whilst in non-occlusive disease there is a 10 per cent mortality. Venous infarction occurs in young patients usually following abdominal surgery. Patients may present with colicky abdominal pain which becomes continuous, associated with vomiting, diarrhoea and rectal bleeding. Bowel gas frequently prevents visualisation of colonic changes which are usually most marked around the splenic flexure. In the initial stages the ischaemic bowel may show increased peristalsis which is then reduced. The bowel wall becomes thickened and nodular and intramural haemorrhage and oedema give rise to areas of reduced echogenicity. Echogenic areas may develop in the bowel wall and these may reflect either areas of infarction, infiltrate or clot. Echogenic areas with shadowing occur because of the presence of intramural gas. Gas may also be detected in the portal vein and this is a poor prognostic sign.

Ultrasonography

Technique

Doppler colour flow imaging is performed after an overnight fast to minimise bowel gas. The patient is usually scanned in a supine position with the head slightly elevated to enable the abdominal viscera to descend. To identify the coeliac axis and superior mesenteric artery the aorta is scanned in the left sagittal paramedian plane starting at the xiphisternum. The superior mesenteric artery is 1 to 2 cm distal to the coeliac axis, however the two may have a common origin. Before Doppler studies on the superior mesenteric artery and coeliac axis a main stream of Doppler velocity signal in the aorta is obtained at the level of the coeliac axis and superior mesenteric artery at a 60 degree angle. The aorta is scanned for atheroma, dissection and aneurysm. Colour flow and spectral analysis is used to detect flow disturbance. The peak systolic aortic velocity is recorded followed by velocity measurements at the coeliac axis and superior mesenteric artery origins. Care should be taken when recording Doppler time–velocity waveforms at the origins of the coeliac axis and superior mesenteric artery so as not to increase the isonation angle beyond 60 degrees. Both the coeliac axis and superior mesenteric artery should be examined both in inspiration and expiration to distinguish extrinsic disease (compression from the median arcuate ligament of the diaphragm on the coeliac axis) from intrinsic disease (atheroma).

Coeliac axis

Colour flow Doppler is effective in demonstrating flow disturbance associated with tortuosity and stenosis at the origin of the coeliac axis. Doppler spectral waveforms in a normal fasting coeliac axis demonstrates a forward flow with an average peak systolic velocity of 123 ± 9 cm/s (age range 48 to 79 years) associated with a significant increase in systolic or diastolic flow velocity following a meal. This increase is also reflected in the hepatic and splenic arteries. The average post-prandial systolic velocity 30 minutes following a meal of 355 Kcal is 132 ± 7 cm/s. In the presence of 60 per cent coeliac axis stenosis the peak velocity is increased to $167-208 \pm 9$ cm/s. With this degree of stenosis colour Doppler demonstrates a high-velocity jet at the stenotic site associated with post-stenotic turbulent flow. The potential for collateralisation between the coeliac axis, superior mesenteric artery and inferior mesenteric artery is remarkable, as a result the reading of peak systolic velocity in the coeliac axis may be lower or much higher than expected when there is concomitant superior mesenteric artery occlusion. This may result in the over-estimation or under-estimation of ischaemic disease.

Superior mesenteric artery evaluation

The fasting superior mesenteric artery demonstrates a low diastolic flow, however following a meal both the peak systolic and end-diastolic velocities show tremendous increase in the absence of arterial stenosis. The normal fasting superior mesenteric artery velocities are recorded at 128 ± 16 cm/s (age range 23 to 42 years). Following a meal the peak systolic velocity increases to 162 ± 11 cm/s with end diastolic velocity in the range of 48 ± 7 cm/s within 15 minutes of ingesting a meal. The peak systolic velocity almost doubles within 45 minutes following a meal. With significant superior mesenteric artery stenosis the peak systolic velocity exceeds 270 cm/s with a concomitant increase in diastolic flow. Colour flow Doppler shows a jet through the stenotic segment with turbulent flow for some distance downstream.

Limitations of Doppler analysis of coeliac axis and superior mesenteric artery ischaemia

1. The extensive potential for collateralisation in splanchnic vessels may make assessment of a single vessel stenosis difficult.
2. There is an increased risk of error when the angle of isonation used is greater than 60 degrees
3. Careful placement of the sample volume is crucial; the superior mesenteric artery unless examined throughout the visualised vessel may result in false negative diagnosis.

3.6.8 COLONIC NEOPLASMS

Adenocarcinoma makes up 98 per cent of large bowel tumours and is responsible for 15 per cent of cancer deaths in the UK. These tumours often arise in polyps. Left-sided tumours tend to encircle the bowel (apple-core lesions) whilst the right colonic lesions tend to be polypoid, particularly in the caecum. Twenty-five to thirty per cent have a significant spread at the time of diagnosis. The 5-year survival rate is 35 to 49 per cent. Local recurrence occurs at the line of anastamosis in 60 per cent within 1 year after resection. Serum carcinoembryonic antigen is related to tumour size and extent of spread. With recent developments and improvements in liver metastasectomy the survival figures in patients with up to four liver metastases have improved.

Sonography

At the present stage sonography cannot replace the barium enema or colonoscopy for diagnosing either polyps or bowel cancers. Neither can ultrasound match the sensitivity of CT for staging bowel cancers. Polyps are often difficult to detect on ultrasound. However a warm-saline-filled bowel lends itself to better real time imaging. A polyp larger than 7 mm may be seen as a lobular hyperechoic mass within the bowel lumen, although an adequate assessment of the bowel thickening may not be possible. Ultrasonography may detect colonic neoplasms which are not palpable and may also be used to locate the site or confirm the presence of a palpable abdominal mass. The false positive diagnosis of an abdominal mass is uncommon but once a mass is demonstrated its appearance is frequently non-specific. Colonic neoplasms give rise to hypoechoic or heterogeneous bowel wall thickening, the target or atypical target sign. The hypoechoic area becomes broader with more wall infiltration. With high resolution scans disruption of the layered bowel pattern may be seen. Malignant lesions are more common in patients with greater wall thickness (mean of 26.22 versus 10.2 mm), asymmetric involvement, loss of stratification, absence of perigut findings and involvement of short segments. When examining the large bowel it should not be forgotten that synchronous carcinoma may be present in 5 per cent of patients. When a colonic lesion is seen, a search for possible lymph node and live metastases should be made. Bowel obstruction is not an unusual mode of colonic carcinoma presentation. With a fluid-filled proximal bowel the obstructive bowel lesion may be directly visualised. The differential diagnosis of a target or atypical target pattern is wide and other possibilities should be considered.

Large bowel lymphoma

Large bowel lymphoma represent 1.5 per cent of all abdominal tumours and only 0.5 per cent of malignant tumours of the colon. Primary colonic lymphomas account for only 4 per cent of all extranodal lymphomas.

Sonography

It is usually indistinguishable from a carcinoma causing an atypical or typical target sign. However the bowel thickness tends to be more hypoechoic in lymphoma than bowel carcinoma.

Colonic masses with thickened bowel wall

Colonic carcinoma.
Inflammatory bowel disease.
Bowel infarction.
Intramural haematoma.
Diverticular mass or abscess.
Metastases.
Lymphoma.

3.7 RECTUM AND ANUS

The rectum and anus are readily accessible by endoscopic ultrasound. The normal ultrasound appearances of the rectum are similar to the more proximal gastrointestinal tract. Five distinct layers are identified. To differentiate these layers a 7 MHz transducer is necessary. A 360 degree radial, linear longitudinal or short-curved linear transverse transducer is usually used in the range of 5 to 12 MHz. For more proximal rectal masses at the rectosigmoid junction transducers mounted on an endoscope are most efficient in reaching the lesion, while rigid-type endorectal transducers are more efficient at probing lesions in the distal rectum and anus. Anatomical location is described as the 6 o'clock position for lesions placed anteriorly, 12 o'clock position for lesions placed posteriorly (towards the coccyx), 9 o'clock position to the left and 3 o'clock position to the right (see Figure 3.3).

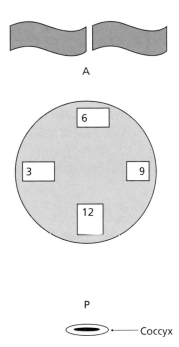

Figure 3.3 Endorectal ultrasound orientation.

Rectum   The five-layered structure is seen as follows.

1. The balloon–mucosa interface is hyperechoic.
2. The mucosa and muscularis mucosa forms a thin hypoechoic line.
3. The submucosa is extremely hyperechoic.
4. The muscularis propria is hypoechoic.
5. The muscularis propria with serosa or perirectal fat is hyperechoic.

Anus   The ultrasonic anatomy of the anus appears to be more complex than that of the rectum.

1. The interface between the transducer and mucosa is hyperechoic.
2. The mucosa is hypoechoic.
3. The subepithelial tissues are hyperechoic.
4. The internal anal sphincter is hypoechoic.
5. The longitudinal muscle separating the internal from the external sphincter is hyperechoic.
6. The external sphincter presents a heterogenous, speckled or streaky appearance.
7. The average thickness of the internal anal sphincter is 2 to 3.5 mm, this is affected by the size of transducer and age of the patient. In normal volunteers aged less than 55 years the mean thickness was 2.56 mm and in those over 55 years the mean thickness was 3.08 mm. Thus it follows that an external sphincter thicker than 4 mm is abnormal for all ages and a 2 mm sphincter may be normal in young patients but not in older patients. The thickness of the external sphincter can be reduced by 30 per cent when the transducer size is increased from 1 to 2 cm. The measurement of the external sphincter is not affected by the transducer size.

   The standard rectal probe used is 1 cm and hence measurements usually apply to this size probe.
8. The external sphincter is less well defined as compared to the internal sphincter. In non-pathological states it measures 5 to 8 mm.

3.7.1 STAGING SYSTEMS FOR COLORECTAL TUMOURS

Modified Duke's staging classification

A   the tumour is in the mucosa only.
B1   Extension into but not beyond the muscularis propria.
B2   Extension beyond the muscularis propria, no nodes involved.
C1   No penetration of the bowel wall but metastases to lymph nodes.
C2   Penetration of bowel wall with metastases to lymph nodes.
D   Distal metastases.

TNM staging classification

Tumours (T)

T0   No tumour is detected.

T1   No invasion beyond the submucosa.

T2   No invasion beyond the muscularis propria.

T3   When serosa is present (the proximal third of the rectum) there is invasion beyond the muscularis propria, into but not beyond the serosa. When serosa is absent (the distal two-thirds of the rectum) there is invasion beyond the muscularis propria.

T4   When serosa is present there is invasion through the serosa into the peritoneal cavity or adjacent organs. When serosa is absent there is invasion of other organs.

Regional nodes (N)

N0   There are no nodal metastases.

N1   Nodal metastases are present.

Distant metastases (M)

M0   There are no distant metastases.

M1   Distant metastases are present.

Staging of rectal carcinoma

On endorectal ultrasound a rectal carcinoma appears as a hypoechoic mass that infiltrates the bowel wall irregularly, growing from the mucosa outwards and invading the layered structure of the rectum. The stratified structure of the rectum is eventually lost. The wall invasion is seen as a hyperechoic thickening associated with loss of definition between the layers. Endoscopic ultrasound is sensitive at determining TNM staging of the tumour with an accuracy rate of 90 per cent. The most important observation is to determine if the tumour is confined to the bowel wall (T1 or T2) or if it has extended beyond the rectal wall. With invasion of perirectal fat (T3), the tumour border becomes irregular.

3.7.2 PITFALLS IN RECTAL WALL ULTRASOUND

Endorectal ultrasound is predisposed to a variety of artefacts, partly because of the limited space available for the transducer–tissue interface in an organ that tends to be tortuous. Limitations are also posed by the use of rigid transducers which have a limited depth of penetration into the rectum.

Artefacts are not unusual because of attenuation differences between a large tumour and adjacent normal tissue. Through transmission attenuation from large tumours may result in over-staging of the tumour.

Balloon inflation

To achieve an optimal acoustic interface between the balloon and the rectal mucosa it is important to fill the balloon with the right amount of water as over-distension causes compression of the rectal wall and may lead to over-staging of the tumour. Under-distension may cause separation of the balloon and rectal wall and technical artefacts. The rectum does not have an even diameter and is wider in the ampullary region where additional water inflation may be needed. To avoid these problems some workers do not use the balloon and fill the rectum with water instead.

Transducer characteristics

High gain settings may obscure the layered bowel structure and may result in over-staging of the tumour. To obtain optimal images when using a side-fire transducer a 90 degree angle should be maintained between the ultrasound probe and rectal wall, this will avoid refraction artefact otherwise over-estimation of the tumour may occur.

Air artefact

Air bubbles trapped within the balloon may cause shadowing thus limiting the field of view. Air bubbles may also be trapped under the edges of ulcerating tumours causing acoustic shadowing and thus limiting visualisation of the stratified layers of the rectal wall. Air–fluid levels within ulcer craters can produce reverberation artefacts.

Refraction artefacts

This is a particular problem when a linear array transducer is used, refraction artefact can occur behind the transverse rectal folds in the form of a narrow shadow behind the fold compromising the evaluation of the bowel wall. This artefact can also be seen at tumour edges compromising accurate staging. The artefact is produced with redirection of the incident beam by an oblique interface and can be eliminated or minimised by keeping the transducer at a right angle to the rectal wall.

Shadowing artefact from faeces

Faeces adherent to the wall of the rectum have a mixed echotexture and may mimic villous adenomas. Faeces adherent to the apex of the tumour also have a similar appearance and may shadow. These artefacts can be avoided by thorough bowel preparation.

Transducer insertion beyond the stricture

If the transducer does not pass the stricture the entire tumour may not be visible. Inadequate evaluation of the depth of rectal stenotic tumours often occurs.

Tumour proximity to the anal verge

Because the balloon on the transducer tip will not pass through the anal canal it has to be deflated before introduction through the anal sphincter. Subsequently tumours very near the anal verge may be missed. It is important from the surgical point of view that an accurate demonstration of the tumour in relation to the internal and external sphincter is made. With involvement of these muscle sphincters a stage T3 carcinoma is diagnosed, thus limiting the operative options available. Replacing the balloon with a hard plastic cap is said to improve resolution at the anal verge.

Rectal wall tumours that may mimic rectal carcinoma

Benign villous adenoma may pose problems, as compression of the tumour against the wall by the balloon and shadowing artefact from air trapped between the villi may result in the over-estimation of tumour penetration. One should concentrate on the submucous layer deep to the muscularis layer, when this layer is intact one can assume that no invasive malignancy is present. However endorectal ultrasound cannot differentiate between T1 cancer and villous adenoma. The ultrasound appearances of a squamous carcinoma are similar to adenocarcinoma. The tumour presents as a hypo-echoic mass that eventually involves all layers. Carcinoids can be similarly assessed for bowel wall invasion or lymph node metastases. Leiomyomas can be reliably differentiated from cancers. Leiomyomas are hypoechoic well-defined tumours that remain within the bowel wall and do not invade beyond the muscularis propria layer.

3.7.3 RECTAL WALL MASSES AND THICKENING

Causes of rectal wall masses and thickening

Adenocarcinoma.
Squamous cell carcinoma.
Villous adenoma.
Carcinoid.
Leiomyoma.
Kaposi's sarcoma.
Rectal varices.
Post-surgical changes.
Post-radiation changes.
Rectal abscess.
Granulation tissue.
Biopsy changes.
Rectal duplication cyst.
Endometriosis.
Inflammatory bowel disease.
Solitary rectal ulcer.
Internal rectal prolapse.
Hereditary internal anal sphincter myopathy.

Perirectal lymph nodes

Normal perirectal lymph nodes are usually less than 3 mm in size and are not seen. When normal glands are seen, as well as being small they are oval and the hilum contains fat. Inflamed or metastatic lymph nodes may be visualised. Metastatic lymph nodes are hypoechoic, more round than oval and usually have well-defined borders. Inflamed nodes vary in size and tend to be hyperechoic with ill-defined margins. However there is considerable overlap between metastatic and inflammatory nodes and therefore if in doubt one should obtain an ultrasound-guided biopsy.

Recurrent rectal carcinoma

The accuracy of endorectal ultrasound at detecting recurrent rectal carcinoma is high and quoted at 85 to 100 per cent and at times it may provide the only evidence of tumour recurrence. The normal stratified structure of the rectum is not visualised at the site of normal scar formation at the anastamotic site. Recurrent carcinoma causes localised wall thickening associated with loss of definition of the wall layers. Anastamotic recurrence may extend into the perirectal fat and may involve lymph nodes. Granulation tissue closely resembles a carcinoma and can be differentiated by biopsy only. Hypoechoic enlargement is strongly suspicious of tumour recurrence while shrinkage or stability suggests a benign process.

Anastamotic rectal complications

Endorectal ultrasound is superior at detecting anastamotic complications or insufficiency as compared to endoscopy or barium studies.

Causes of rectal wall thickening post-surgery

Recurrent rectal carcinoma.
Post-biopsy changes.
Granulation tissue.
Sequelae of local sepsis.
Postoperative scarring.
Post-radiation therapy changes.
Rectal varices.

Radiation therapy

Endorectal ultrasound is not reliable at restaging rectal wall tumours following radiotherapy. Following radiotherapy there is inflammation of the rectal wall associated with thickening. The wall becomes hyperechoic with loss of wall stratification. The border between the rectal wall and perirectal tissues becomes indistinct. Radiation usually results in fibrosis which appears hyperechoic, however the residual tumour remains hypoechoic. Some metastatic lymph nodes are no longer visible whilst others may become hyperechoic. Some hypoechoic malignant lymph nodes do not change following radiation treatment.

Rectal wall varices

Endorectal ultrasound is superior to endoscopy at detecting rectal varices as a result of portal hypertension. They seldom cause symptoms but it is important to differentiate them from rectal carcinoma. Rectal wall varices seldom bleed. Sclerotherapy for haemorrhoids has been carried out using Doppler guidance and has been reported to have a better success rate than sclerotherapy without guidance.

3.7.4 CONGENITAL ANORECTAL ANOMALIES

Endorectal ultrasound has been used in the investigation of Hirschsprung's disease, idiopathic megacolon and imperforate anus to locate normal anal sphincters. Endorectal ultrasound is useful in identifying the optimum location for fashioning a pull-through procedure.

3.7.5 INFLAMMATORY AND INFECTIVE ANORECTAL DISORDERS

Anorectal abscesses may occur as a result of an infected anal gland or as a complication of inflammatory bowel disease, diabetes mellitus, AIDS, colorectal cancer, blood dyscrasias and trauma. Fistulous or sinus tracts may occur. The majority of fistulous tracts occur in the intersphincteric space while a minority involve the external sphincter or extend above the sphincters. From the prognostic viewpoint it is important to know the extent of sphincter damage if any. Fistulous tracts are seen as hypoechoic linear spaces which may extend into the external sphincter. With sphincter involvement there is irregular hypoechoic thickening. A rectal abscess has a heterogeneous appearance with bright shadowing echoes due to air. Inflammatory disorders may widen the intersphincteric space.

3.7.6 FAECAL INCONTINENCE

The external anal sphincter has a vital role in maintaining continence. The morphology of the external sphincter can be readily studied by endorectal ultrasound although traditionally defecatory disorders tend to be studied by manometry, electromyography and defecography. A good correlation has been found between electromyography and endorectal ultrasound in characterising external sphincter abnormalities. One major change that may occur within the external sphincter, which affects continence, is replacement of the striated muscle by abnormal, usually homogeneous, echogenicity, while a generally symmetrical sphincter complex ensures normalcy. Endorectal ultrasound can identify external sphincter abnormalities due to traumatic causes such as childbirth in 85 per cent of patients. In nearly half of such patients internal sphincter abnormalities can also be detected.

Solitary rectal ulcer syndrome is characterised by abnormal defecation, with clinically occult rectal prolapse in some cases, endorectal ultrasound may demonstrate irregular thickening of the third layer, while the muscularis mucosa is usually not affected. In some instances internal sphincter hypertrophy has been recorded. The presence of internal sphincter hypertrophy when seen by ultrasound changes the management from surgical to conservative.

In myotonic muscular dystrophy abnormal defecation is associated with sonographically demonstrable decreased anal sphincter thickness.

Hereditary internal sphincter myopathy is a rare cause of defecation disorder, which is associated with an abnormally thickened internal anal sphincter. These patients may respond to internal anal sphincter strip myomectomy.

3.8 FURTHER READING

Alexander JE, Williamson SL, Seibert JJ, Golladay ES, Jimenez JF: The ultrasonographic diagnosis of typhlitis (neutropenic colitis). Pediatr Radiol *18*:200–204, 1988.

Aliotta A *et al.*: Ultrasonic signs of sliding gastric hiatal hernia and their prospective evaluation. J Ultrasound Med *14*:457–461, 1995.

Aliotta A *et al.*: Doppler ultrasonographic evaluation of blood flow in the superior mesenteric artery in celiac patients and healthy controls in fasting conditions and after saccharose ingestion. J Ultrasound Med *16*:85–91, 1997.

Avila NA *et al.*: Symptomatic wall thickening in an HIV-infected patient caused by Interleukin-2 therapy. Am J Roentgenol *169*:499–500, 1997.

Avunduk C *et al.*: Endoscopic sonography of the stomach: findings in benign and malignant lesions. Am J Roentgenol *163*:591–595, 1994.

Barnard GF *et al.*: Endoscopic ultrasound appearance of watermelon stomach. Abdom Imaging *20*:26–28, 1996.

Barr LL *et al.*: Enteric duplication cysts in children: are their ultrasonographic wall characteristics diagnostic. Pediatr Radiol *20*:326–328, 1990.

Benya EC *et al.*: Abdominal complications after bone marrow transplantation in children: sonographic and CT findings. Am J Roentgenol *161*:1023–1027, 1993.

Bloom RA *et al.*: The ultrasound appearances of intramural gas: the 'bright ring' appearance and effervescence bowel: a report of three cases. Br J Radiol *65*:585–588, 1992.

Bozkurt T *et al.*: Ultrasonography as a primary diagnostic tool in patients with inflammatory disease and tumours of the small intestine and large bowel. J Clin Ultrasound *22*:85–91, 1994.

Chen S *et al.*: Sonographic features of colovesical fistula. J Clin Ultrasound *18*:589–591, 1990.

Chintapalli KN: Gastric bezoar causing intramural pneumatosis. J Clin Gastroenterol *18*:264–265, 1994.

Connally B, O'Halpin D: Sonographic evaluation of the bowel in Henoch–Schönlein purpura. Clin Radiol *49*:320–323, 1994.

Danse EM *et al.*: Early diagnosis of acute intestinal ischaemia: contribution of color Doppler sonography. Acta Chir Belg *97*:173–176, 1997.

Davis RJ *et al.*: Ultrasound in the diagnosis of gallstone ileus. Clin Radiol *43*:282–284, 1991.

Downey DB, Wilson SR: Pseudomembranous colitis: sonographic features. Radiology *180*:61–64, 1991.

Geller A *et al.*: Diagnosis of foregut duplication cysts by endoscopic ultrasonography. Gastroenterology *109*:383–384, 1995.

Goerg L *et al.*: Gastrointestinal lymphoma: sonographic findings in 54 patients. Am J Roentgenol *155*:795–798, 1990.

Hanquinet S *et al.*: Gastric outlet obstruction: unusual ultrasonographic findings in pyloric and antral regions. Paediatr Radiol *25*(suppl. 1):S163–S166, 1995.

Hashimoto BE *et al.*: Applications of ultrasound of the rectum and anus. Ultrasound Quarterly *13*:179–196, 1995.

Hsu TT *et al.*: Sonographic characteristics of a large gastric lipoma: report of a case. J Med Ult 5:148-151, 1997.

Ido K *et al.*: Sonographic diagnosis of small intestinal anisakiasis. J Clin Ultrasound 26:125-130, 1997.

Itagaski A *et al.*: Double target signs in ultrasonic diagnosis of intussuscepted Meckel's diverticulum. Pediatr Radiol 21:148-149, 1991.

Jeffrey RB *et al.*: Sonographic diagnosis of acute appendicitis: interpretative pitfalls. Am J Roentgenol 162:55-59, 1994.

Katz DS *et al.*: Diverticulitis of the right colon: revisited. Am J Roentgenol 171:151-156, 1998.

Kenney IJ *et al.*: Ultrasound in intussusception: a false cystic lead point. Paediatr Radiol 20:348, 1990.

Khaw KT *et al.*: Ultrasonic patterns in inflammatory bowel disease. Clin Radiol 43:171-175, 1991.

Kohzaki S *et al.*: Case report: 'the aurora sign' - a new sonographic sign of pneumatosis cystoides intestinalis. Br J Radiol 67:1275-1277, 1994.

Kruskal JB *et al.*: Pitfalls and sources of error in staging rectal cancer with endorectal ultrasound. Radiographics 17:600-626, 1997.

Lambrecht L *et al.*: Ultrasonic evaluation of gastric clearing in young infants. Paediatr Radiol 18:314-318, 1988.

Lee DH *et al.*: Sonographic detection of pneumoperitoneum in patients with acute abdomen. Am J Roentgenol 154:107-109, 1990.

Lim HK *et al.*: Appendicitis: usefulness of color Doppler ultrasound. Radiology 201:221-225, 1996.

Lim HK *et al.*: Assessment of pancreatic invasion in patients with advanced gastric carcinoma: usefulness of the sliding sign on sonograms. Am J Roentgenol 172:815-818, 1999.

Lim JH: Colorectal cancer: sonographic findings. Am J Roentgenol 167:45-47, 1996.

Long MA, Boultbu JE: The transabdominal ultrasound appearances of colovesical fistula. Br J Radiol 66:465-467, 1993.

Lowe GM *et al.*: Gastric pneumatosis: sign of biliary stent-related perforation. Radiology 174:1037-1038, 1990.

Malde HM, Chadha D: Roundworm obstruction: sonographic diagnosis. Abdom Imaging 18:274-276, 1993.

Mandell GA, Finkelstein M: Gastric pneumatosis secondary to an intramural feeding catheter. Pediatr Radiol 18:418-420, 1988.

Marcus PS *et al.*: Abnormally thickened rectal wall on transrectal sonography: rectal Kaposi sarcoma. J Ultrasound Med 12:179-181, 1993.

McAlister WH *et al.*: Sonography of focal foveolar hyperplasia causing gastric obstruction in an infant. Pediatr Radiol 18:79-81, 1988.

Neal MR *et al.*: Neonatal ultrasonography to distinguish between meconium ileus and ileal atresia. J Ultrasound Med 16:263-266, 1997.

Neumyer MM *et al.*: Ultrasonic assessment of mesenteric and renal ischaemia. Ultrasound Quarterly 12:89-103, 1994.

Nicholson DA, Shorvon PJ: Endoscopic ultrasound of the stomach. Br J Radiol 66:487-492, 1993.

Ozsvath RR *et al.*: Pyloric volume: an important factor in the surgeon's ability to palpate the pyloric 'olive' in hypertrophic pyloric stenosis. Pediatr Radiol 27:175-177, 1997.

Palavesa F de la *et al.*: Appendiceal stump abscess. Abdom Imaging 21:65-66, 1996.

Patriquin HB *et al.*: Appendicitis in children and young adults: Doppler sonographic–pathologic correlation. Am J Roentgenol 166:629-633, 1996.

Pear BL: Pneumatosis intestinalis: a review. Radiology *207*:13–19, 1998.

Peck RJ *et al*.: Ultrasound of coeliac disease with demonstration of response to treatment. Clin Radiol *52*:244–245, 1997.

Quillin SP, Siegel MJ: Appendicitis: efficacy of color Doppler sonography. Radiology *191*:557–560, 1994.

Quillin SP, Siegel MJ: Gastrointestinal inflammation in children: color Doppler ultrasonography. J Ultrasound Med *13*:751–756, 1994.

Quillin SP, Siegel MJ: Diagnosis of appendiceal abscess in children with acute appendicitis: value of color Doppler sonography. Am J Roentgenol *164*:1251–1254, 1995.

Rettenbacher T *et al*.: Adult celiac disease: ultrasound signs. Radiology *211*:389–394, 1999.

Rossi P *et al*.: Meckel's diverticulum: imaging findings. Am J Roentgenol *166*:567–573, 1996.

Saverymuttu SH *et al*.: Thickened stomach – an ultrasound sign of portal hypertension. Clin Radiol *41*:17–18, 1990.

Shirahama M *et al*.: The value of colour Doppler ultrasonography for small bowel involvement of adult Henoch–Schönlein purpura. Br J Radiol *71*:788–791, 1998.

Sidhu MK *et al*.: Intramural duodenal haematoma after blunt abdominal trauma. Am J Roentgenol *170*:38, 1998.

Simonovsk V: Ultrasound in the differential diagnosis of appendicitis. Clin Radiol *50*:768–773, 1995.

Stephenson CA *et al*.: Intussusception: clinical and radiographic factors influencing reducibility. Paediatr Radiol *20*:57–60, 1989.

Takaya J *et al*.: Ménétrier's disease evaluated serially by abdominal ultrasonography. Pediatr Radiol *27*:178–180, 1997.

Taniura H, Satou I: Sonography of pedunculated exogastric leiomyoblastoma. Am J Roentgenol *166*:725, 1996.

Tous F, Busto M: Assessment of abdominal sonography in the diagnosis of tumours of the gastrointestinal tract. J Clin Ultrasound *25*:243–247, 1996.

Truong M *et al*.: Sonographic appearance of benign and malignant conditions of the colon. Am J Roentgenol *170*:1451–1455, 1998.

Tsai CY *et al*.: Endoscopic ultrasonographic diagnosis of gastric lymphangioma. J Clin Ultrasound *25*:333–335, 1996.

Van Oostayan JA *et al*.: Doppler sonography evaluation of superior mesenteric artery flow to assess Crohn's disease activity index, and alpha 1 antitrypsin clearance in feces. Am J Roentgenol *168*:429–433, 1997.

Wada M *et al*.: Uncomplicated acute diverticulitis of the colon and ascending colon: sonographic findings in 18 patients. Am J Roentgenol *155*:283–287, 1990.

Walter DF *et al*.: Colonic sonography: preliminary observations. Clin Radiol *47*:200–204, 1993.

Weinberger E *et al*.: Sonographic diagnosis of intestinal malrotation in infants, importance of the relative positions of the superior mesenteric vein and artery. Am J Roentgenol *159*:825–828, 1992.

Westra SJ *et al*.: Ultrasound diagnosis of gastro-oesophageal reflux in infants and young children. J Clin Ultrasound *18*:477, 1990.

Winckel MV *et al*.: 'Whirlpool sign' not always associated with volvulus in intestinal malrotation. J Clin Ultrasound *24*:367–370, 1996.

Wu C: Sonographic spectrum of giant intramural duodenal haematoma: identifying a case simulating traumatic pancreatic pseudocyst. J Clin Ultrasound *20*:352–355, 1992.

Yacoe ME, Jeffrey RB: Degenerated uterine leiomyoma mimicking acute appendicitis: sonographic diagnosis. J Clin Ultrasound 23:473–475, 1995.

Yoshikane H et al.: Carcinoid tumours of the gastrointestinal tract: evaluation with endoscopic ultrasonography. Gastrointest Endosc 39:375–383, 1993.

Zerbey AL 3rd et al.: Endoscopic sonography of the upper gastrointestinal tract and pancreas. Am J Roentgenol 166:45–50, 1996.

4

Urinary tract and adrenal glands

4.1 URINARY TRACT

Anomalies of the genitourinary tract are common and are found in 10 per cent of infants. The high incidence of anatomical variants is explained by the complex embryology of the region. The genitourinary tract develops from the urogenital ridges on the posterior abdominal wall. Three pairs of renal structures form in early foetal life, the pronephros (forekidney) and the mesonephros (midkidney) involute but the metanephros (hindkidney) which begins to form during the fifth week of life persists to form the definitive kidney, producing urine from the eleventh week of life. The large number of anatomical variants occur due to anomalies of growth and fusion of the metanephric duct which forms the renal collecting system and ureter, and the metanephric mesenchyme which forms the nephrons. The kidneys initially form in the pelvis but differential rates of growth in the length of the trunk cause them to migrate into the abdomen. The renal hilum, which is initially directed anteriorly, rotates medially as the kidney ascends. Whilst in the pelvis the kidney derives its blood supply from the sacral and iliac vessels but as they ascend into the abdomen they derive their blood supply from the aorta. This changing vascular anatomy accounts for the high incidence of variants encountered in a quarter of the human population who have three or more renal arteries.

4.1.1 RENAL ANATOMY

The kidneys lie obliquely in the retroperitoneum, on the posterior abdominal wall. The average renal weight is 150g in males and 135g in females. The kidneys are usually 10 to 11 cm long, 5 cm wide and 3 cm thick, though renal size depends upon the patient's size and build. The kidney is bean shaped with a hilum on its medial border, this receives the renal vein, artery and pelvis from anterior to posterior. Small vessels may pass around the renal pelvis and upper ureter and may not follow this anatomical relationship. The kidneys are highly vascular organs and together receive 25 per cent of resting cardiac output, which approximates to 1250 ml of blood per minute. The renal substance is divided into outer cortex and inner medullary pyramids. Projections of cortex, the columns or septae of Bertin, lie between the pyramids. The collecting system, vessels, nerves, fat and connective tissue lie in the centre of the kidney.

The urinary bladder forms from the cloaca which divides into the urogenital sinus anteriorly and the rectum posteriorly. The urogenital sinus gives rise to the bladder and urethra and is continuous superiorly with the allantois. The allantois is a diverticulum on the caudal wall of the yolk sac, it extends from the bladder into the placenta and though it normally involutes it may give rise to cysts, fistulae and even tumours such as embryonal rhabdomyosarcoma.

Sonographic appearance of renal anatomy

The sonographic appearance of internal renal anatomy is remarkably similar to the appearance of the cut sections of a kidney at post mortem. Cortical thickness is usually uniform but may be lobulated particularly in a neonate. The renal cortex is normally hypoechoic relative to hepatic or splenic parenchyma whilst the renal pyramids are hypoechoic relative to the renal cortex. The corticomedullary junction is demarcated by the arcuate arteries, which are seen as small echogenic foci. The collecting system, vessels and connective tissue at the centre of the kidney are seen as the echogenic 'central echo complex' which is the most echogenic part of the kidney. The echogenicity of the central echo complex increases with age and in conditions such as renal fibrolipomatosis. Its echogenicity is reduced in neonates and conditions with reduced total body fat such as starvation.

4.1.2 RENAL ANOMALIES

Anomalies of the kidney and ureter are common affecting 4 per cent of the population.

Most people have two kidneys but unilateral renal agenesis occurs at a rate of 1 in 1000 of the population. It should be remembered that an empty renal fossa might contain bowel loops which may be mistaken for a kidney, abscess or calculus. The adrenal gland is relatively large in the neonate and may be mistaken for a small kidney.

If a kidney cannot be found search for an ectopic kidney and consider a Tc-99m DMSA scan.

Unilateral renal hypoplasia is more common than agenesis. The kidney is small, but of normal echopattern and configuration. The main differential diagnosis is ischaemic atrophy but identical appearances can occur with growth retardation due to infection, thus renal hypoplasia should not be diagnosed until the urinary tract has been fully evaluated.

Unilateral renal agenesis is frequently associated with other anomalies, particularly in women. Fifty-eight per cent of cases have other congenital anomalies and 48 per cent of these are of the genital tract, for example bicornuate uterus, unicornuate uterus and uterine and vaginal septations.

Rotational anomalies of the kidney are uncommon. Rotation normally occurs as the kidney ascends from the pelvis and thus the majority of cases are associated with low or ectopic kidneys.

Ectopic kidneys usually lie in the pelvis because of failure to ascend. These kidneys may be malformed from a lack of pressure from adjacent organs during growth.

Crossed renal ectopia occurs when a kidney crosses the midline during ascent. In these cases the ureter enters the bladder on the side from which the kidney originated.

Renal fusion across the midline results in the formation of a horseshoe kidney. This is found in 1 in 400 to 1 in 600 of the population and in over 90 per cent of cases the renal fusion is at the lower poles. The mesenteric vessels arrest ascent of the horseshoe kidney and thus they lie lower in the abdomen than normal. The isthmus joining the two kidneys is often hidden by bowel gas and thus diagnosis of horseshoe kidney is easily missed on sonography, though the kidney may be noted to have more vertical axes than normal. Duplication of the renal collecting system and ureter are common affecting 1 in 70 of the population. They occur because of varying degrees of division of the ureteric bud (metanephric diverticulum) as it grows into the urogenital ridge. There is a great variation in the degree of division resulting in a spectrum of changes from a completely duplicated collecting system with two ureters, to a slightly bifid collecting system draining to a single ureter. In mild cases the kidneys appear normal sonographically but more prominent cases are associated with increased renal length and division of the central echo complex into two parts on longitudinal sections. Oblique sections through a normal kidney, renal cyst or renal columnar hypertrophy may mimic this appearance. When the two renal moieties drain by separate ureters and the ureter draining the lower collecting system inserts into the bladder at the normal site, it has a shortened intramural course and is prone to reflux. The ureter draining the upper half of the kidney inserts into the bladder distal to the normal site and may insert ectopically into the vagina, urethra, seminal vesicles, etc. These ureters are prone to ureterocoele formation and obstruction. Ectopic ureteric insertion without ureteric duplication is rare.

Supernumerary kidneys resulting from the formation of extra ureteric buds are extremely rare.

4.1.3 NORMAL RENAL LOBULATION

Foetal lobulation is the term applied to lobulation of the renal contour to renal lobular architecture. This is most prominent in neonates and *in utero* and decreases with age. It may be visible when the kidney is swollen.

Dromedary hump is lobulation of the lateral aspect of the left kidney at the site of impression by the lower pole of the spleen, it occurs because of pressure *in utero* during renal development and is seen more frequently on sonography than urography because of the increased number of sections taken.

Hypertrophy of the renal sinus margin shows as a prominent renal sinus margin usually seen on transverse sections.

Anterior indentation on sagittal sections is seen at the level of the renal hilum on sagittal sections and should not be mistaken for pyelonephritic scarring.

Oblique sections through the kidney may give the appearance of variation in renal parenchymal thickness. The true nature of this appearance is usually evident on further sections.

4.1.4 RENAL EXAMINATION

Renal location

Locating the kidneys is not always easy particularly in patients with spinal deformity. Do not assume that an atypical structure in the renal bed is a kidney, it may be a bowel loop. If a typically reniform structure is not seen in the renal bed search for ectopic kidneys. When in doubt perform a Tc-99m DMSA scan.

When the kidney is located assess its

- position
- mobility
- size
- contour
- parenchymal echopattern
- central echo complex, the collecting system
- adjacent structures including the renal artery, vein, pelvis and perinephric space.

Renal size

Renal size may be measured visually or by direct measurement. The bipolar diameter is the most frequently used parameter measuring from the upper to the lower poles. If the sections taken are oblique the bipolar diameter will underestimate the renal length. The greatest measurement obtained for each kidney is the closest estimation of true renal length. Renal size is related to age, weight and body surface area.

Renal size in children

- Average renal length in babies less than 1 year of age is 4.98 + (0.155 × age in months) cm.
- Average renal length in children less than 1 year of age is 6.79 + (0.22 × age in years) cm.

In infants less than 1 year of age renal size correlates most closely with body weight and length and thus small babies can be expected to have small kidneys. At birth the two kidneys are approximately the same length but as they grow the left kidney becomes slightly longer and thinner than the right. In older children renal length correlates better with height, weight and surface area than age.

Renal size in a single functioning kidney in children exceeds the size-established standards for bilateral functioning kidneys. Compensatory hypertrophy of a single functioning kidney occurs *in utero*.

Renal size in adults

Chronicity of renal failure is assessed by renal length measurements. Unlike x-rays sonography does not suffer from magnification. The normal renal length reported by Brandt *et al.* (1982) is

- right kidney = 10.74 ± 1.35 cm
- left kidney = 11.0 ± 1.15 cm

Table 4.1 Renal length (cm)

Age	Percentile		
	5 per cent	50 per cent	95 per cent
Birth	4	5	6
1 year	5	6.5	8
5 years		8	
10 years	7	9	10.5
Adult	9.5	11	12.5

and reported by Emamian *et al.* (1993) is

- right kidney = 10.9 cm (median length)
- left kidney = 11.2 cm (median length).

Renal parenchymal thickness

Normal values for parenchymal thickness are not available but in end stage renal failure it is less than 1.5 cm.

Renal volume

$$\text{Renal volume} = \text{width} \times \text{length} \times \text{thickness} \times 0.5233 \, \text{cm}^3$$

The renal volume of a child's kidneys increases as the child grows:

- birth – 20 cm^3
- 1 year – 30 cm^3
- 18 years – 155 cm^3.

Causes of renal parenchymal thickness less than 1.5 cm

Renal parenchymal thickness is less than 1.5 cm in patients with chronic renal disease due to

glomerular sclerosis
extensive chronic inflammatory infiltrate
tubular atrophy.

Patients with these conditions have shorter kidneys and thinner renal parenchyma compared to patients with other chronic renal diseases.

Renal parenchyma

The renal parenchymal echopattern is compared with adjacent organs. Renal cortex is normally less echogenic than liver parenchyma except in the newborn. For the first 6 months of life the renal cortex may be as echogenic as liver parenchyma, and 50 per cent of neonatal left kidneys are as echogenic as the spleen. It has been said that normal neonatal renal cortex is never more echogenic than liver though there are reports of very echogenic cortex in the kidneys of preterm infants. If there is doubt about the normality of the parenchyma of a neonatal kidney it should be followed up as 90 per cent of infants' kidneys show an adult pattern of echoes by 4 months of age.

Aetiology of increased cortical echogenicity in neonatal kidneys

Glomeruli occupy a greater percentage of renal cortex in neonates (18 per cent in neonates, 8.6 per cent in adults).

There is a greater proportion of cellular component in the glomerular tuft in neonates than in adults.

Twenty per cent of loops of Henle lie in the cortex in the neonate rather than in the medulla.

Metanephric mesenchyme persists in the renal cortex for the first 6 months of life.

The renal pyramids should remain hypoechoic relative to the renal cortex regardless of age.

When a renal parenchymal abnormality is identified it should be assessed with regard to

- its distribution – unilateral or bilateral
- whether it is focal or diffuse
- whether it affects the cortex, the medulla or both
- whether or not there is loss of corticomedullary differentiation
- the renal size
- the presence of perirenal or distant anomalies.

Absent kidneys on intravenous urography

No kidney found on sonography
Renal aplasia.
Renal ectopia.
Small scarred kidney – infection, trauma, calculi, etc.

Liquid pattern in the renal bed
Hydronephrosis.
Polycystic disease.
Necrotic tumour (rare).

Solid kidney identified
Small – severe renal scarring, for example chronic pyelonephritis, renal ischaemia.
Normal – renal ischaemia, nephritis, acute obstruction with minimal collecting-system dilatation.
Large – tumour, renal vein thrombosis, acute obstruction with minimal collecting-system dilatation.

Non-visualised kidney on ultrasonography

When a kidney is absent bowel may lie in the renal fossa and mimic a renal abscess or hydronephrosis. The adrenal is relatively large in the neonate and can be mistaken for a small kidney if the kidney is absent.

Renal agenesis.
Renal ectopia.

A small kidney may be difficult to visualise particularly if the parenchyma is echogenic.

Replaced kidney – the renal parenchyma is replaced by an infiltrative process for example neoplasia or xanthogranulomatous pyelonephritis.

A horseshoe kidney is often low in the abdomen and obscured by bowel gas.

A pancake kidney is a flat kidney in the lower abdomen. The deformity results from a lack of normal pressure from adjacent structures *in utero*.

A hydronephrotic sac may be mistaken for fluid-filled bowel loops.

Calcified kidney, for example tuberculous auto-nephrectomy.

Juxta-renal fluid-acoustic enhancement because of adjacent fluid may make the kidney difficult to recognise.

4.1.5 INTRINSIC RENAL DISEASE

Echogenicity in renal disease is assessed by comparison to adjacent liver or spleen. Normal parenchymal renal echogenicity is usually less than that of the liver or spleen (assuming that the hepatic or splenic echogenicity is normal!). Echogenicity equal to, or greater than, the liver or spleen is considered abnormal. Rosenfield *et al.* classified renal parenchymal disease into two types.

Rosenfield type 1 renal parenchymal changes

Type 1 changes are a diffuse increase in cortical echogenicity with preservation of corticomedullary differentiation so that the pyramids become abnormally prominent. These changes are observed in the following conditions.

Acute or chronic glomerulonephritis.
Hypertensive nephrosclerosis.
Diabetic nephrosclerosis.
Transplant rejection.
Chronic renal parenchymal disease.
Lupus nephritis.
Some patients with acute tubular necrosis.
Lipoid nephrosis.
Bilateral renal vein thrombosis.
Leukaemia – the only malignancy causing type 1 changes.
Amyloid.
Beckwith–Wiedmann syndrome.
Myoglobinuric renal failure.
AIDS nephropathy.
Cortical nephrocalcinosis.

Kawasaki disease.
Early polycystic disease.
Alport's disease.

Rosenfield type 2 renal parenchymal changes

Type 2 changes are a loss of corticomedullary differentiation either focally (as with scars, masses or infarcts) or globally as in acute pyelonephritis, acute renal vein thrombosis and end stage renal disease. They are seen in the following conditions.

Acute bacterial nephritis.
Chronic pyelonephritis.
Chronic glomerulonephritis.
Healing infarcts.
Infantile polycystic disease.
Adult polycystic disease.
Glomerular polycystic disease.
Medullary cystic disease.

Problems with Rosenfield's classification

The appearances in normal people are variable, for example the pyramids may not be recognised.
It assumes that liver and splenic echogenicity is normal.
Patients with histological and clinical evidence of renal failure may have a normal renal echogenicity.
It is a cumbersome classification which does not offer a working diagnosis.
Seventy-two per cent of patients with renal echogenicity equal to that of the liver have a normal renal function.
With renal echogenicity greater than that of the liver, the specificity of detecting renal abnormality is high at 96 per cent but sensitivity is poor at 20 per cent.
With no difference in the echogenicity between the liver and renal parenchyma, the renal parenchyma may still be abnormal.
The degree of renal echogenicity correlates poorly with the extent of disease.
Echogenicity relates well with interstitial disease but not glomerular disease.
Renal echogenicity correlates with a variety of histological criteria particularly global sclerosis, tubular atrophy, hyaline casts, focal leukocyte infiltration, glomerular sclerosis, arteriosclerosis and oedema. Thus renal echogenicity is non-specific but correlates somewhat with histological features and functional changes of chronic renal failure whatever the cause.

Focal area of increased echogenicity

Chronic infarction.
Acute bacterial focal nephritis.
Angiomyolipoma.
Haemangioma.
Oncocytoma.
Malignancy, for example renal cell carcinoma, sarcoma, metastases.

Focal depression of the renal cortex

Scan artefact.
Foetal lobulation.
Splenic impression.
Focal scar.
Infarct.

Diffuse increase in renal echogenicity

Neonates
Normal.
Infantile polycystic disease.
Renal vein thrombosis.
Cortical nephrocalcinosis.
Early stages of adult polycystic disease.
Glomerulocystic disease.
Congenital/neonatal nephrotic syndrome.
Amyloid deposition.
Infections.
Bile nephrosis.
Storage disease.
Leukaemia.
Solid tumours.
Laurence–Moon–Biedle syndrome – large echogenic kidneys with loss of cortico-
    medullary differentiation. Renal disease is a cardinal feature. Other features
    include obesity, polydactyly, mental retardation, hypogonadism and pigmented
    retinal dystrophy.

Adults
Acute glomerulonephritis.
Chronic glomerulonephritis.
Ethylene glycol poisoning.
Renal amyloid.

Leukaemia.
Renal fatty infiltration (diffuse) in multiple angiomyolipomas.

NB There is generally diffuse parenchymal echogenicity with preservation of corticomedullary differentiation, although corticomedullary differentiation may be lost.

Echogenic renal pyramids in children

Nephrocalcinosis – the single most frequent cause
Iatrogenic – frusemide, vitamin D.
Non-iatrogenic – idiopathic hypercalcaemia, Williams' syndrome, Kenny–Caffey syndrome, absorptive hypercalcaemia, renal tubular necrosis, tubular necrosis or dystrophic calcification, chronic glomerulonephritis, malignancy, Sjogren's syndrome.

No nephrocalcinosis
Protein deposits – proteinuria (dehydration), toxic shock syndrome, sepsis, degenerative leucoencephalopathy, hypotensive or hypovolaemic shock.
Vascular congestion or occlusion – sickle cell disease.
Systemic infection – bacterial septicaemia, *Candida* spp., cytomegalovirus, AIDS (*Mycobacterium avium intracellulare.*)
Metabolic causes – Gout–Lesch–Nyhan syndrome, glycogen storage disease, hypokalaemia primary aldosteronism, pseudo-Bartter syndrome, Wilson syndrome, Fanconi's syndrome, tyrosinosis, cholestatic jaundice, oxalosis, alpha antitrypsin deficiency.
Fibrosis – renal pyramidal fibrosis (this usually forms a part of a generalised parenchymal abnormality), congenital hepatic fibrosis.
Unknown causes – pyloric stenosis, metabolic alkalosis, tubular ectasia (infantile and juvenile polycystic kidneys), intrarenal reflux, Crohn's disease.
Cystic medullary disease – medullary sponge kidney.

Echogenic pyramids and hyperechoic rings in the periphery of renal pyramids in adults

Nephrocalcinosis – most common cause
Hypercalcaemia.
Hypercalciuria.
Papillary necrosis – analgesic nephropathy, diabetes mellitus, obstructive uropathy, acute pyelonephritis, sickle cell disease.
Medullary sponge kidney.
Oxalosis.
AIDS-related *Mycobacterium avium intracellulare.*

No nephrocalcinosis

Renal tubular ectasia.
Medullary sponge kidney.
Congenital hepatic fibrosis.
Sarcoidosis.
Hyperuricaemia.
Glomerulonephritis.
Rheumatoid arthritis with amyloid.
Analgesic nephropathy.
Hypocalcaemia.
Hypokalaemia.
Hyperuricaemia.
Addison's disease (normal calcium, potassium, uric acid).
Renovascular hypertension.
Normal variant.

Hypoechoic renal sinus

Fibrolipomatosis (rare).
Prominent column of Bertin.
Duplex kidney.
Transitional cell or renal cell carcinoma.
Parapelvic cyst.
Caliectasis.
Varix.
Arteriovenous malformation.
Aneurysm.

Echogenic focus with thinning of overlying renal parenchyma

Normal variant.
Focal infarct.
Pyelonephritic scar.
Tuberculous scar.
Renal papillary necrosis.

4.1.6 THE CAUSES OF 'SNOWSTORM' KIDNEYS: TINY ECHOGENIC FOCI WHICH MAY OR MAY NOT SHADOW

AIDS-related infections – systemic *Pneumocystis carinii*, cytomegalovirus, *Mycobacterium avium intracellulare*, histoplasmosis, aspergillus, *Candida albicans*.

These infections are associated with echogenic foci in the liver, spleen, bowel and pleura. Renal foci may shadow after treatment because of calcification.

Pseudoxanthoma elasticum – several cases of pseudoxanthoma elasticum have been reported as showing fine highly reflective echoes in the renal parenchyma mostly at the corticomedullary junction.

Renal transplant – appearances similar to pseudoxanthoma elasticum have been reported with transplant rejection.

Hypercalciuria – appearances indistinguishable from pseudoxanthoma elasticum have been reported with hypercalciuria with no functional renal abnormality.

Hypercalcaemia – hyperparathyroidism, hypervitaminosis D, all causes of nephrocalcinosis.

4.1.7 ACUTE GLOMERULONEPHRITIS

Acute glomerulonephritis is usually caused by the presence of circulating immune complexes or autoimmune disease, causing renal damage. The main use of sonography in these patients, who may present with rapidly failing renal function, is to exclude obstructive uropathy and other surgically treatable causes of renal failure. Initially the kidney appears normal or enlarged. As the disease progresses the renal parenchyma becomes echogenic, though less often oedema causes a reduction in parenchymal echogenicity. In children renal oedema may cause increased echogenicity because of disruption of tissue interface.

4.1.8 CAUSES OF UNILATERAL SMALL KIDNEY

Developmental – congenital hypoplasia, multicystic dysplastic kidney (adult).

Vascular – renal infarction, renal artery stenosis, radiation nephritis, multiple renal emboli, post-traumatic atrophy.

Inflammatory – renal tuberculosis, unilateral chronic pyelonephritis or reflux.

Miscellaneous – Postobstructive atrophy, heminephrectomy.

4.1.9 CAUSES OF BILATERAL SMALL KIDNEYS

Developmental – medullary cystic disease, hereditary chronic nephritis (Alport syndrome).

Arterial – acute renal hypoperfusion, hypertensive nephrosclerosis, arterial emboli (for example atrial fibrillation), bilateral renal infarction (late), arteritis (for example polyarteritis nodosa), scleroderma (late), diabetic nephropathy, renal cortical necrosis.

Inflammatory, infectious and metabolic – gout nephropathy, hyperparathyroidism (late), chronic glomerulonephritis, chronic pyelonephritis, papillary necrosis (late), chronic lead poisoning, renal amyloid (late).

Postobstructive atrophy – bladder outlet obstruction, retroperitoneal fibrosis.

NB   Any longstanding renal parenchymal disease may result in bilateral small kidneys.

4.1.10 RENAL FIBROLIPOMATOSIS

The presence of excess fat in the renal sinus enlarges the central echo complex so that the renal parenchymal tissue appears relatively narrow. Occasionally the enlarged central echo complex is anechoic but usually the excess fat is of high echogenicity. The fatty nature of the tissue in the renal sinus may be confirmed by CT. When the sinus fat is hypoechoic the appearances may be mistaken for parapelvic cysts, hydronephrosis or transitional cell carcinoma.

4.1.11 RENAL SINUS MASS

Neoplastic masses

Benign – lipoma, fibroma, neurofibroma, myoma, haemangioma.
Malignant – transitional cell carcinoma, metastases, renal cell carcinoma, lymphoma, plasmacytoma, myeloid metaplasia, renal medullary carcinoma (sickle cell trait or disease), leiomyosarcoma.

Miscellaneous masses

Renal fibrolipomatosis.
Parapelvic cysts.
Aneurysm, arteriovenous malformation, varices.
Fungus ball.
Pus.
Haematoma.
Calculi (usually shadow).

4.1.12 RENAL OEDEMA

Renal oedema usually causes a reduction in renal echogenicity. This is particularly prominent in the renal pyramids which appear anechoic and may be mistaken for cysts. The renal capsule may appear unusually prominent. Less commonly renal oedema causes a transient increase in parenchymal echogenicity because of disruption of tissue interfaces.

Aetiology of renal oedema

Acute glomerulonephritis.
Acute pyelonephritis.

Nephrotic syndrome.
Transplant rejection.
Renal contusion.

4.1.13 RENAL CALCIFICATION

Small calcific nodules are seen as very echogenic foci. As these foci enlarge they cause distal acoustic shadowing. When the kidney is densely calcified it may be difficult to recognise and may be indistinguishable from gas-filled bowel loops.

Renal parenchymal calcification

Medullary calcification.
Cortical calcification.
Calcification in a cyst wall, usually a complicated cyst (3 per cent of renal cysts show wall calcification).
Calcification in a renal tumour is usually amorphous but can be ring-like and mimic cyst wall calcification (6 per cent of tumours show calcification).

Medullary calcinosis

Medullary calcinosis accounts for 95 per cent of all renal parenchymal calcification and occurs in the distal convoluted tubules in the loop of Henle. It can result from literally any cause of hypercalcaemia or hypercalciuria. The margins of the pyramids are echogenic whilst the centre of the pyramids remain echolucent. The pyramids may be densely echogenic and may shadow. This may be evident on sonography before it is seen on plain-film radiography.

Aetiology of medullary calcinosis

Hypercalcaemic causes

Non-renal causes – hyperparathyroidism, paraneoplastic syndrome, bony metastases (including myeloma), sarcoidosis, prolonged immobilisation (for example in Paget's disease), hyperthyroidism, Cushing's disease, diabetes insipidus, idiopathic hypercalcaemia and hypercalcuria.
Renal causes – renal tubular acidosis, Bartter syndrome, medullary sponge kidney.
Iatrogenic causes – milk-alkali syndrome, hypervitaminosis D, beryllium poisoning, furosemide (frusemide) therapy in infants, prolonged vitamin E therapy, excess ingestion of calcium, prolonged ACTH treatment

Non-hypercalcaemic/hypercalciuric causes

Oxalosis – oxaluria is a rare autosomal recessive condition which causes recurrent calculi and nephrocalcinosis. Oxalate may be deposited in bone, bone marrow, heart, blood vessels, cartilage, etc. The condition may cause early death in childhood. Secondary oxaluria may rarely occur with a blind loop syndrome, ileal resection or bypass and increased ingestion of oxalates. Sonography reveals diffusely echogenic kidneys.

Hyperuricosuria – gout, Lesch–Nyhan syndrome.

Urinary stasis – pyelocalyceal diverticulum.

Dystrophic calcification – papillary necrosis.

Renal cortical calcification

Renal cortical calcification, which makes up only 5 per cent of the renal calcinosis causes increased cortical echogenicity with complete shadowing in severe cases. Secondary pyramidal fibrosis may occur.

Aetiology of renal cortical calcification

Acute cortical necrosis.

Chronic glomerulonephritis.

Alport's syndrome.

Oxalosis – this may cause medullary calcinosis or both cortical and medullary calcification.

Rejected renal transplant.

Chronic paraneoplastic hypercalcaemia.

Nephrocalcinosis and nephrolithiasis in children

64 per cent of cases are associated with an underlying structural renal lesion or urinary tract infection.

10 per cent are associated with hypercalcaemia or hypercalciuria.

6 per cent are associated with cystinuria.

20 per cent are idiopathic (up to 50 per cent in some series), oxalosis and miscellaneous conditions.

4.1.14 RENAL ENLARGEMENT

Nephromegaly with a normal echotexture

Acute processes – acute pyelonephritis, interstitial nephritis, renal tubular necrosis, renal vein thrombosis.

Chronic processes – compensatory hypertrophy, amyloid, leukaemic infiltration, lymphoma – diffuse infiltration or reactive changes, metastatic infiltration, malakoplakia – 75 per cent of cases show multifocal changes but 25 per cent show diffuse disease which may not be detectable.

Unilateral renal enlargement

Normal variant, for example duplex collecting system.
Duplication.
Compensatory hypertrophy – nephrectomy, contralateral disease.
Hydronephrosis.
Adult polycystic disease – one kidney may be larger.
Multicystic dysplastic kidney.
Neoplasia – primary or metastatic.
Renal vein thrombosis.
Pyonephrosis.
Xanthogranulomatous pyelonephritis.
Acute renal artery thrombosis – infarction.
Malakoplakia.

Focal renal enlargement

Primary or metastatic malignancy.
Renal cyst.
Renal abscess.
Acute lobar nephritis or acute lobar nephronia.
Enlarged septum of Bertin.
Dromedary hump.
Haematoma.
Renal lobe supplied by an aberrant artery.
Focal xanthogranulomatous pyelonephritis.
Focal malakoplakia.
Pseudo-mass lesion.

Bilateral renal enlargement

Multiple simple cysts.
Polycystic disease.
Bilateral duplex kidneys.
Bilateral outflow obstruction or hydronephrosis.
Acute glomerulonephritis.
Bilateral acute bacterial nephritis.
Diabetic nephropathy.
Nephrotic syndrome.
Acute oedema – acute tubular necrosis, acute cortical necrosis.

Acute infarction.

Bilateral renal vein thrombosis.

Systemic disease – vasculitides.

Amyloid.

Myeloma.

Lymphoma.

Leukaemia.

Bilateral neoplasms – primary or metastatic.

Gaucher's disease.

Acromegaly.

Tuberous sclerosis with hamartomas.

Acute uric acid nephropathy.

Total parenteral nutrition.

Renal lymphangioma.

Nephroblastomatosis.

Beckwith–Wiedmann syndrome.

Xanthogranulomatous pyelonephritis.

Glycogen storage disease.

Haemophilia.

Fabry disease.

Sickle cell disease.

Physiologic response to fluids or diuretics – beer drinker's kidneys.

4.1.15 URINARY TRACT INFECTIONS

Urinary tract infections are common in both adults and children and remain a major cause of morbidity with further risk of renal scarring causing hypertension and chronic renal failure. As a safe non-invasive investigation renal sonography is the initial investigation of choice in cases of urinary tract infection.

Aims of sonography in urinary tract infections

- To demonstrate the presence of two kidneys.
- To exclude an underlying abnormality, for example hydronephrosis.
- To assess complications such as abscess or scarring.

Intravenous urography and sonography are insensitive detectors of renal scarring, although sonography is more sensitive than urography but less sensitive than CT and Tc-99m DMSA scanning. A Tc-99m DMSA scan is the most sensitive means of detecting scarring.

The term 'acute renal infections' encompasses a spectrum of pathologic processes involving the renal parenchyma that may vary in severity from an acute pyelonephritis to a renal abscess which can spread to the perirenal space. The terminology applied to renal tract infections has been confusing. The terms acute pyelonephritis, focal pyelonephritis, lobar nephronia, carbuncle, pseudo-abscess state, preabscess state and phlegmon are encountered with no universal agreement amongst radiologists on their use. The Society of Uroradiology has recommended a simplified nomenclature based on the time-honoured term 'acute pyelonephritis', which may be focal or diffuse, unilateral or bilateral. An acute pyelonephritis may completely regress or progress to a renal and/or extrarenal abscess or emphysematous pyelonephritis. Pyonephrosis may complicate an obstructive uropathy. Renal abscesses may complicate an acute pyelonephritis or develop from haematogenous spread of infection.

Acute pyelonephritis is a bacterial infection of the renal parenchyma. Ninety per cent of cases occur in women and predisposing conditions include pregnancy, diabetes mellitus, obstructive uropathy, steroids and immunosuppression. The affected kidney is oedematous with inflammatory cell infiltrate and streaks of pus in the parenchyma.

Urographic signs of acute pyelonephritis

The role of intravenous urography is to rule out the presence of obstructing calculi, pyonephrosis and the most serious complications of acute pyelonephritis. The results are normal in 76 per cent of cases while 24 per cent show the following.

Diffuse, patchy or focal attenuation of the nephrogram.
Normal or a diffuse or focal increase in renal size.
Mild calyceal dilatation or blunting.
Narrowing of the calices because of spasm.

When an abscess complicates an acute pyelonephritis, nephrotomography may show the abscess cavity as a low attenuation ill-defined, round or triangular lesion with a mass effect.

Sonographic signs of acute pyelonephritis in adults

The kidney may appear normal on sonography despite the presence of inflammation shown on CT.
Focal or diffuse renal enlargement associated with increased parenchymal thickness.
Reduction or disappearance of the renal sinus.
Decreased echogenicity with focal areas that may appear almost anechoic.
Rarely hyperechoic areas may be seen due to gas or haemorrhage.
An abscess may be seen as a hypoechoic mass with low level echoes, the intensity of the echoes is related to the debris as well as the amount of gas produced by the bacteria. A fluid–fluid level may be seen as an abscess. The margins of an abscess remain ill defined.

Ultrasound may demonstrate an extrarenal fluid collection with perinephric extension of infection, although ultrasound has poor sensitivity at showing increased thickness of the septa.
Power Doppler may show focal or multifocal areas of hypoperfusion.

The majority of affected kidneys do not have an underlying abnormality. Performing intravenous urography during an acute infection can result in a poor-quality examination and thus ultrasonography has replaced urography as the initial investigation of choice in cases of acute pyelonephritis. Ultrasonography will also demonstrate complications such as perinephric abscess that are not evident on urography.

Renal scarring

Severe infections cause destruction of renal parenchyma leading to atrophy and fibrosis with thinning of the parenchyma and alteration of the echopattern. Sonography and urography only show these changes at a late stage of evolution. Sonography may show scars on the anterior and posterior renal surface which are not visible at urography, while urography may show calyceal deformity associated with scarring more clearly than sonography. Isotope scanning with Tc-99m DMSA is a much more sensitive means of detecting early renal scars than urography or sonography. Acute pyelonephritis can result in permanent renal damage but it is often difficult to diagnose in children as clinical findings may be limited and varied. Enhanced CT and Tc-99m DMSA have been shown to be capable of visualising the renal changes that occur with acute pyelonephritis. Sonography is usually the first technique used, it is considered a poor technique but the addition of power Doppler improves sensitivity.

Sonographic signs of acute pyelonephritis in children

Normal kidneys in 33 per cent of children.
Thickening of the renal pelvis.
Renal enlargement.
Mild pelvicalyceal dilatation.
Increased cortical echogenicity.
Hyperechoic fat.
Thickening of the bladder wall.
Rounded hypoechoic areas, these are uncommon but most occur in infants' lesions that are not yet suppurative.
Power Doppler, triangular areas of hypovascularity are identified with acute pyelonephritis, peripheral interlobular arteries are compressed by adjacent oedematous parenchyma, appearing curvilinear rather than straight and could be com-

pared with a claw of a bird of prey. Power Doppler seems significantly more sensitive than conventional ultrasound for detecting acute pyelonephritis in children. In normal children power Doppler shows a straight course of interlobular arteries around the pyramids, on both axial and longitudinal scans.

Flow within the interlobular arteries appears as a blush beneath the renal cortical surface.

4.1.16 RENAL HYPOPERFUSION ON POWER DOPPLER

Focal hypoperfusion – pyelonephritis, renal tuberculosis, xanthogranulomatous pyelonephritis, abscesses, infarction, avascular tumour.

Splaying of intrarenal vasculature on power Doppler suggests a mass effect consistent with an abscess or tumour.

Multifocal hypoperfusion – pyelonephritis, abscesses, infarction, multifocal tumours (metastases or lymphoma).

Global hypoperfusion – renal artery occlusion (renal transplantation).

Cortical hypoperfusion – acute cortical necrosis, acute interstitial nephritis, unilateral cortical ischaemia (this is rare and may result from infiltrative processes such as perirenal fibrosis or tumour).

4.1.17 VESICOURETERIC REFLUX

Although ultrasonography is not a sensitive detector of vesicoureteric reflux the authors routinely perform pre- and post-micturition renal sonography. This also allows measurement of the residual volume of urine in the bladder after micturition.

Sonographic features of reflux

Transient visualisation of the ureters seen during ultrasound examination may be caused by either reflux or by transient ureteric dilatation during the passage of a wave of peristalsis. More prominent reflux may lead to permanent dilatation but this may be difficult to differentiate from other causes of upper tract dilatation such as obstruction. If the renal collecting system is seen to be dilated but the ureters are not visualised then the appearance may be mistaken for pelviureteric junction obstruction.

Reflux is common in children, being found in 25 per cent of neonates and infants. The incidence decreases with age and the majority of children have ceased to reflux by the age of 2 years. Bladder wall oedema during lower urinary tract infection may predispose to reflux, as do abnormalities of the vesicoureteric junction such as 'hutch diverticulum' and ectopic ureters. Reflux with upper tract infection may be the presenting signs of either bladder outlet obstruction or neurogenic bladder, and bladder function should be carefully assessed prior to surgical implantation of the ureters as a treatment for reflux.

4.1.18 POSTNEPHRECTOMY ABSCESS

A postnephrectomy abscess gives the appearance of a fluid collection in the renal bed although the presence of echogenic microbubbles may give a solid appearance. Identical appearances may occur with fluid-filled bowel loops lying in the renal bed.

4.1.19 PERIRENAL FLUID COLLECTIONS

Non-obstructive urinoma – blunt or penetrating trauma, surgery, infection, calculus erosion.

Obstructive urinoma – ureteral obstruction (calculus, surgical ligature, neoplasm), bladder outlet obstruction (posterior urethral valves).

Haematoma – trauma, renal biopsy, percutaneous stone removal, renal tumour rupture, renal cyst rupture, hepatic tumour rupture (right renal collection), anticoagulant therapy, aortic aneurysm rupture.

Infection – perinephric abscesses, sinus or fistula related to xanthogranulomatous pyelonephritis, renal mucomycosis (zygomycosis).

Lymph collection – lymphocoeles, lymphatic collection from trauma or malignant obstruction.

Pseudocyst – a pseudocyst may cause retroperitoneal fluid collections or free fluid from an acute pancreatitis.

Fluid mimic – malignant infiltration, particularly lymphoma which may cause a pre-renal hypoechoic collar mimicking a fluid collection.

4.1.20 RETAINED SURGICAL SWABS

Retained swabs give the appearance of a densely echogenic mass which, at high gain settings, may show linear folds. Swabs totally soaked in fluid without any gas present may actually give a woven pattern.

4.1.21 INFLAMMATORY RENAL PSEUDO-TUMOURS

Focal pyelonephritis (focal lobar nephronia).
Chronic pyelonephritis with areas of hypertrophy.
Focal xanthogranulomatous pyelonephritis.
Renal tuberculosis.
Pyonephrosis.
Echinococcus multilocularis.

Malakoplakia.
Renal aspergilloma.

4.1.22 CHRONIC AND COMPLEX RENAL INFECTIONS

Renal tuberculosis

The vascular nature of the kidneys allows haematological spread of tuberculosis from distant sites, usually the lungs. The bacilli are arrested in or around the glomeruli and give rise to multiple caseating granulomatous foci. At this stage the foci are microscopic and the kidney appears normal. The majority of foci heal but some enlarge and spread to the medulla. These may rupture into the calyces giving rise to cavities which communicate with the collecting system. Bacilluria is common in renal tuberculosis but despite this the majority of patients do not develop symptoms or signs of renal tuberculosis.

Sonography
Sonography is not as informative as an intravenous urogram or CT because of problems with identifying calyceal, pelvic or ureteric abnormalities.

- The kidney may appear entirely normal in early stages.
- Hypoechoic cystic masses communicating with the collecting system may be seen.
- Large abscesses may distort the renal contour and may mimic tumours and cysts. Fibrosis and scarring may give an appearance identical to chronic pyelonephritis or multiple renal infarcts. Calcification is common in late stages and varies from punctate foci to dense calcification of the whole kidney associated with hydronephrosis or atrophy (tuberculous autonephrectomy).

Bladder tuberculosis causes fibrosis and mucosal thickening leading to thick-walled small volume bladder with vesicoureteric reflux. Large granulomatous lesions in the ureters or bladder wall may mimic transitional cell lesions.

Chronic pyelonephritis

The typical intravenous urography finding is cortical scar opposite a blunted calyx. With severe scarring uninvolved areas of the kidney may enlarge forming pseudo-masses, this is best confirmed by a Tc-99m DMSA scan.

Chronic pyelonephritis causes areas of increased echogenicity associated with parenchymal thinning, reduced renal size and calyceal blunting. Similar renal parenchymal changes also occur in hypertensive nephrosclerosis, focal infarction and chronic glomerulonephritis.

Xanthogranulomatous pyelonephritis

This is a chronic granulomatous disease precipitated by recurrent renal infections. The process may be global (a non-functioning kidney) or focal mimicking a renal tumour. There is a frequent association with renal calculi and infection with *Proteus* spp. and *Escherichia coli*. The kidney is replaced by sheets of inflammatory and 'foam' cells. Diagnosis is difficult and sonographic and radiographic findings may mimic a renal tumour. Sonography shows an enlarged kidney with a thin parenchyma containing hypoechoic or anechoic masses. Calculi are frequently present and appear as central echogenic foci with shadowing.

Malakoplakia

Malakoplakia is a granulomatous disease associated with chronic *E. coli* infections. The bladder is the most common site affected but the kidney can be involved. Most occur in middle-aged women and by far the majority are unilateral and multifocal. Sonography shows an enlarged kidney associated with distortion and compression of the central echo complex by ill-defined solid or cystic masses. When unifocal a non-specific echogenic mass can be seen. Calcification is unusual.

Cholesteotoma

Chronic urinary tract infections, particularly tuberculosis, may cause squamous metaplasia of the epithelium of the urinary collecting system. Shedding of the squamous epithelium may form a keratinous ball within the renal pelvis or collecting system, called a cholesteotoma. This may manifest itself as a filling defect with a laminated or mottled appearance on an intravenous urography or retrograde pyelography. Computed tomography shows a high attenuation mass. Calcification may occur. It has no malignant potential. Ultrasound appearances have not been described.

Pyonephrosis

Infection in an obstructed or hydronephrotic kidney may lead to an accumulation of pus within the collecting system. Clinically a pyonephrosis may be suspected if a urinary tract infection proves difficult to treat or if the patient suffers recurrent episodes of septicaemia despite antibiotic treatment.

Sonography
Appearances may be identical to uncomplicated hydronephrosis despite the presence of thick pus in the collecting system. When in doubt, aspirate the pus under local anaesthesia.

There may be debris or dependent echoes in the collecting system. The urine in the collecting system may appear anechoic but distal acoustic enhancement may be markedly reduced.

Renal and perirenal abscesses

A renal abscess develops when focal pyelonephritis progresses to parenchymal necrosis. Most renal abscesses occur as a result of incomplete antibiotic treatment of urinary tract infections. The causative organisms in most cases are either *E. coli* or *Proteus mirabilis* although some cases of haematogenous spread may be due to *Staphylococcus aureus* infection. Many renal abscesses have extrarenal extension at presentation.

Sonography

A renal abscess may give a spectrum of appearances varying from that of a simple cyst to a debris and air-filled collection. The main features include the following.

1. Initially the affected area has a hypoechoic semi-solid appearance. This may resolve with treatment or progress.
2. There is a hypoechoic or anechoic mass with variable amounts of internal debris with enhanced through transmission.
3. A focal, primarily cystic, collection can be seen but through transmission is generally less than that of a cyst, the walls are usually thick with ill-defined margins.
4. Hyperechoic shadowing foci representing stones or gas may be present.

Ultrasound may underestimate perinephric extension of renal infection.

A chronic renal abscess may mimic a renal cell carcinoma, both clinically and on imaging. Aspiration under ultrasound guidance allows diagnosis.

Emphysematous pyelitis and pyelonephritis

Renal emphysema is gas in or around the kidney. The clinical presentation of emphysematous pyelonephritis is similar to pyonephrosis. When caused by an infection of renal parenchyma by gas forming organisms, the clinical outcome is potentially grave. It causes densely echogenic areas with 'dirty' distal shadowing/comet tail reverberation echoes. The kidney may be completely obscured by gas in the perinephric space

Aetiology of renal emphysema
Urological surgery.
Instrumentation – surgical.
Radiological intervention – nephrostomy, renal embolisation.

Acute pyelonephritis, particularly in diabetics and immune compromised patients.

Fistula with bowel – Crohn's, xanthogranulomatous pyelonephritis, diverticulitis, colonic carcinoma, ileal conduit, etc.

Penetrating trauma.

Differential diagnosis of renal emphysema

Stage horn calculi.

Renal calcification.

Fat-containing tumours.

Xanthogranulomatous pyelonephritis.

Anomalous position of the colon.

Fungal infections

The urinary tract can be infected by *Candida albicans*, *Cryptococcus* spp., *Coccidioides* spp., *Mucor* spp. (*zygomycosis*) and *Blastomyces* spp. especially in immune compromised individuals. The renal tract may be infected in isolation or more commonly it may be associated with a disseminated fungal infection. Acute pyelonephritis or multiple microabscesses may develop. The infection may invade the perinephric spaces. *C. albicans* may infect the urinary tract in an ascending manner. Most fungal infections are acute but some may turn chronic. A fungus ball may form in the renal collecting system. Renal aspergillomas are rare and are usually limited to the renal parenchyma or renal pelvis. They are uncommon in AIDS patients because phagocytic cell function is relatively preserved. Predisposing factors for urinary aspergillosis include diabetes mellitus, leukaemia, lymphoma and ureteral obstruction. Renal aspergillosis has a favourable prognosis if treated promptly.

Mucormycosis belongs to the subclass *Zygomycetes* that belongs to the order *Mucorales*. These fungi form non-septate hyphae with irregular branching. They exclusively infect the immunocompromised. The kidney is involved in 22 per cent of patients usually in the context of systemic mucormycosis. Isolated renal involvement is rare. The mortality is high. The final diagnosis of fungal urine infection rests on urine cultures.

Sonography

1. There is renal enlargement.
2. The microabscesses are too small to resolve but they may cause a 'snowstorm' appearance (see p. 314).
3. Multiple abscesses may make the kidney echogenic or hypoechoic.
4. Bezoars of debris and fungus balls form echogenic non-shadowing masses within the collecting system.

5. Fermentative gases may be produced by the fungi that are detectable on plain abdominal radiographs and ultrasound.
6. In renal mucormycosis the kidney is enlarged with a heterogeneous echopattern. Usually no normal renal tissue is identified and the cortico-medullary differentiation is lost. A small perirenal fluid collection is present. Colour Doppler sonography shows no flow within the mass.
7. The ultrasound features in renal aspergillosis have been described as single or multiple multiloculated cystic masses, however a solid renal mass due to a conglomerate of hyphae and necrotic tissue may be seen. Fungus balls causing pelviureteric junction or ureteric obstruction may ensue. A renal aspergilloma may mimic a tumour on sonography.

AIDS-related nephropathy

Renal disease in AIDS is an important cause of mortality and morbidity. It is associated with an almost 100 per cent mortality within 6 months of onset of uraemia despite the use of dialysis, although acute renal complications can be reversible with prompt assessment and management directed at correcting hydration, preventing sepsis and the careful monitoring of drugs. Renal infections are common and result in variable proteinuria and renal insufficiency. The following pathological changes have been reported

- segmental glomerulosclerosis
- interstitial fibrosis
- mononuclear cell infiltrate
- dilated tubules containing casts
- tubular atrophy
- acute tubular necrosis
- focal nephrocalcinosis.

NB *These pathological changes may also occur in heroin-associated nephropathy.*

A variety of renal diseases may cause nephromegaly due to renal oedema as a result of haemodynamic factors and toxins.

In fifty-eight per cent of AIDS patients with deteriorating renal function, the cortical echogenicity is equal to or greater than the liver. This non-specific appearance is related to a variety of glomerular and tubular abnormalities.

The incidence of acute and recurrent urinary tract infections in AIDS patients is as much as 50 per cent. Sonography may reveal enlarged oedematous kidneys with localised foci of increased or decreased echogenicity. Complications such as renal or perirenal abscesses may be identified.

Focal echogenic densities may develop, these may be well defined or have ill-defined margins, some of these are related to punctuate calcification which may or may not shadow. Similar densities may be present in the liver, spleen, pancreas and the adrenal glands. Inflammatory masses caused by mycobacteria and aspergillosis may produce hypoechoic masses indistinguishable from lymphomas.

Hydronephrosis may develop as a result of vesicoureteral reflux or obstruction from fungus balls

Non-Hodgkin's lymphoma and Kaposi's sarcoma may present as single or multiple hypoechoic masses that need to be distinguished from opportunistic infections. The kidney may be enlarged and diffusely infiltrated or it may be invaded from an adjacent organ. Lymphadenopathy may displace and obstruct the kidney. Renal cell carcinoma has been reported in a relatively young AIDS patient.

Renal hydatid disease

Hydatid disease occurs due to infection with *Echinococcus granulosus* or *E. multilocularis*. The liver is the most commonly affected organ but the kidney may also be involved. Granulosus infection usually has a cystic appearance, which initially is similar to a simple cyst but becomes more complex with time developing an endocyst and membranes. Separation of endocyst may give rise to the 'floating lily' sign of floating septae. As with the liver, renal hydatid cysts may be multiloculate, complex or solid, however a solid cyst is more common in multilocularis infection, which tends to be ill defined and infiltrative. Cyst-wall calcification results in a densely echogenic shadowing mass.

4.1.23 HYDRONEPHROSIS

The renal collecting system forms part of the echogenic central echo complex and is frequently not identifiable as a separate structure. Visualisation of the collecting system depends upon the rate of urine formation and the rate of urine drainage. The latter depends upon the system dispensability, ureteric peristalsis, the degree of bladder fullness and other mechanical factors. Slight collecting system dilatation is a common normal finding during a diuresis or when the bladder is quite full. In these cases the dilatation resolves when the bladder is emptied. Hydronephrosis is simply a dilatation of the renal collecting system. This is not always caused by an obstruction and similarly an obstruction does not always cause hydronephrosis. Hydronephrosis is seen as anechoic fluid in the renal collecting system and pelvis separating the central sinus echoes. Longstanding cases may show secondary thinning of the renal parenchyma. Dilated calyces lose their sharp angular margins and become blunted. When the hydronephrosis is marked, the entire collecting system is outlined as a series of connected fluid-filled channels.

Mimics of hydronephrosis

Normal variants – full bladder, extrarenal pelvis, congenital megacalyces, lucent pyramids, calyceal diverticula, distensible collecting system.

Increased diuresis – over-hydration, diuretics, diabetes insipidus, contrast media, osmotic load, non-oliguric renal failure.

Inflammatory disease – acute pyelonephritis (generalised collecting system dilatation), chronic pyelonephritis (calyceal blunting), tuberculosis and other cavities, papillary necrosis, postinfective calyceal distortion, reflux nephropathy.

Renal cystic disease.

Postobstructive residual dilatation.

Renal cachexia in oncological patients (treated or untreated cancer patients).

The presence of blood vessels mimicking grade 1 hydronephrosis.

Intrarenal varices.

Hydronephrotic type of multicystic dysplastic kidney in children.

Pancreatic pseudocyst.

Calyceal diverticula.

Lucent renal pyramids.

Renal artery aneurysm.

Arteriovenous malformation.

Renal sinus lipomatosis (rare lucent form).

Sonolucent renal masses.

Anterior lumbar meningocoele.

Parapelvic cysts.

Parapelvic cysts

One to three per cent of cysts originate either from the central sinus or parapelvic renal parenchyma. Although they can occasionally resemble a dilated pelvis the remaining sinus echoes appear normal, a false diagnosis of renal obstruction is seldom a problem. Occasionally excretory urography may be needed to exclude pelvicalyceal dilatation. An isotope renogram will also exclude an obstructive uropathy.

4.1.24 URINARY TRACT OBSTRUCTION: FALSE NEGATIVE DIAGNOSIS

Acute obstruction – upper tracts are not yet dilated, increased intracalyceal pressure may drastically reduce glomerular filtration rate.

Dehydration.

Intermittent obstruction.

Ruptured collecting system.
Bladder outflow obstruction.
Spontaneous decompression of an obstructed system (back flow).
Staghorn calculus – obscures dilated collecting system.
Multiple parapelvic cysts with superimposed obstruction.
Misinterpretation of hydronephrosis as polycystic disease.
Caliectasis – dilated calyces can be mistaken for prominent renal pyramids.
Retroperitoneal fibrosis – the degree of renal failure is far greater than the degree of urinary dilatation.
Technical factors – obesity, overlying bowel loops, etc.
Obstructed moiety in a duplex kidney – it may be atrophic and difficult to visualise.

4.1.25 THE KIDNEY IN PREGNANCY

The renal collecting system may dilate in pregnancy during the third trimester. Dilatation is most marked at 28 weeks and is usually more prominent on the right than the left. This is associated with an increased risk of urinary tract infection.

4.1.26 CALIECTASIS

Localised caliectasis

Pyelonephritis
Compound calyx.
Calyceal diverticulum.
Congenital megacalyx.
Localised obstruction or postobstruction.
Focal tuberculosis.
Papillary necrosis.
Infundibular calculus.
Trauma.

Generalised caliectasis

Postobstructive atrophy.
Congenital megacalyces (the renal pelvis is usually of normal size).
Obstructive uropathy.
Non-obstructive dilatation.

4.1.27 COLLECTING SYSTEM MASSES

Masses are easier to identify in a dilated than a non-dilated collecting system. The mass may be the cause of the dilatation, a secondary effect or an incidental finding.

Calculus pattern

Echogenic mass with or without shadowing.
Calculus.
Tumour with surface calcification.
Gas.
Calcification in adjacent renal artery.
Surgical stent or drain.
Tuberculosis autonephrectomy.

Soft-tissue pattern

Transitional cell tumour.
Squamous cell carcinoma.
Blood clot.
Adenocarcinoma of the renal pelvis (rare).
Medullary carcinoma of the renal pelvis (associated with sickle cell trait).
Pyonephrosis – debris or sludge.
Fungus ball.
Sloughed papilla.
Leukoplakia or cholesteotoma.
Malakoplakia.

Renal calculi

Renal calculi give rise to densely echogenic foci with distal shadowing unless they are narrower than the ultrasound beam. Non-shadowing calculi are easily lost in the central echo complex if the collecting system is not dilated.

4.1.28 RENAL CYSTIC DISEASE

Renal cysts are a common incidental finding on ultrasonography but they may also form part of a specific disease process. Differentiation of the pattern of cystic disease is necessary for diagnosis.

Classification of renal cystic disease

Renal dysplasia
Multicystic dysplastic kidney (Potter 2).
Focal and segmental renal dysplasia.
Familial renal dysplasia.
Multiple cysts associated with lower urinary tract obstruction.

Polycystic disease
Autosomal recessive (Potter 1).
Autosomal dominant (Potter 3).
Glomerulocystic disease.

Cortical cysts
Tuberous sclerosis.
Trisomy 13–15, 17–18.
Potter type 4 – small cortical cysts with obstructive hydronephrosis.
Multilocular cysts.
Chronic dialysis.

Medullary cysts
Medullary sponge kidney.
Familial juvenile nephronophthisis – medullary cystic disease complex.
Medullary necrosis.
Pyelogenic cysts.

Miscellaneous cysts
Inflammatory cysts – abscesses.
Tuberculosis.
Echinococcus granulosis.
Calculus disease.
Haematoma.

Cystic neoplasms
Cystic renal cell carcinoma.
Cystic Wilms' tumour.

Extraparenchymal cysts
Parapelvic – outside the renal capsule but adjacent to the renal pelvis.
Perinephric cysts.

Simple renal cysts

The exact aetiology of simple renal cysts is uncertain, they may be retention cysts caused by an obstruction or they may arise in embryonic rests. They are uncommon in children (found in 2 to 4 per cent of paediatric post mortems) but they occur with increasing frequency with age and are found in 50 per cent of adults over 50 years old. Simple cysts are usually asymptomatic unless complicated by

- haemorrhage or infection
- size – a mass effect
- position – those that arise in a parapelvic position may compress part of the renal collecting system.

Sonography

1. The cyst is entirely echofree.
2. Good sound transmission gives rise to distal acoustic enhancement.
3. The cyst has a smooth outline without a demonstrable wall.
4. Small cysts may only appear echofree when they are in the focal zone of the ultrasound beam because of a partial volume effect, and very small cysts (less than 3 mm in diameter) cannot be identified in the parenchyma.

Ultrasonography is more accurate than CT at visualisation of internal septae and the demonstration of internal cyst morphology. If there is any doubt about the nature of a cyst identified at sonography then a follow up scan or cyst aspiration should be performed. If the appearances are classically those of a simple cyst then no further action need be taken.

Simple renal cyst aspirate contents

Fluid is straw coloured.
Cyst fluid should not contain fat.
Cyst fluid LDH level should be less than the serum LDH level at the same time.
The cyst should not contain blood or altered blood products.

NB Sonography cannot reliably differentiate simple cysts from those complicated by infection and aspiration may yield pus even though the cysts appear anechoic.

Characteristics of atypical renal cysts

Shape

The cyst is not entirely circular or has irregular margins.

Cyst wall

An irregular outline may be due to cyst collapse, haemorrhage or infection, but elevations and irregularities of a cyst wall may also be caused by a tumour.

Cyst wall calcification is uncommon in simple cysts. It also occurs in tumours and does not differentiate benign from malignant cysts.

Fluid contents

Internal echoes are usually caused by intracyst haemorrhage or, less often, infection. Tumours rarely undergo sufficient necrosis to mimic simple cysts. Necrotic tumours usually have a complex appearance. Fine internal septations are usually due to previous haemorrhage or infection.

Causes of atypical renal cysts

Collapsed old benign cysts.
Septated benign cysts.
Haemorrhagic benign cysts.
Cysts with intracystic carcinoma.
Echinococcal cysts.
Renal abscesses.
Cystic nephroma.
Necrotic tumour.
Tumours in cyst wall.
Cystic degeneration in an adenoma.
Focal xanthogranulomatous pyelonephritis.

Complex renal masses

Complex renal masses may have both cystic and solid elements but one needs to exclude reverberation echoes at the near wall which may artificially give rise to a solid appearance near the cyst wall closest to the ultrasound probe.

Renal tumours (primary) – necrotic tumour, adenoma (cystic degeneration), multilocular cystic nephroma, Wilms' tumour, clear cell sarcoma.
Renal tumours (metastases).
Complicated simple cysts – infected, haemorrhagic, multiple, multiloculated.
Inflammatory masses – abscesses, echinococcal cysts, duplication with obstruction, pyonephrosis, focal xanthogranulomatous pyelonephritis.
Traumatic causes – haematoma, hemorrhagic infarct.
Miscellaneous masses – arteriovenous fistula, polycystic (a conglomerate of cysts may mimic a complex cyst).

Calcified renal cysts

Simple cyst (rare).
Adult polycystic disease.
Tumour.
Calcium deposition in a calyceal diverticulum or hydrocalyx.

Echinococcal cysts.
Old multicystic dysplastic kidney.
Healed abscesses.

Haemorrhagic cysts

Haemorrhage into a simple cyst.
Liquefied haematoma.
Focal infection.
Focal infarction.
Cystic degeneration in a tumour – appearances are variable and may be identical to
a simple cyst or may show irregular borders and internal echoes.

Lesions that mimic renal cysts

Prominent renal pyramids.
Intrarenal aneurysm, arteriovenous malformation.
Haematoma.
Abscesses.
Focal hydronephrosis.
Pyonephrosis.
Calyceal diverticula.
Tuberculous cavities.
Duplication.
Necrotic tumour.
Urinoma.
Lymphoma and hypoechoic masses – on high gain settings these deposits may show
internal echoes and less distal enhancement than cysts.

4.1.29 INTRARENAL FLUID COLLECTIONS

Cysts including polycystic disease.
Calyceal diverticula.
Renal papillary necrosis.
Calyceal dilatation.
Dilated moiety of a duplex kidney.
Hydronephrosis.
Abscesses.
Tuberculous cavities.
Necrotic carcinoma or metastases.
Echinococcal cysts.
Renal artery aneurysm.
Haematoma.

4.1.30 CONGENITAL CYSTIC DILATATIONS OF THE UPPER URINARY TRACT

Malformations of the upper urinary tract are frequently found, probably as a result of the complicated development of the ureteral bud. The ureteral bud grows cephalad and branches repeatedly for fifteen generations. The branches evolve into the ureter, renal pelvis, calyces and the collecting tubules. Cystic dilatations of the collecting system may be considered as an anomalous growth disturbance at various stages of the development of the ureteral bud.

Primary megaureter

This is a developmental anomaly in which ureteral dilatation occurs above a short adynamic extravesical distal ureteral segment. This narrowing is unassociated with vesicoureteral reflux or bladder outlet obstruction. When examined fluoroscopically about 1.5 cm of extravesical distal segment of the ureter appears as a narrow band which does not transmit a peristaltic wave. This may be because of a muscle anomaly, collagenous infiltration or an aganglionic segment of ureter analogous to Hirschsprung's disease of the bowel. Above this narrowed segment the distal one-third or half of the ureter is dilated in up to 50 per cent of patients whilst in the other half the whole ureter is dilated. Ureteral drainage is invariably delayed. In children the male to female ratio is 4 : 1, bilateral disease is exclusively found in boys (20 per cent incidence). In adults the abnormality is 2.5 times more frequent on the left. There is a 40 per cent association with other urogenital anomalies

- pelviureteric junction obstruction in 25 per cent
- contralateral vesicoureteral reflux in 6 to 8 per cent
- contralateral renal agenesis in 4 to 15 per cent
- contralateral ureteral duplication in 2 to 6 per cent
- contralateral calyceal diverticulum in 4 per cent
- contralateral ureterocoeles in 3 per cent of cases.

On the ipsilateral side cryptorchism, megacalyces and ectopic ureterocoeles have been recorded. Patients may present with urinary tract infection or calculus disease. Primary megaureter needs to be differentiated from secondary megaureter due to reflux, organic obstruction or obstruction masked by reflux.

Multicystic dysplastic kidney

Multicystic dysplastic kidney is the commonest cause of an abdominal mass in the neonate and accounts for 50 to 65 per cent of renal masses in the same age group. It is a developmental anomaly caused by atresia of the upper third of the ureter. In most cases there is concomitant atresia of the renal pelvis and infundibula. The underlying obstruction usually occurs at or before 8 to 10 weeks of life. Obstruction occurring at a later stage gives rise to a rarer combination of renal dysplasia and hydronephrosis. In 33 per cent of patients there are contralateral renal anomalies such as multicystic dysplastic kidney, pelviuteric junction obstruction, hypoplasia and rotational anomalies. When ureteric duplication is encountered on the contralateral side, one of the ureters may be atretic with associated segmental renal dysplasia.

Sonography

Sonographic appearances are of a large unilateral renal mass with 10 to 20, but sometimes up to 50, cysts of varying sizes. There may be islands of dysplastic renal tissue between the cysts but no normal tissue is seen. Sonography can differentiate between multicystic dysplastic kidney, hydronephrosis, Wilms' tumour, neuroblastoma, mesoblastic nephroma and adrenal haemorrhage.

Pelviureteric junction obstruction

The most common congenital urinary tract obstruction occurs at the pelviureteric junction. The site of obstruction is at the first bifurcation of the ureteral bud and is invariably seen in the ampullary type of renal pelvis rather than the bifid type. There is great variation in disease severity and age at presentation and the obstruction evolves over a period of time. It may be bilateral (30 per cent) or unilateral though in bilateral cases the kidneys may be affected at different times. The left kidney is affected slightly more often than the right. Associated upper urinary tract anomalies occur in 16 to 19 per cent of cases, these include ipsilateral reflux, ipsilateral duplex, horseshoe kidney, solitary kidney and contralateral multicystic dysplastic kidney.

Sonography

Dilatation of the renal collecting system and pelvis without ureteric dilatation. In severe cases there may be marked parenchymal thinning until the kidney eventually becomes 'a bag of water'. Pelviureteric junction obstruction may be intermittent and may only occur during the stress of diuresis, thus in uncertain cases repeat the examination after oral fluids with or without intravenous diuretics.

NB Reflux coexists with pelviureteric junction obstruction and may cause ureteric dilatation. Urine may reflux into an obstructed pelvis as the obstruction is usually only in the normal direction of flow.

Pyelocalyceal diverticulum

Pyelocalyceal diverticula are developmental, smooth-walled uroepithelium-lined outpouchings of the renal pelvis or calyces that lie within the renal parenchyma. They can be classified into Type I, the more common variety connected to the calyceal cup, and Type II, these are interpolar and communicate directly with the renal pelvis. They are thought to result when a generation of ureteric bud divisions is not assimilated into the wall of the collecting system. The most common presentation is with urinary tract infections and calculus formation. Rarely they may be complicated by transitional cell carcinoma. They are readily identified by intravenous urography though the isthmus may not be identified. Sonography may reveal cystic lesions at the corticomedullary junction that are indistinguishable from simple cysts apart from the location. They must be distinguished from acquired diverticula as a result of a calculus or an infection causing stenosis of an infundibulum. A hydrocalyx can be differentiated by its location which is the normal position of a calyx.

Congenital megacalyx

Congenital megacalyx refers to a non-obstructive enlargement of the calyces. These calyces are polygonal in shape and are found in increased numbers compared to anatomically normal kidneys. The cortical thickness is normal although the medullary pyramids are decreased in thickness. The polycalyces, the presence of a normal cortex and the polygonal shape of the calyces exclude pathological states. There is an association of mega-ureter with megacalyces, which may lead to an erroneous diagnosis of hydronephrosis.

The renal pelvis is of normal size and configuration, the infundibula are short and broad and the renal pyramids are short in radial length.

Medullary sponge kidney

Medullary sponge kidney is thought to represent dysplastic, cylindrical or saccular dilatation of the papillary collecting ducts. These dilated collecting ducts result in enlargement of the papilla associated with widening and deepening of the calyceal cups. Presentation usually occurs in the second to fourth decades with abdominal pain, haematuria and pyelonephritis. Thirty per cent of patients also have hypercalciuria and small calculi usually form in the dilated papillary collecting ducts. The condition is of variable severity and may affect a single lobe of one kidney or it may be found throughout both kidneys. Intravenous urography may show radial strands or cystic collections of contrast medium in the papillae in the majority of cases associated with spherical or cylindrical calcification in the distribution of the papilla in 10 to 15 per cent of patients.

Sonography
Sonographically the kidneys may appear normal or may show increased pyramidal echogenicity because of the presence of multiple small calculi. Occasionally small cysts are seen.

Familial juvenile nephronophthisis and medullary cystic disease complex (JN-MCD)

Juvenile nephronophthisis and medullary cystic disease both cause severe medullary cystic disease, and both are known as autosomal inherited renal diseases with similar clinical characteristics. Although some authors distinguish between juvenile nephronophthis as a recessive disorder which manifests itself in childhood, whilst medullary cystic disease is autosomal dominant which typically presents in adults, most workers prefer the term JN-MCD to describe these diseases with overlapping manifestations. Presentation is with renal failure, hypertension, proteinuria and occasionally salt losing nephropathy.

Sonography
Sonographically the kidneys are small and hyperechoic with loss of corticomedullary differentiation associated with medullary cysts. However renal medullary cysts are not a prerequisite for diagnosis of JN-MCD as they are present only in two-thirds of patients presenting with terminal uraemia. It has been postulated that the increasing numbers of acystic cases seen lately is possibly related to early detection by sonography before cysts are large enough to be detected by ultrasound and patients become symptomatic. The cysts may be single or multiple, tiny or large. Single large cysts may mimic simple renal cysts.

Autosomal recessive polycystic kidney disease

Also known as infantile polycystic disease, this is thought to occur as a result of dysplasia of the upper collecting system or collecting tubule resulting in cysts of varying sizes. Microdissection studies have shown fusiform sacculations and cystic diverticula of the distal portions of collecting tubules and collecting ducts whilst the proximal collecting tubules show diffuse dilatation. The condition is inherited in an autosomal recessive manner and usually presents in infancy or childhood though it may be diagnosed *in utero* by ultrasonography. Disease severity is usually greater in cases which present early. Renal involvement is bilateral but may be asymmetric.

There is an association with hepatic fibrosis and ductal hyperplasia, that may cause portal hypertension. In the context of autosomal recessive polycystic renal disease death is usually caused by renal failure in the youngest children and by hepatic failure in the older children. The disease may be subdivided by age at presentation

- prenatal form – this presents in infants, is rapidly fatal, 90 per cent of renal tubules are involved
- infantile form – 60 per cent of tubules are involved, the child has uraemia but survives longer than those with the prenatal form
- young children – presentation with hypertension and chronic renal failure, 25 per cent of the renal tubules are involved
- late presentation (juvenile form) – symptoms are usually related to hepatic fibrosis, portal hypertension and gastrointestinal haemorrhage, small cysts can sometimes be seen in the renal cortex.

Sonography

The kidneys are diffusely enlarged with generalised increase in echoes produced by the innumerable fluid–tubular wall interfaces. There is poor definition of the renal borders and loss of corticomedullary differentiation. Increased echogenicity of the liver is frequently seen. The peripheral cortex may be spared as the peripheral cortex does not have collecting ducts. This feature is found in infants who do not have severe disease and are likely to survive infancy. However in severely affected infants there may be a peripheral sonolucent halo that may represent markedly dilated ectatic tubules near the renal surface. With high-resolution probes a radial array of ectatic dilated tubules 1 to 2 mm in diameter are seen. *In utero* the normal combined renal circumference is 27 to 30 per cent of the abdominal circumference. In infantile polycystic disease this increases to 60 per cent allowing prenatal diagnosis.

Glomerulocystic disease

Glomerulocystic disease is an unusual sporadic condition characterised by cystic dilatation of the space of Bowman and the proximal convoluted tubule in the absence of urinary obstruction. The renal medulla is normal as the loop of Henle and collecting ducts are spared. These cysts are usually 2 to 3 mm in diameter but may be up to 1 cm and occasionally even larger. The majority of visible cysts occur in the cortex and may be accompanied by interstitial renal disease. Glomerulocystic disease does not usually show Mendelian inheritance but may occur in association with tuberous sclerosis, trisomy 13, cerebrohepatorenal syndrome, Zellweger syndrome, orofaciodigital syndrome or renal retinal dysplasia. Generally renal failure occurs and the prognosis is poor.

Sonography

The sonographic appearance is that of bilateral enlarged echogenic kidneys with normal renal outline but loss of corticomedullary differentiation. Tiny peripheral subcapsular cortical cysts are seen, the entire cortex may be involved. No cysts are seen in the medulla in contrast to ADPCKD (autosomal dominant polycystic kidney disease) in which cysts are seen both in the renal cortex and the medulla. Inflammatory changes and fibrosis may occur in the medulla secondary to glomerulocystic disease leading to increased medullary echogenicity. Eventually the kidney size may decrease in relation to body size and age. Punctate calcification in the thin peripheral renal tissue surrounding the cortical cysts has been reported on follow-up scans and would tend to increase the echogenicity of cyst walls. If no cysts are seen in enlarged echogenic kidneys differentiation from autosomal recessive polycystic kidney disease (ARPKD) may not be possible.

Adult polycystic kidney disease (ADPCKD)

Adult polycystic kidney disease is transmitted as an autosomal dominant condition which affects approximately 1 in 1000 of the population. The cysts arise from the nephrons and the collecting tubules. Islands of normal parenchymal renal tissues are interspaced between the cysts. Microdissection reveals that the cysts directly communicate with the nephrons and collecting tubules. Presentation is usually with hypertension and progressive renal failure after the third decade. Uncommonly it presents in children and has rarely been seen in neonates. Thirty to forty per cent of cases are associated with hepatic cysts, 10 per cent with pancreatic cysts, 5 per cent with splenic cysts and uncommonly pulmonary cysts occur. These extrarenal manifestations are not found in cases in neonates and children.

Sonography

Sonography is a valuable screening test in cases of suspected polycystic disease. In children most cases have a normal scan at birth. In neonates that are severely affected the kidneys are large and echogenic with loss of corticomedullary differentiation indistinguishable from ARPCKD. When cysts are seen they are of varying sizes scattered throughout the cortex including the medulla and subcapsular location, by contrast in ARPCKD the peripheral cortex is spared in mild disease. Sequential examinations usually demonstrate an increase in these cysts over a period of years resulting in calyceal distortion and irregularity of the renal outline. The cysts may have irregular walls and may show internal echoes if they have been complicated by haemorrhage or infection. Surviving islands of renal parenchyma may be seen between the cysts. Calcification of cyst walls may be seen later in life.

When screening for evidence of ADPCKD, if the kidney shows no evidence of cysts or parenchymal abnormality by the age of 19 years the patient is extremely unlikely to be affected.

Differential diagnosis

- Any cause of multiple intrarenal fluid collections.
- Hydrocalycosis, particularly if the renal pelvis is not dilated.
- Multiple hypo- or anechoic nodes, for example lymphoma.

Multilocular renal cyst

This condition is synonymous with benign multilocular cystic nephroma, cystic Wilms' tumour, hamartoma, cystic adenoma, polycystic nephroblastoma, Perlman tumour and segmental multicystic kidney. These confusing terms indicate the uncertainty of its aetiology, whether the lesion is dysplastic, neoplastic or hamartomatous. Morphologically it forms a well-defined bulky mass arising at the lower pole or between poles of an otherwise normal-looking kidney. The mass has a fibrous capsule which may contain smooth muscle and cartilage. The tumour mass itself has multiloculated non-communicating cysts separated by fibrous tissue. The tumour often protrudes into the renal pelvis and approximately 50 per cent of tumours calcify. It has been postulated that a focal failure of a ureteral branch to organise this segment of the metanephric blastema would give rise to this appearance. The presence of undifferentiated mesenchymal tissue within the various constituents of the fibrous capsule supports the postulate that this tumour is a renal dysplasia.

Sonography

Sonographically the appearance is that of a bulky renal mass with a conglomerate of cysts separated by thick septa protruding into the renal pelvis. Calcification is detected in some masses.

Differential diagnosis of multicystic dysplastic kidney

Gross hydronephrosis.
Multicystic cyst.
Cystic nephroma.
Cystic hamartoma.
Cystic lymphangioma.
Multilocular renal cyst.
Multiple simple cysts (very rare in children).

4.1.31 RENAL FAILURE

Renal failure is a degree of renal insufficiency which causes substantial alteration in plasma biochemistry. The main uses of ultrasonography in renal failure are the exclusion of obstruction to urine drainage, demonstration of renal parenchymal abnormalities and guided biopsy. Acute renal failure results from obstruction to drainage in only 5 per cent of cases. Sonography can reliably exclude dilatation of the urinary tract but this does not entirely exclude obstruction, particularly if the patient is dehydrated. In cases of doubt antegrade pyelography should be performed. Polyuric renal failure may cause distension of the urinary tract particularly if the patient is scanned with a full bladder and this may be mistaken for obstruction.

Causes of renal failure

Poor perfusion – prerenal failure
Major vessel disease – renal artery avulsion, renal artery embolus, congestion (renal vein thrombosis).

Renal disease
Acute tubular necrosis.
Acute glomerulonephritis.
Interstitial nephritis.
Small blood vessel disease – malignant hypertension, haemolytic uraemic syndrome, etc.
Multiple renal infarcts
Polycystic disease
Infection

Metabolic disorders
Diabetes.
Amyloid.
Gout.
Dysproteinaemia
Myoglobinuria.
Radiation nephritis.
Renal tubular disease – tubular acidosis.

Urinary tract obstruction – bladder
Outlet obstruction – prostatism.
Bilateral ureteric obstruction.

4.1.32 MYOGLOBINURIA

Myoglobinuria occurs when muscle necrosis allows myoglobin to enter the blood stream. Severe cases cause acute renal failure. Sonographically the kidneys appear swollen with increased cortical echogenicity with preservation of the corticomedullary junction.

4.1.33 THE TRANSPLANTED KIDNEY

The transplanted kidney is usually situated in the iliac fossa on the opposite side from which it was derived. It is superficial and thus accessible to examination with high-frequency probes. A base line scan is often taken around 5 days post-transplant to assess renal size, shape, volume and echopattern. Immediately after the operation the kidney appears normal. It than becomes oedematous making the pyramids appear sonolucent relative to the central sinus. There is frequently slight fullness of the collecting system, this should not be assumed to be caused by obstruction. After transplantation the kidney hypertrophies with renal volume increasing by around 22 per cent by the end of the third week. A greater increase in renal volume suggests rejection.

NB   In the transplanted kidney the renal pelvis is usually anterior with the renal artery and vein lying posteriorly.

Acute tubular necrosis in a renal transplant

Acute tubular necrosis usually occurs within 72 hours after transplantation presenting with oliguria. Usually there are no constitutional symptoms. Improvement may take from a few days to 6 weeks. Predisposing factors in transplant acute tubular necrosis include cadaveric transplant, transplanted kidneys with more than one renal artery and prolonged interval in harvesting the kidney and transplantation.

Sonography
Sonography reveals enlargement of the transplanted kidney associated with a transient rise in the resistive index.

Acute renal transplant rejection

Rejection is a dynamic process, not an all-or-nothing phenomenon. Rejection occurs in most transplanted kidneys to some degree. It may be affected by many factors particularly by immunosuppressive drugs. Acute rejection may rarely be hyperacute occurring minutes after transplantation, accelerated rejection that occurs within a few days, but more commonly within

5 days to 6 months. This results in a wide spectrum of disease severity, which in turn gives a spectrum of sonographic changes.

Ultrasonography of acute renal transplant rejection

Sonography has a 30 to 50 per cent negative predictive value.

There is an increase in renal size because of oedema.

There is an increased renal volume more than 20 per cent in 5 days, more than 25 per cent in 14 days, more than 30 per cent in 21 days. (Renal volume is approximately equal to renal length × width × depth × 0.49.)

Increased cortical thickness is seen.

There are large sonolucent pyramids and increasing corticomedullary differentiation.

Conversely renal parenchyma can also be sonolucent reducing corticomedullary differentiation.

Renal pyramid length × pyramid width ÷ by cortical thickness = 4.6 (normal value). During acute rejection renal pyramidal swelling increases this index to around 7.5.

There is reduced echogenicity of the central echo complex, which may eventually be reduced to a small group of echogenic foci. Thickening of the pelvoinfundibular wall.

Areas of haemorrhage and infarction may give rise to a heterogeneous echopattern.

Renal haematoma.

Renal vein thrombosis.

Renal rupture.

Perinephric fluid collections occur early after transplant rejection in up to 50 per cent of patients (non-specific).

Doppler sonography has a higher accuracy in diagnosing rejection. The hallmark of acute transplant rejection is diminished diastolic flow in the intrarenal arteries due to increased vascular resistance. Calculating the resistive index can increase the diagnostic accuracy. Initially there may be a decrease in resistive index, but with increasing severity of rejection the resistive index increases. A resistive index greater than 0.90 has a 100 per cent positive predictive value and 26 per cent sensitivity for renal transplant rejection.

Duplex sonography lacks specificity in the diagnosis of renal transplant rejection as high vascular impedance can be encountered in acute tubular necrosis, pyelonephritis, renal vein obstruction and extrarenal compression besides acute rejection. However most non-rejection complications can be diagnosed clinically and although some overlap is encountered, acute vascular renal transplant rejection remains the major cause of higher vascular impedance.

Chronic renal transplant rejection

Initially the kidney is normal in size but cortical echogenicity increases because of periglomerular cellular infiltration and cortical fibrosis. The kidney slowly reduces in size and the pyramids become increasingly echogenic causing loss of corticomedullary differentiation. Appearances are eventually the same as any end stage renal parenchymal disease. Chronic rejection still needs a biopsy for reliable diagnosis.

Acute post-transplant renal failure

Acute tubular necrosis.
Acute rejection.
Arterial obstruction.
Renal vein thrombosis.
Ureteric obstruction.
Pyelonephritis.
Cytomegalovirus infection.

Renal allograft complications

Systemic complications

Despite improvements in immunosuppressive therapy opportunistic infections remain a problem. The organisms involved are similar to those seen in AIDS patients. Malignant tumours of all kinds occur more frequently after renal transplantation, lymphomas being the commonest. There is also a higher incidence of cardiovascular disease. There is an increased incidence of acquired cystic disease in the native kidney with 1 per cent risk of renal cell carcinoma. Pancreatitis occurs in 2.3 per cent of renal transplant patients with a mortality rate of up to 80 per cent following pseudocyst formation.

Transplant hydronephrosis: aetiology

Ureteric oedema.
Ureteric stricture.
Ureteric ischaemia.
Extrinsic compression – lymphocoele, haematoma, urinoma, abscesses.
Calculi.
Clot in the collecting system.
A functional obstruction may occur as a result of over-distension of the bladder.
Ureteric obstruction occurs in 2 to 7.5 per cent of patients. Hydronephrosis is readily seen on ultrasound. However a degree of calyceal dilatation is fairly common after transplantation but increasing calyceal dilatation suggests obstructed renal drainage.

Perinephric fluid collections

Perinephric fluid collections occur in 50 per cent of patients. The significance of fluid collection around the transplanted kidney depends upon its size and location. A thin rim of fluid around a transplanted kidney is common and should not be assumed to be pathological. Ultrasound with guided aspiration and drainage is the primary method of diagnosis in most perinephric fluid collections with a success rate of 80 per cent.

Haematomas

Haematomas often appear as complex collections which usually occur immediately after surgery or following a percutaneous biopsy, but they may follow rejection as complication of hypertension.

Urinomas

Urinomas are found in 3 to 10 per cent of kidney transplants and can cause loss of a kidney. Leaks can result from the anastamotic site at the vesicoureteric junction or from the ureter following vascular injury. Late urinomas may be due to biopsy, trauma, infection or ischaemia. Drainage of urinoma and percutaneous nephrostomy with stenting is successful in many cases.

Abscesses

Perirenal abscesses form complex collections. The presence of air within a perinephric collection of fluid is highly suggestive of an abscess. Guided aspiration allows diagnosis and provides aspirate for culture and sensitivity.

Lymphocoeles

Lymphocoeles form in 18 per cent of renal transplant patients because of division of lymphatics at surgery. The kidneys produce as much lymph each day as they do urine (1.5 to 2.0 L) thus the occurrence of lymphocoeles is not surprising. They usually present 2 to 6 weeks postoperatively but may be exacerbated by rejection. They tend to be large and are usually situated adjacent to the lower pole of the transplant, where they can obstruct the ureter or compress the bladder or vascular structures.

Sonography The sonographic appearances are those of a large multiseptate fluid collection, but fine needle aspiration may be necessary for diagnosis. Aspiration alone is not a successful form of treatment because of the recurrence of the lymphocoele. More successful forms of treatment include external drainage, transperitoneal marsupialisation or peritoneal venous shunting.

Renal artery stenosis

This is seen in about 10 per cent of postrenal transplant patients and is the most important cause of treatable hypertension. The site of stenosis is not at the anastamotic site in the majority of patients. Duplex and colour

Doppler ultrasound has had a great impact on the diagnosis of renal artery stenosis. The most reliable Doppler criteria for stenosis are a high-velocity jet and distal turbulence.

Renal vein thrombosis

Renal vein thrombosis is possibly caused by compression of the renal vein from the adjacent graft. A higher incidence has also been reported when ciclosporin is used in the immunosuppressive regime. Renal vein thrombosis is often secondary to iliac vein thrombosis. On Doppler ultrasound the thrombus itself may be directly visualised. There is usually complete absence of venous flow. There is a high vascular resistance within the graft. The arterial signal may show a sharp systolic peak with a notch on the reverse diastolic component resembling an inverted 'M'.

Acute tubular necrosis

See p. 335.

4.1.34 CAUSES OF PERIRENAL FLUID COLLECTIONS

Abscesses.

Loculated ascites.

Urinoma – anechoic fluid collection usually without septae or debris unless complicated by infection or haemorrhage. Most cases are secondary to obstruction, calculi, trauma, surgery or radiological intervention.

Haematoma – this may appear solid or fluid depending upon the stage of formation or liquefaction.

Lymphocoele see pp. 324, 349, 523.

Pancreatic or cerebrospinal fluid pseudocysts may track into the perinephric spaces.

Malignant infiltration around the kidney may be remarkably hypoechoic and may be mistaken for fluid collection. Lymphoma may completely encircle a kidney, giving rise to a hypoechoic mantle.

4.1.35 THE URETERS

The ureters lie on the anterior surface of the psoas near its medial edge. In the pelvis they cross anterior to the common iliac vessels in front of the sacroiliac joints. They turn forwards at the level of the ischial spines and in the female the ureter passes close to the lateral fornix of the vagina. The normal ureter is of small calibre and not usually visualised. When dilated the ureters may be identified as a tubular fluid-filled structure continuous with the renal pelvis or lying behind the bladder. A dilated ureter may indent a partially filled bladder and mimic a ureterocoele.

4.1.36 MEGAURETERS IN CHILDREN

Classification

Primary   These are non-obstructive and non-refluxing.
Secondary   These are caused by reflux, obstruction or obstruction masked by reflux.

The patient usually presents with urinary tract infection. The upper ureter is dilated though dilatation of the renal collecting system and lower ureter is variable. The underlying abnormality is lack of transmission of peristalsis in a short segment of ureter which may be narrowed. This may be because of muscle anomaly, collagenous infiltration or an aganglionic segment of ureter analogous to Hirschsprung's disease of the bowel.

4.1.37 PRUNE BELLY SYNDROME (EAGLE–BARRETT SYNDROME)

This syndrome comprises deficiency of the abdominal musculature, cryptorchidism and urinary tract abnormality. The eventual prognosis depends upon the degree of underlying renal dysplasia and malformation. There is an intrinsic ureteric defect, which gives rise to elongated tortuous ureters with upper tract dilatation. Ureteric dilatation is often massive and far greater than calyceal dilatation. Mild cases show fluid-filled flank masses representing dysplastic kidneys with ureteric dilatation.

4.1.38 RETROPERITONEAL FIBROSIS

Retroperitoneal fibrosis fixes the ureters and prevents peristalsis leading to functional obstruction though the ureteric lumen is not obliterated and a retrograde catheter can be introduced via the bladder. Fibrosis may be secondary to autoimmune disease (inflammation), retroperitoneal haemorrhage, malignancy or drug toxicity. The degree of renal failure is far greater than that suggested by the degree of upper tract dilatation, which may be slight. A soft-tissue mass may be present around the great vessels. Unlike para-aortic lymphadenopathy the mass does not usually distort the great vessels.

4.1.39 RENAL VASCULAR DISEASE

Renal vein thrombosis

This is an uncommon condition occurring most frequently in neonates usually secondary to dehydration caused by diarrhoea, vomiting or sepsis.

It is also associated with the nephrotic syndrome, glomerulonephritis, tumour, trauma and pregnancy. In adults tumour extension into the renal vein is the commonest cause. The left renal vein is affected three times as much as the right as it is longer and is compressed between the aorta and the superior mesenteric artery. Thrombosis begins in the arcuate and inter-lobular veins and extends to the renal veins. Most cases are unilateral. Intra-venous urography shows impaired renal function with a delayed and prolonged nephrogram.

Sonography

On ultrasonography the kidney is initially enlarged in the acute phase with reduced cortical echogenicity. Haemorrhage may distort the central echo complex. A thrombus may be seen in the distended renal vein or distended inferior vena cava on colour Doppler. Although Doppler ultrasound may show flow in the segmental and collateral veins overlying the renal hilum, mimicking renal vein patency. When flow can be detected on Doppler ultra-sound it is steady or less pulsatile as compared to the normal side. In the subacute phase (7 to 14 days) the cortex becomes echogenic with preser-vation of corticomedullary differentiation because of cellular infiltration. Hypoechoic areas may persist because of focal haemorrhage. The thrombus may be visible within the renal vein as intraluminal echoes and Doppler-scanning shows reduced or absent flow. In neonatal renal vein thrombosis a snowstorm appearance of diffuse echogenicity or a 'patchwork' appear-ance of mainly hyperechoic areas (haemorrhage) and hypoechoic (oedema and/or resolving haemorrhage) may be seen in the subacute stage. Devel-opment of collateral venous drainage may allow the kidney to return to normal or it may atrophy producing a small echogenic kidney in which cor-ticomedullary differentiation may be preserved or lost. In the chronic phase the kidney may become small and echogenic. Linear branching calcification due to calcified thrombus may be detectable. In patients with renal cell car-cinoma colour Doppler is fairly accurate in assessing tumour extension or thrombus into the renal vein.

Renal ischaemia

Ultrasound technique

Ultrasound of the renal vasculature and renal parenchyma requires high resolution ultrasound with low-frequency pulsed Doppler capable of 4 to 17 cm depth. An overnight fast is desirable to reduce abdominal gas. The patient is usually examined with the head propped up 30 degrees to allow the abdominal viscera to settle down into the pelvis. The aorta is located in the long left paramedian location at the level of the origin of the superior mesenteric artery. Morphological changes in the aorta such as an aneurysm, dissection or atheroma are noted. At this level a peak systolic aortic velocity is recorded at a 60 degree angle of insonation with respect to the blood flow vector. The ultrasound probe is then orientated so the aorta is imaged transversely. The renal artery should be located just distal to the superior mesenteric artery. The renal examination may be simplified by using a lateral decubitus position and a flank or translumbar approach to interrogate the renal hilum. The use of colour Doppler facilitates identification of renal vasculature. Time–velocity waveforms are then recorded at three points starting at the origin of the renal artery followed by measurements at the mid-point and finally at the hilum. These measurements are usually recorded at an angle of 60 degrees. When interrogating the renal artery special attention is paid to flow disturbance or high-velocity flow signals.

Renal artery stenosis

Renal artery stenosis is found in 2 per cent of hypertensive patients, 25 per cent of patients with difficult to control hypertension and approximately 45 per cent of patients with peripheral vascular disease. Atheromatous disease is the commonest cause (60 to 90 per cent) whilst 10 to 30 per cent of patients have fibromuscular dysplasia.

The diagnosis of renal artery stenosis is based on systolic and diastolic velocity changes throughout the length of the renal artery. Renal artery flow patterns can be classified into four categories

1. normal
2. diameter-reducing stenosis less than 60 per cent
3. diameter-reducing stenosis greater than 60 per cent
4. renal artery occlusion.

The peak systolic velocity in normal renal arteries averages 120 ± 12 cm/s, with an average peak systolic aortic velocity of 60 ± 15 cm/s, both velocities decrease with age. The kidneys offer a low-resistance vascular bed, thus the Doppler spectral waveform from the normal kidney is that of a constant forward diastolic flow. In renal parenchymal disease there is increased vascular resistance which in turn causes a decrease in the diastolic flow component and increased pulsatility of the Doppler spectral waveform. Parenchymal diastolic flow velocities less than 20 per cent of the peak systolic velocity are consistent with renal parenchymal disease.

In renal artery stenosis the peak systolic velocity shows an increase of more than 150 cm/s for angles less than 60 degrees, or 180 cm/s for angles greater than 70 degrees. There may be post-stenotic spectral broadening with or without flow reversal. Flow may be absent during diastole in stenoses over 50 per cent. A ratio of the peak systolic renal artery velocity to the aortic peak systolic velocity greater than or equal to 3.5 is said to be predictive of a greater than 60 per cent diameter-reducing renal artery stenosis.

Renal artery stenosis = peak systolic renal artery velocity:aortic peak systolic velocity ≥ 3.5

Certain indirect Doppler ultrasound signs have been described for renal artery stenosis. One such sign is the presence of tardus-pavus pulse demonstrated by a gradual slope of Doppler waveform during systole (pulse time rise greater than 0.07 to 0.12 s) and attenuated Doppler waveform amplitude (peak systolic velocity less than 20 to 30 cm/s).

The acceleration index is determined by dividing the slope of the systolic upstroke (kHz/s) by the carrier Doppler frequency and an acceleration time is the time interval between the onset of systole and the initial peak. The acceleration index in renal artery stenosis is greater than or equal to 3 m/s^2. The resistive index in renal artery stenosis is usually less than 0.56. The early systolic peak may be absent in renal artery stenosis. Colour flow Doppler may demonstrate disorganised flow patterns and high-velocity flow stream associated with haemodynamically significant stenosis. A false negative diagnosis may occur with an accessory renal artery whilst a false positive diagnosis may be made with coarctation of aorta.

Limitations of Doppler ultrasound in the diagnosis of renal artery stenosis

Patient-related factors – bowel gas, obesity, respiratory renal movements and poor patient compliance.

Anatomical factors – multiple renal arteries (16 to 28 per cent) variation of renal veins (used as imaging landmarks), horseshoe kidneys and crossed ectopia.

Technical factors – false positive examinations caused by sub-optimal angles, variation in operator experience, incomplete examination as complete renal evaluation is cumbersome, the need to visualise the entire length of artery and transmitted cardiac or aortic pulsation may obscure renal waveforms and different emphasis put on variable parameters.

Pathologic factors – false tracings may be recorded from large collateral vessels and reconstituted main renal artery, variable causes of renal artery stenosis affect different sites (atheroma, fibromuscular hyperplasia, vasculitis, arteriovenous fistula, retroperitoneal fibrosis, neurofibromatosis, etc.).

Renal artery thrombosis

Renal artery thrombosis is rare in children and is usually secondary to dehydration, maternal diabetes, umbilical artery catheters or emboli via a patent ductus arteriosus. In adults it is usually secondary to severe atheroma, trauma, arteritis, aneurysm or fibromuscular hyperplasia.

Sonography

If visualised the artery shows internal echoes with decreased or absent flow on duplex and colour Doppler studies. Focal infarction may give rise to echogenic or hypoechoic areas which may have a mass effect. Echogenic infarcts usually become hypoechoic over a few days. Eventually the infarct atrophies causing parenchymal thinning. If the whole kidney is ischaemic it may appear normal or enlarged but becomes hypoechoic and then atrophies giving rise to a small scarred kidney. Renal artery trauma gives rise to similar appearances and although Doppler studies can confirm reduced or absent arterial flow, a normal ultrasound scan does not exclude renal artery damage or thrombosis.

Renal cortical necrosis

This unusual condition occurs more frequently in children than adults. It results from severe hypotension or hypoxia, which is usually secondary to dehydration, sepsis, blood loss, hypoxia, haemoglobinopathy or the haemolytic or uraemic syndrome. In the acute stage the kidney is either normal in size or enlarged. There is a subcapsular rim of reduced echogenicity. In sub-acute and long-standing cases this area of cortex becomes echogenic and may calcify. Secondary medullary fibrosis may also occur.

Acute tubular necrosis

Acute tubular (medullary) necrosis occurs as a result of secondary to severe compromise to renal perfusion or hypoxia.

Sonography

Sonographic appearances are variable as tubules are found both in the medulla and the cortex. The kidney frequently appears normal but a variable increase in the pyramidal echogenicity may occur though the renal pyramids usually remain well defined. Increased pyramidal echogenicity may be associated with a variable increase in cortical echogenicity. The renal pyramids may appear swollen and this may give the central echo complex a scalloped outline. Uncommonly the pyramids are of reduced echogenicity.

Renal trauma

Renal trauma is common in both adults and children and ultrasonography is valuable in detecting many of its complications such as haematomas, lacerations and contusions. Though Doppler studies may confirm arterial flow they cannot exclude arterial damage, and intravenous urography, CT, isotope studies or angiography may be necessary to confirm perfusion and function. When assessing the kidney in trauma cases adjacent organs should also be evaluated as renal damage may be associated with hepatic or splenic injury. In cases of trauma renal damage is more likely if there is underlying renal pathology such as hydronephrosis.

Renal contusion

Appearances are variable depending upon the state of the blood within the contusion or haematoma. Initially blood is hypoechoic but it rapidly becomes echogenic as it clots. Later the haematoma liquefies and the collection becomes hypoechoic, anechoic or complex. A contusion may be seen as a defect in the renal contour.

Renal haematoma

Subcapsular haematomas spread around the kidney giving rise to an echogenic rim. Focal subcapsular haematomas may depress the cortex. As the haematoma resolves fibrosis may occur which may compress the kidney resulting in hypertension. Intrarenal haematomas are more frequently hypoechoic than renal contusion and subcapsular haematoma. Echogenic haematomas may be lost in the central echo complex. Renal haematomas may enlarge and thus they should be followed up as they may cause delayed rupture of the kidney.

Perirenal haematoma

These haematomas initially appear anechoic but rapidly become moderately echogenic. Perirenal haematomas do not usually change the renal shape but may expand into the anterior or posterior space. Large collections may appear septate and may contain both blood and urine.

4.1.40 SOLID RENAL MASSES

Renal pseudo-tumours

Felson and Moskowitz defined renal pseudo-tumours as 'a real or simulated renal mass roentgenologically resembling neoplasms but histologically consisting of normal renal parenchyma'. The concept of renal pseudo-tumours now includes extrarenal normal structures that radiologically mimic renal tumours.

Developmental pseudo-masses

Large column of Bertin Columnar hypertrophy or septum of Bertin gives rise to projection of cortex between the medullary pyramids. A large column of Bertin may displace adjacent papilla, infundibula and calyces and produce the appearances of an intrarenal mass. A large column of Bertin is usually found in abortive or actual renal duplication and commonly found near the junction of the middle and upper poles of the kidney. The problem usually arises with intravenous urography. These masses are usually less than 3 cm in diameter, ellipsoid and isoechoic placed between the upper and middle poles of the kidney and they do not distort the renal contour. There is splaying of the adjacent renal sinus referred to as 'the split sinus sign', other ultrasound signs include lateral contiguity with normal renal cortex, an echogenic linear rim and close proximity to the renal vein. The most sensitive test to confirm the diagnosis in case of doubt is a Tc-99m DMSA isotope scan.

Lobar dysmorphism This is of similar genesis as the column of Bertin, in which not only the cortex but also the medulla is found deep within the kidney complete with its own diminutive calyx. Ultrasound appearances are those of an isoechoic ill-defined mass with no evidence of neovascularity on colour or power Doppler. A DMSA scan may confirm the diagnosis in case of doubt.

Foetal lobulation The persistence of cortical lobulation as a result of incomplete fusion of the foetal lobes beyond the age of 5 years occurs in almost 50 per cent of adults. Usually the anterior calyces are involved which may be unilateral or bilateral. The indentation, unlike renal scars, occurs in between the calyces. Foetal lobulation seldom gives rise to difficulty on imaging particularly on ultrasound which shows isoechoic cortical lobulation.

Dromedary hump This refers to a triangular bulge of the lateral renal cortex of the left kidney with an elongated middle calyx. Most authors now agree that this bulge is not secondary to splenic impression but a developmental variant. It may be confused with a renal mass, on an intravenous urography when a rounded hump or a triangular-shaped mass is produced on the lateral aspect of the kidney just below the splenic impression. Confusion seldom occurs with ultrasound, when an isoechoic thickened cortex is seen on the lateral border of the left kidney, below the splenic tip.

Polar hypertrophy or hilar lip Polar hypertrophy or hilar lip represents a supra- or infrahilar bulge on the medial aspect of the kidney. This is a congenital hyperplasia usually confined to a single pole, with an increased distance between the margin of the hilar lip and adjacent calyx. Polar hypertrophy is readily identified on ultrasound as an isoechoic bulge on the medial renal border above or below the hilum. In equivocal cases a Tc-99m DMSA scan offers a simple diagnostic method.

Pseudo-tumours following partial nephrectomy
Pseudo-tumours may mimic tumour recurrence after partial nephrectomy or enucleation of small renal tumours.

Splenic migration With left partial nephrectomy or enucleation, the spleen may migrate into the renal defect and mimic a mass or recurrence. This pseudo-mass is usually echogenic and of uniform echogenicity. With meticulous technique it is usually possible to demonstrate continuity with the spleen. If further clarification is required a Tc sulphur colloid scan may be helpful as the splenic tissue would concentrate the radionuclide.

Pseudo-tumour to fatty flap A fatty flap filling the surgical defect in the kidney may appear as an echogenic mass. A CT or magnetic resonance scan will confirm the presence of fat within the pseudo-mass (differential diagnosis: angiomyolipoma).

Inflammatory pseudo-masses

Focal compensatory hypertrophy Nodular focal compensatory hypertrophy may occur in response to extensive renal scarring as a result of chronic pyelonephritis, trauma, infarction, mal-development or surgery. The persistence of normal residual renal parenchyma and compensatory hypertrophy may mimic tumours. Problems often arise with intravenous urography when these areas of normal parenchyma or compensatory hypertrophy show a mass effect by distorting the calyces or renal outline. An ultrasound usually reveals a non-necrotic ill-defined isoechoic mass. Colour Doppler shows an avascular mass.

Inflammatory pseudo-tumours in children and young adults
Inflammatory pseudo-tumours are rare benign masses. The majority of these have been reported in the lungs but a number of cases have now been reported at extrapulmonary sites. Inflammatory pseudo-masses may clinically and radiologically mimic malignant neoplasia particularly lymphoma and sarcoma. When in the kidney ultrasound may reveal a well-defined hypoechoic, hyperechoic complex mass lesion. Tissue diagnosis is required for confirmation.

Inflammatory masses

Focal compensatory hypertrophy See above.

Focal hydronephrosis Focal hydronephrosis may result from a multitude of causes but particularly from tuberculosis. Focal hydronephrosis may mimic a mass on intravenous urography; this difficulty seldom arises with ultrasound, moreover ultrasound replaces more invasive techniques in guiding aspiration biopsy or antegrade pyelography which may help confirm the diagnosis.

Reflux or repeated infections in a duplicated lower pole may cause considerable atrophic changes in the lower pole so much so that only a small 'nubbin' of renal tissue remains at the lower renal pole. This may mimic a mass protruding from the lower pole of a normal non-duplicated kidney. Sonography may show focal parenchymal loss of tissue at the lower renal pole associated with increased echogenicity. If there is functioning residual tissue intravenous urography or a MAG-3 scan may show the presence of two collecting systems.

Acute focal bacterial nephritis Acute focal bacterial nephritis, a chronic renal abscess or an infected cyst may mimic a renal tumour. There is controversy regarding whether to use CT or ultrasound as the first imaging modality in complicated acute pyelonephritis, the authors prefer ultrasound. Acute focal bacterial nephritis appears as a relatively hypoechoic mass, rather ill defined but with scattered low-level echoes and disruption of the corticomedullary junction. When complicated by haemorrhage the mass may appear hyperechoic.

The ultrasound findings in a renal abscess depend upon its maturity, the presence of gas, haemorrhage, necrosis and internal debris. As the abscess matures it becomes more echolucent and better defined because of liquefaction and encapsulation. Some abscesses have good through transmission, however they seldom become as sonolucent as a simple cyst. The presence of gas within a renal mass is specific for an abscess. Abscesses may at times mimic necrotic tumours both on CT and ultrasound, and will require aspiration biopsy.

A simple cyst may become infected through a haematogenous route, vesicoureteric reflux, surgery or percutaneous intervention. Most patients are symptomatic with fever and flank pain, however occasionally the patient may be completely asymptomatic. The ultrasound appearances in the acute phase are no different to those of a simple cyst, however if the infection becomes chronic the appearance may resemble an abscess or necrotic tumour. As with a renal abscess an aspiration biopsy may be required to confirm the diagnosis.

Xanthogranulomatous pyelonephritis See p. 326. Focal xanthogranulomatous pyelonephritis may mimic a tumour and many cases present a difficult diagnostic problem. Ultrasound usually shows a solid mass of varying echogenicity, which may be ill defined or well defined and difficult to differentiate from a tumour preoperatively on any modality.

Bacille Calmette-Guerin (BCG) granulomatous renal mass BCG delivered intravesically is occasionally used as a treatment for superficial bladder cancer. A renal granuloma has been described as one of the complications of this form of therapy, probably as a result of vesicoureteric reflux. These granulomas have been reported as small intrarenal hypoechoic masses.

Renal tuberculosis On urography it may be difficult to differentiate between a tuberculoma and focal hydronephrosis as they both represent masses that show opacity with iodinated contrast. On ultrasound a tuberculoma appears as a solid mass with diminished through transmission whilst hydronephrosis is identified as a fluid-filled structure. However there is a diffuse infiltrative type of renal tuberculosis described where the kidney might appear normal on ultrasound.

Inflammatory pseudo-tumours in children and young adults Inflammatory pseudo-tumours are rare benign masses. The majority of these occur in the lungs but extrapulmonary sites may be involved. Inflammatory pseudo-tumours may mimic malignant tumours such as lymphomas and sarcomas, both clinically and radiologically. On sonography these pseudo-tumours appear as well-defined hypoechoic, hyperechoic or complex masses. Preoperative diagnosis is difficult as no characteristic imaging features have been described. Biopsy yields are similarly not fruitful.

Non-neoplastic, non-inflammatory renal masses
Multilocular renal cyst – see p. 344.
Intrarenal haematoma – see p. 356.
Renal infarction – see p. 373.

Benign renal tumours

Angiomyolipoma
Angiomyolipoma is composed of fat, vascular tissue and smooth muscle elements. It is not a hamartoma by definition as fat and smooth muscles are not normal constituents of renal parenchyma. Two types are described.

Isolated angiomyolipoma This occurs sporadically, is often solitary and makes up 80 per cent of the tumours. The mean age of occurrence is 43 years with an age range from 27 to 72 years. It is four times as common in females than males.

Angiomyolipoma associated with tuberous sclerosis (20 per cent)

These tumours are larger, often bilateral and multiple. Angiomyolipoma occurs in 80 per cent of patients with tuberous sclerosis. There is an equal sex distribution.

Angiomyolipoma

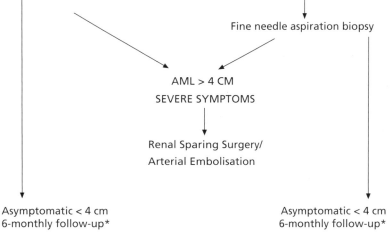

History and imaging diagnostic of AML   Imaging and history non-diagnostic

Fine needle aspiration biopsy

AML > 4 CM
SEVERE SYMPTOMS

Renal Sparing Surgery/
Arterial Embolisation

Asymptomatic < 4 cm   Asymptomatic < 4 cm
6-monthly follow-up*   6-monthly follow-up*

Counselling regards possible complications

Angiomyolipoma is considered benign but extension into the renal vein or inferior vena cava and deposits in the regional lymph nodes have been reported. The latter is possibly related to multicentric disease. Most small lesions are asymptomatic but 40 per cent may present with a palpable abdominal mass, haematuria and flank pain. The solitary sporadic tumours may present as an acute abdomen and shock as a result of spontaneous haemorrhage within the tumour. The most characteristic sonographic feature is a very echogenic mass that may shadow. The echogenic appearance is said to be related to fat content and multiple tissue interfaces. This appearance is not pathognomonic and has been described in renal cell carcinoma and other tumours. If an anechoic rim and/or intratumoural cysts are seen in a hyperechoic mass, this suggests a diagnosis of renal cell carcinoma. Not all angiomyolipomas are hyperechoic as the tumour constituents are variable and fat content may be low, besides haemorrhage, necrosis and dilated calyces may alter the echogenicity of the tumour. Fatty attenuation seen in the tumour on CT is virtually diagnostic of angiomyolipoma. However it should be remembered that angiomyolipoma is not the only renal tumour that may contain fat. Fat has been reported in renal lipoma, liposarcoma, Wilms' tumour, teratoma, xanthogranulomatous pyelonephritis, oncocytoma (engulfing of renal sinus fat) and rarely, but most importantly, in a renal cell carcinoma due to invasion of perinephric fat or metaplasia within the tumour. Since the tumour is common in tuberous sclerosis and not all tumours are angiomyolipoma and most are asymptomatic the question of follow up is important, particularly as renal cell carcinoma has an incidence of 3 per cent and in nearly half the patients they are bilateral. An approach based on the evaluation of the natural history has been devised:

Adenoma

There is considerable debate about the existence of a renal adenoma because histological patterns similar to an adenoma are seen in renal cell carcinoma. Some clinicians have applied size criteria with an upper limit of 3 cm used to define a benign adenoma. Unfortunately there is considerable overlap, imaging is not specific and management is therefore surgical.

Oncocytoma, oxyphilic adenoma, proximal tubular adenoma

These tumours represent 3.1 to 6.6 per cent of all renal tumours. The age group affected is 26 to 94 years (median 65) with a male to female ratio of 2:1. They are usually asymptomatic but occasionally patients present with hypertension, haematuria or flank pain. The tumours can be very large, up to 20 cm in size. Rarely they may be multiple and bilateral. In a quarter of the patients sonography reveals a branching hypoechoic area thought to represent a central scar. However a central scar is not specific for oncocytoma. Generally the mass is solid and usually isoechoic but can show necrotic areas. Calcification, although rare, can be seen. Percutaneous biopsy is usually not adequate as renal cell carcinoma has areas within it which have characteristics of an oncocytoma. Management therefore remains surgical. However if characteristic imaging features are seen the surgeon should be alerted so that renal-saving surgery is considered.

Mesenchymal tumours

Mesenchymal tumours are rare, they include juxtaglomerular tumours, lipoma, fibroma, myoma, angioma, liposarcoma, fibrosarcoma, myosarcoma and angioendothelioma. Most of the benign mesenchymal tumours are small, asymptomatic and usually not detected. The larger tumours and the malignant neoplasia are difficult to differentiate from renal cell carcinoma on imaging.

Renal capsular leiomyoma, renal capsular leiomyoma with myxomatous degeneration and capsulomas These are benign mesenchymal tumours which arise from the renal capsule. The tumour is composed of fibrous tissue, smooth muscle and fat in varying proportions. Most are not detectable on imaging because of their small size (1 to 5mm), although these tumours are found at 6.2 per cent of autopsies. When seen on sonography they are exophytic tumours indenting the renal contour and are moderately echogenic.

Juxtaglomerular tumour (reninoma) Juxtaglomerular tumour (reninoma) is a very rare tumour of the juxtaglomerular cells; none the less it is an important and potentially curable cause of hypertension in young adults usually less than 21 years of age, this condition shows a female predilection. On sonography reninoma is usually an echogenic mass because of the many tissue interfaces between juxtaglomerular cells and the small vascular channels of the tumour. Areas of necrosis and haemorrhage may alter the echogenicity. The CT findings are non-specific and the tumour may not be seen on non-contrast scans. Needle biopsy has been successfully used to diagnose this tumour. Diagnosis can also be achieved by demonstrating a normal renal artery, and hypovascular renal mass using angiography, in combination with elevated renin levels.

Mesoblastic nephroma or congenital Wilms' tumour Mesoblastic nephroma is seen primarily in neonates and young infants, it is seen uncommonly in older children and is very rare in adults. The tumour occurs at a younger age than Wilms' tumour but has similar sonographic appearances. The tumour is usually benign but can be malignant and gives rise to a solid renal mass which may be quite large (a renal mass in a child less than 1 year old is more likely to be a mesoblastic nephroma than a Wilms' tumour). The tumour has a relatively homogeneous pattern of low-level echoes though haemorrhage and necrosis can give rise to anechoic areas. The reniform shape of the kidney is maintained because of its infiltrative growth pattern.

Arteriovenous malformation

Arteriovenous malformations are frequently too small to visualise though small lesions may still cause significant haemorrhage. When visible they are seen as small hypoechoic lesions. The renal artery and renal vein may be enlarged.

Haemangioma

Haemangioma (benign cystic cystadenoma or cystic hamartoma) have a multilocular appearance though careful scanning will show solid intracystic areas.

Malignant renal tumours

Renal cell carcinoma

Renal cell carcinoma is a relatively common malignancy accounting for 90 per cent of primary renal malignancies. It is a primary epithelial neoplasm which arises from the proximal convoluted tubule. Nearly all cases occur in adults although it has been recorded in children less than 10 years of age. Early cases are seen as small cortical-based masses which enlarge and invade the renal parenchyma. Late cases may present with a classic triad of loin pain, flank mass and haematuria. Five per cent of patients have bilateral tumours though these are not usually simultaneous. Predisposing factors include smoking, phenacetin overuse, von Hippel–Lindau disease, haemo-dialysis and acquired cystic disease of renal failure.

Sonography Renal cell carcinoma gives a wide spectrum of appearances depending upon the size of the tumour. It may be solid, cystic or complex. Solid tumours transmit sound waves poorly so that acoustic transmission is either unchanged or decreased when compared with that of a normal kidney. The commonest appearance is that of increased echogenicity which corresponds to areas of increased vascularity on angiography. Small tumours particularly are more echogenic so that small angiomyolipomas cannot be distinguished on ultrasound. However small hyperechoic renal cell carci-noma may show a hypoechoic rim caused by a tumour pseudo-capsule which may contain small anechoic areas because of necrosis features that are absent in angiomyolipoma. There is no true capsule and the margins of the tumour are irregular. The larger tumours tend to be hypoechoic. Six to twenty per cent show evidence of calcification (up to 3 per cent of renal cysts show calcification, peripheral calcification in cysts and tumours may obscure the true internal echopattern) and punctuate calcification within a mass occurs almost exclusively in tumours. Growth of the tumour mass may be rapid or slow but when large the mass may completely replace the kidney. The renal veins, inferior vena cava, para-aortic region, retroperitoneal space, liver and contralateral kidney should be inspected for evidence of tumour spread. Extension of the tumour into the renal vein occurs in 4 to 30 per cent of patients. Tumour within the renal vein causes internal echoes within the lumen of the vein that may or may not dilate. Sonography is less accurate than CT or MRI in tumour staging but the use of duplex Doppler increases its sensitivity, particularly for showing proximal inferior vena caval and right atrial tumour extension. Sonography is superior to CT for the rela-tionship of right upper pole tumour to the liver. Percutaneous renal biopsy of a solid mass is usually not performed because of a sampling error. However biopsy may be fruitful when the imaging features are atypical. Differentiation between metastases, lymphoma or renal cell carcinoma has obvious therapeutic advantages.

Lymphoma

Renal lymphoma is usually associated with disease elsewhere and occurs most frequently in long-standing cases. There is 33 to 63 per cent involvement at autopsy series. Although renal involvement is common only 2.7 to 6 per cent is detected on imaging. The reason for this low detection rate is that the majority of these patients are asymptomatic and renal involvement does not usually affect renal function.

Sonography

1. Hypoechoic multiple bilateral renal masses, small lesions may be confused with medullary pyramids.
2. Direct infiltration from the retroperitoneum and perirenal space is infrequent. The kidney may be diffusely echopoor, but with focal involvement differentiation from a renal cell carcinoma may be difficult.
3. Diffuse involvement of the kidney results in renal enlargement associated with a diffuse and homogeneous increase in renal echogenicity. This phenomenon is called 'hepatisation' and can be confused with other renal parenchymal disease.
4. Perirenal lymphoma is rare. It is characterised by a hypoechoic collar surrounding the kidney, ultrasound unlike CT shows a clear discrimination.

Metastatic tumours

Renal metastases are common in patients with advanced malignancy and are found in up to 45 per cent of large autopsy series. The primary sites include the lung, breast, melanoma, stomach, cervix, colon, pancreas, prostate and kidney, although renal metastases can arise from almost any primary site in the body. As most renal metastases are asymptomatic their clinical detection is rare, as small lesions are the rule. Sonographically they may give rise to isoechoic, hypoechoic or hyperechoic masses. The majority are hypoechoic. Differentiation from renal cell carcinoma may very difficult on imaging.

Leukaemia

Renal abnormality is common in childhood leukaemia; the kidneys are the most frequently involved organs apart from the liver, spleen, marrow and lymph nodes. Renal involvement is found in about 65 per cent of leukaemia patients at autopsy. Cellular infiltration of the renal interstitium occurs, though this is not necessarily by leukaemic cells and may be a secondary inflammatory infiltrate. This results in bilateral renal enlargement.

Although leukaemic infiltration is usually diffuse focal masses may occur. This may particularly occur in acute myeloblastic leukaemia, where poorly differentiated myeloid cells form a granulocytic sarcoma (chloroma). Such focal lesions may be mistaken for renal cell carcinoma. With the more common diffuse involvement the renal cortex may appear normal or it may show increased or decreased echogenicity. Renal changes may be associated with hepatosplenomegaly and lymphadenopathy. Similar renal changes may occur in renal vein thrombosis, pyelonephritis, lymphoma and glomerulonephritis.

Other renal tumours

Other renal tumours are rare, diagnosis is usually made at surgery or biopsy as these tumours rarely have any specific imaging characteristics. Several histological types of renal sarcomas have been reported including leiomyosarcoma, haemangiopericytoma, fibrosarcoma, osteogenic and rhabdomyosarcoma. However most sarcomas involving the kidneys originate in the retroperitoneum. Renal plasmacytoma rarely involves the kidney and may present as a diffuse infiltration or a more focal mass. Wilms' tumour is rarely seen in adults but when it occurs it can become quite large, although histologically similar to childhood Wilms' tumour the prognosis in adults is quite poor. Carcinoid tumours can occasionally involve the kidney, but with no specific imaging characteristics differentiation from renal cell carcinoma can be difficult. Sonographically any of these tumours can be isoechoic, hyperechoic, hypoechoic or complex and therefore on ultrasound, as with any other imaging, differentiation from a renal cell carcinoma can be difficult.

Urothelial tumours

Benign – papilloma, inverted papilloma, neurofibroma.
Malignant – transitional cell carcinoma (85 to 90 per cent), squamous cell carcinoma (6 to 10 per cent), small cell undifferentiated carcinoma (less than 1 per cent), carcinosarcoma (extremely rare).
Malignant – metastatic.

Sonography

The primary role of sonography in the diagnosis of collecting-system tumours is the differentiation from radiolucent calculi and blood clot. The diagnosis of calculi is usually straightforward, however high grade transitional cell carcinomas can be densely echogenic and mimic calculi. The increased echo density in these tumours has been attributed to squamous metaplasia within the tumour with the formation of keratin pearls which can be very echogenic but do not usually shadow. The most common sonographic appearance of transitional cell carcinoma (TCC) is a hypoechoic renal collecting-system mass splitting the central echo complex with varying degrees of infundibular dilatation. Focal hypoechogenicity of adjacent renal cortex reflects local invasion. Occasionally the central echo complex may only be segmentally amputated. There are no specific ultrasound features of TCC and renal cell carcinoma, leukaemia or metastases may cause appearances similar to TCC. The detection of a centrally placed renal pelvic mass on ultrasound should prompt further studies such as antegrade or retrograde pyelography.

4.1.41 RENAL MASSES IN CHILDREN

Renal masses in neonates

Multicystic dysplastic kidney
See pp. 338–339.

Congenital mesoblastic nephroma
See p. 363.

Renal vein thrombosis
See pp. 351–352.

Autosomal recessive polycystic disease
See p. 341.

Renal masses in toddlers

Wilms' tumour
Wilms' tumour is the commonest renal neoplasm in childhood. Eighty per cent of cases present at less than 5 years of age with a mean age at presentation of 3 years. The tumour usually presents as a rapidly growing, painless, abdominal mass. Microscopic haematuria, fever and leucocytosis may occur and the blood pressure is elevated in 50 per cent of cases. Tumours are bilateral in 10 to 15 per cent of cases although the second tumour may be a metastasis. There is an increased incidence of Wilms' tumour in sporadic aniridia, nephroblastomatosis, hemihypertrophy, horseshoe kidney, Beckwith–Wiedemann syndrome, chromosomal abnormalities, Drash syndrome and Perlmann syndrome. Renal involvement is usual but rare extrarenal variants have been reported both within the abdomen and at distal extra-abdominal sites. Any solid renal mass in a young child should be assumed to be Wilms' tumour until proven otherwise.

Sonography

1. Sonography is the primary modality for evaluating the site or organ of origin and the size, extent and architecture of the tumour.
2. The mass is solid and quite large at presentation, usually over 10 cm in size.
3. Echogenicity is variable, generally echogenic but 'cysts' within the tumour contribute to its complexity. These 'cysts' may be caused by tumour necrosis, deposits of mucin or trapped calyces.
4. Calcification is uncommon, it is usually irregular and amorphous.
5. Intense echogenic foci within the tumour may be related to fat deposition.
6. The inferior vena cava should be imaged to the level of the right atrium for tumour extension.
7. Inferior vena cava tumour extension may be shown on real time ultrasound and if necessary confirmed by Duplex or colour Doppler. Tumours on the right may compress the inferior vena cava and make its visualisation difficult, though the inferior vena cava may be patent.
8. The contralateral kidney should always be examined because 10 to 15 per cent of tumours are bilateral at presentation and their detection alters primary therapy.
9. Anomalies that could alter surgery such as contralateral renal agenesis, horseshoe kidney and pelviureteric junction obstruction must be excluded.

NB   An imaging review indicates that the addition of other imaging to plain abdominal radiographs and ultrasound do not alter patient outcome.

Renal blastema and nephroblastomatosis

These are inter-related conditions closely related to Wilms' tumour. The persistence of primitive renal blastema beyond infancy (4 months) is abnormal except in small microscopic rests. Larger amounts of primitive blastema remaining in sheets in the cortex or in more discrete nodules are termed nephroblastomatosis. A small number progress to Wilms' tumours and others may form the less malignant epithelial nephroblastoma. Its recognition is important since it is associated with bilateral Wilms' tumours. Sonographic detection is possible but lacks the sensitivity of CT and MRI. On ultrasound the affected kidney may be enlarged and lobulated with multiple hypoechoic areas. There may be loss of corticomedullary differentiation. Once discovered, frequent ultrasound examinations are carried out to detect progression to malignant change, which is suggested by the rapid growth of any of the hypoechoic rests.

Epithelial nephroblastoma

Epithelial nephroblastomatosis or cystic Wilms' tumour is less malignant than Wilms' tumour and may appear cystic or papillary. In its very benign form it gives rise to a multilocular cystic renal disease. Ultrasonography and CT cannot predict the degree of malignancy.

Clear cell sarcoma

Clear cell sarcoma is a distinct histological entity, making up 4 per cent of the renal tumours in childhood. These tumours cannot usually be differentiated from Wilms' tumour on imaging. There is no association with any other somatic abnormality, but overall prognosis is poor as compared to Wilms' tumour.

Rhabdoid tumour of the kidney

The term rhabdoid is derived from the microscopic appearance of the tumour cells that resemble muscle cells. Rhabdoid tumours make up around 2 per cent of the renal neoplasms, which are more frequent in infancy than in any other period. An association with brain tumours, especially medulloblastoma, has been described. The brain tumours may precede, or appear several years after, the detection of this tumour. The prognosis of rhabdoid tumour of the kidney is much worse as compared to other renal tumours in this age group. This tumour, as other neonatal masses, can be diagnosed *in utero*. In the neonate detection may follow presentation with an abdominal mass, hypertension or hypercalcaemia. The age at presentation overlaps with congenital mesoblastic nephroma. The clinical and imaging characteristics are similar to congenital mesoblastic nephroma, clear cell sarcoma and Wilms' tumour; specific diagnosis is therefore usually not possible. One important differentiating point is that clear cell sarcoma of the kidney and rhabdoid tumour of the kidney is invariably unilateral.

Multilocular cystic nephroma

See p. 344.

Intrarenal neuroblastoma

Neuroblastoma within the abdomen usually develops in the retroperitoneum; most arise from an adrenal gland displacing a kidney inferomedially. Rarely, however, a neuroblastoma may mimic a Wilms' tumour arising from tissues within the kidney or invasion of the kidney by neuroblastoma. To make things complicated neuroblastomas may rarely manifest other features more typical of Wilms' tumour such as inferior vena cava extension and lung metastases.

Renal masses in older children

Autosomal dominant polycystic kidney disease

See pp. 343–344.

Renal cell carcinoma

Renal cell carcinoma is usually a tumour of adults in their forties and fifties but paediatric cases occur comprising 5% of paediatric renal tumours. The prognosis in children is worse than Wilms' tumour. It is difficult to differentiate renal cell carcinomas from other renal tumours on imaging. On sonography renal cell carcinomas appear as a hypoechoic or mixed echogenicity mass with calcification in up to 10%.

4.1.42 SONOGRAPHIC CHARACTERISTICS OF SOLID RENAL MASSES

General characteristics

1. They distort renal architecture.
2. They have a mass effect.
3. They absorb sound.
4. Usually they show internal echoes.
5. A very uniform mass may appear anechoic.
6. A hyperechoic mass is often very vascular.
7. If far wall echoes are present they are less prominent than cysts.

Inflammatory masses

They are almost exclusively echopoor, inhomogeneous, a small number may enhance or shadow but the majority do not affect sound transmission.

Lymphomas

Eighty per cent are homogeneously hypoechoic and have no effect on sound transmission, a minority are inhomogeneous, while a small number shadow.

Metastases

They are predominantly hypoechoic but may be isoechoic or hyperechoic. They may be homogeneous or inhomogeneous in equal numbers, similarly half show acoustic shadowing, 25 per cent acoustic enhancement and 25 per cent may have no effect on sound transmission.

Angiomyolipoma

The majority are hyperechoic and shadow, exceptionally they are hypoechoic.

Adenomas

They are predominantly hypoechoic, homogeneous with no effect on sound transmission, a small number are isoechoic whilst a minority may shadow.

Multifocal solid renal masses

Benign neoplasms – angiomyolipoma, renal adenoma.
Malignant neoplasms – renal cell carcinoma, metastases, lymphoma, oncocytoma (potentially malignant), Wilms' tumour.
Infections – renal abscesses, multifocal bacterial nephritis, multifocal xanthogranulomatous pyelonephritis, renal malakoplakia, hydatid cysts.
Infiltrative processes – lymphatic leukaemia, lymphatoid granulomatosis, amyloid (focal), sarcoidosis.
Vascular – multiple renal infarcts, multiple arteriovenous malformations.

Neonatal renal masses

Unilateral – multicystic kidney (15 per cent), pelviureteric junction obstruction hydronephrosis (25 per cent), hydronephrotic upper moiety, renal vein thrombosis, mesoblastic nephroma, Wilms' teratoma (rare).
Bilateral – hydronephrosis, polycystic disease, multicystic kidney with contralateral hydronephrosis, nephroblastomatosis, bilateral multicystic kidney.

Renal masses in the older child

Solitary – Wilms' tumour, multilocular cystic nephroma, focal hydronephrosis, traumatic cyst, renal abscess, renal cell carcinoma, clear cell sarcoma, rhabdoid tumour of the kidney, intrarenal neuroblastoma.
Multiple – nephroblastomatosis, multiple Wilms' tumours, angiomyolipoma, lymphoma or leukaemia, adult polycystic disease, abscesses.

Paediatric cystic renal masses

Hydronephrosis
Duplication with obstructed moiety.
Multicystic dysplastic kidney.
Adult polycystic disease.
Cystic Wilms' tumours.
Multiseptate urinoma.
Multilocular cystic nephroma.
Haematoma.
Abscesses.

Paediatric solid renal masses

Wilms' tumour.
Hamartoma.
Nephroblastomatosis.
Mesoblastic nephroma.
Infantile polycystic disease.
Rhabdomyosarcoma.
Leiomyosarcoma.
Angiomyolipoma.
Haemangioma.
Haemangiopericytoma.
Mucosal epithelial tumours.
Clear cell sarcoma.
Renal cell carcinoma.
Metastases.
Lymphoma.
Leukaemia.
Rhabdoid tumour of the kidney.
Pseudo-tumours.

Hyperechoic renal masses

Malignant tumours – renal cell carcinoma, liposarcoma, atypical Wilms' tumour, oncocytoma (malignant potential), lymphoma, angiosarcoma, undifferentiated sarcoma, metastasis (usually echopoor).

Benign tumours – angiomyolipoma, hamartoma, angioma, lipoma, oncocytoma, cavernous haemangioma, renal capsular leiomyoma, renal capsular leiomyoma with myxomatous degeneration, juxtaglomerular tumour.

Cystic lesions – mature hydatid cysts, abscess with microbubbles, complicated renal cyst, calcified renal cyst.

Vascular lesions – calcified renal artery aneurysm, haematoma, renal infarct scar.

Miscellaneous lesions – renal sinus lipomatosis (particularly the focal form), fat-filled postoperative cortical defects, focal renal dysplasia, extramedullary haematopoiesis.

Hypoechoic renal masses

Renal pseudo-tumour.
Renal malignancy.
Metastasis.
Acute bacterial nephritis.
Early abscess.

Infarct.
Contusion.
Haematoma.
Lymphoma.
Arteriovenous malformation.
Benign tumours (exceptional).
Xanthogranulomatous pyelonephritis.

Renal enlargement with a heterogenous echopattern

Tumours – renal cell carcinoma, Wilms' tumour, sarcoma, transitional cell carcinoma.
Malakoplakia (nodular form).
Xanthogranulomatous pyelonephritis (nodular form).
Multiple abscesses.
Leukaemia or lymphoma – focal deposits.
Contusion or intrarenal clot.

NB Most of the causes of an echogenic renal mass may give it a heterogeneous appearance.

Tumours within the inferior vena cava

Renal malignancy.
Phaeochromocytoma.
Malignant melanoma.
Choriocarcinoma.
Angiomyolipoma.
Wilms' tumour (rare).
Caval leiomyosarcoma.

Patterns of tumours within the inferior vena cava
A mass with low level echoes within the inferior vena cava lumen.
Inferior vena cava is widened.
Complete inferior vena cava thrombosis with collateral vessels.
Foci of thrombus and tumour adhering to the inferior vena cava wall.
No flow demonstrated on Duplex or colour Doppler ultrasound.

4.1.43 RENAL SURVEILLANCE

Ultrasonography is of value in long-term follow up of patients who have had nephrectomy for a carcinoma. It is also of value in the surveillance of patients with a high risk of renal tumours provided it is performed at regular intervals, for example every 2 to 3 months.

4.1.44 CONDITIONS ASSOCIATED WITH AN INCREASED RISK OF RENAL NEOPLASMS

Previous neoplasm.
Hemihypertrophy (may present after tumour diagnosis).
Aniridia.
Beckwith–Wiedemann syndrome.
Tuberous sclerosis.
Von Hippel–Lindau syndrome.
Long-term renal dialysis.
Polycystic disease.

4.1.45 THE URINARY BLADDER

The urinary bladder is extraperitoneal and lies in the pelvis though it is primarily an abdominal organ until 6 years of age. The ureters pass obliquely through the bladder wall, the intramural course being 6 to 16 mm long. The bladder wall thickness is usually between 3 and 6 mm when the bladder is distended. The bladder wall is made up of (from the mural surface outwards)

- transitional epithelium
- submucous layer
- muscle (detrusor)
- subserous layer
- serous or peritoneal lining.

Sonography

Sonographically the bladder is seen as an anechoic sac of fluid in the anterior pelvis. Its shape, size and wall thickness is very variable depending upon the degree of distension.

Bladder volume

Assessment of post-voiding bladder volumes allows therapeutic decisions to be made regarding bladder function and outlet obstruction. Given the variable shape of the bladder, in practice using the formula for an ellipsoid can make only approximate volume measurements

$$L \times D \times W \times 0.523 = \text{Volume}$$

L = length, D = depth, W = width (there is a 15 to 20 per cent error when using this formula).

With 3D ultrasound more accurate volume measurements can be achieved because it permits accurate tracking of bladder borders. Accurate measurements can be obtained even with irregular shapes, moreover the walls of the bladder can be excluded from volume measurements.

4.1.46 BLADDER ABNORMALITIES IN CHILDREN

Variants – pseudo-ectopic insertion of the ureter

The sonographic 'jet' phenomenon is related to a difference in specific gravity of urine between that in the bladder and the urine being propelled from the ureter into the bladder. This is a normal phenomenon unrelated to vesicoureteric reflux. On CT and intravenous urography films the 'jet' phenomenon may mimic an ectopic insertion of the ureter. This phenomenon is unlikely to be misinterpreted on real-time sonography and color Doppler ultrasound.

Variants – pseudo-ureterocoele

An artefact may be produced because of the introduction of air during catheterisation for voiding cystourethrography. The air produces a filling defect within the contrast when the patient is placed in an oblique position, mimicking a ureterocoele. After voiding the air may cause small filling defects at the bladder base. These artefacts are less likely to occur with ultrasound.

Ureterocoele

A ureterocoele is a dilatation of the distal ureter which has herniated through the bladder wall into the bladder lumen. This usually occurs secondary to a distal ureteric stenosis which causes obstruction and dilatation of the distal ureter.

Orthoptic (simple) ureterocoele   This is sited at the normal vesicoureteric junction.

Ectopic ureterocoele   These occur at sites of ectopic insertion of the ureter into the bladder, urethra, vagina, perineum, etc. They usually arise at the ectopic insertion of the upper moiety ureter of a duplex kidney though a ureter from a non-duplex kidney can have an ectopic insertion.

Ureterocoeles may be small or they may be large enough to fill the entire bladder. They are dynamic structures which change shape depending upon the rate of urine production and degree of bladder distension.

Sonography

On sonography a ureterocoele is seen as an anechoic cyst-like fluid-filled structure with a thin echogenic wall bulging into the bladder lumen. Continuation with the dilated ureter is frequently evident. At times, particularly in boys, a large simple ureterocoele may prolapse into the urethra and cause obstruction of the bladder outlet. Calculi may either form within the ureterocoele or migrate from the kidney. These are seen as highly echogenic foci within the ureterocoele, that most often cast a shadow. Ectopic ureterocoeles have a varied appearance. The usually anechoic ureterocoele can become echo intense when complicated by infection or by the precipitation of solutes.

Endoscopic ureterocoele incision

Endoscopic ureterocoele incision is advocated in neonates with an infected or obstructed collecting system, in older children with obstructing simple ureterocoeles and in patients with antenatally diagnosed ureterocoeles with no symptoms.

Postoperative appearances of endoscopically resected ureterocoeles

Pseudo-mass.

Focal mucosal thickening.

Residual ureterocoele with decrease in size.

Ureterocoeles can evert during bladder filling and mimic a diverticulum – both intact and incised ureterocoeles can evert or intussuscept during bladder filling mimicking a bladder diverticulum.

Persistent ureterocoele.

No residual abnormality.

Urachal anomalies

The most common urachal abnormality is the presence of a cavity of variable size within the urachal remnant arising from the dome of the diaphragm. These cysts or diverticula contain clear fluid, however they may become traumatised and fill with blood products or become infected.

Sonography

Sonography is used to look at the internal architecture of these cysts and to exclude other cystic structures at this location, such as duplication and mesenteric and ovarian cysts. With sagittal scanning one should be able to define the relationship of the bladder and the umbilicus.

Congenital bladder diverticula

Congenital diverticula (not associated with bladder outlet obstruction) may be single or bilateral. These are usually asymptomatic and an incidental finding but they can be associated with stasis, infection, calculus formation, bladder outlet obstruction, ureteral obstruction, vesicoureteric reflux and inferior vena cava obstruction.

Differential diagnosis of multiple bladder diverticula

Bladder outlet obstruction.
Menke's syndrome.
Williams syndrome.
Prune belly syndrome.
Ehlers–Danlos syndrome.
Cutis laxa.

Rhabdomyosarcoma

The most frequently encountered bladder tumour in children is a rhabdomyosarcoma. The tumour may arise in the bladder base or adjacent structures such as the prostate, vulva or vagina.

Sonography

Sonography can be used to establish the intravesical extent of the tumour at diagnosis and to assess the bladder lumen in response to treatment. The tumour appears to be of homogeneous echogenicity similar to muscle but areas of necrosis and haemorrhage may appear hypoechoic. The tumour may show increased vascularity on duplex or colour Doppler. Rhabdomyosarcoma may manifest itself as a solitary polyp indistinguishable from inflammatory or other polyps.

Pseudo-tumoral cystitis

Also known as eosinophilic cystitis this is an uncommon inflammatory process seen both in children and adults. In children it is a self-limiting condition which resolves spontaneously and usually requires no treatment. Recognition is therefore important.

Sonographic signs of pseudo-tumoral cystitis

Broad-based intravesical masses with smooth or irregular outline.
Mass confined to bladder mucosa with preservation of the muscle layers.
Trigone primarily involved with variable extension.
Generalised bladder wall thickening with mucosal irregularity.

Unilateral or bilateral hydronephrosis as a result of mucosal thickening or obstruction at the vesicoureteric junction.

Primary lymphoma

Primary lymphoma of the bladder has no characteristic ultrasound features. The tumour may infiltrate the bladder wall or present as a polyp. Tissue diagnosis is usually required.

Differential diagnosis of a polypoid bladder mass in children
Inflammatory polyp.
Nephrogenic adenoma.
Collapsed ureterocoele.
Incised ureterocoele.
Rhabdomyosarcoma.
Transitional cell carcinoma.
Cavernous haemangioma.
Neurofibroma.

Vesicoureteric reflux

Primary   This is related to incompetence of the vesicoureteric junction as a result of abnormal tunnelling of the distal ureter through the bladder wall. It is found in 10 per cent of babies and in 30 per cent of children with a first episode of urinary tract infection. Reflux may be unilateral or bilateral. The lower moiety of a duplex kidney is commonly involved when two ureters are present. Nearly half of the children with reflux develop renal scarring. In 80 per cent of children there is spontaneous resolution of reflux.

Secondary   Secondary or acquired reflux may accompany paraureteric diverticulum, duplication with ureterocoeles, bladder outlet obstruction, cystitis and prune belly syndrome.

Grading of vesicoureteric reflux
Grade I – reflux into distal ureters.
Grade II – reflux into the renal sinus but with no calyceal dilatation.
Grade III – I and II associated with mild pelvicalyceal dilatation.
Grade IV – I, II and III associated with moderate pelvicalyceal dilatation.
Grade V – I to IV associated with marked tortuosity of the ureters.

The grading is based on voiding cystourethrography.

Sonography
There has been a lot of controversy as to the role of ultrasound in the detection of vesicoureteric reflux. Earlier work shows that the sensitivity of ultra-

sound is low. However recent work with colour Doppler and the use of echo enhancers has shown ultrasound to be as good as voiding cysto-urethrography (VCUG). In neonates 87 per cent of patients with reflux show at least one of the following sonographic abnormalities.

Sonographic signs of vesicoureteric reflux

Intermittent dilatation of the renal collecting system.

In a neonate renal pelvic dilatation above 7 mm on a transverse scan.

Pelvic and ureteral wall thickening.

Absence of corticomedullary differentiation.

Signs of renal dysplasia (small kidney, thin hyperechoic cortex and cortical cysts).

Large thin-walled urinary bladder.

A midline to ureteric orifice distance greater than 7 to 9 mm.

Reflux is diagnosed when hyperechoic floating microbubbles appear in the ureters or renal pelvises after the introduction of galactose-based microbubbles into the bladder.

Colour Doppler signals from the bladder to the ureter during the course of bladder filling and during micturition.

4.1.47 BLADDER DIVERTICULA ASSOCIATED WITH BLADDER-OUTLET OBSTRUCTION

Bladder diverticula occur as protrusions of the bladder mucosa between the bundles of detrusor muscle. They are very variable in size and as they have no muscle in their walls they may increase in size during micturition. Most diverticula are secondary to bladder-outlet obstruction. Congenital diverticula are rare.

Sonography

Diverticula are difficult to see when small but large diverticula are seen as anechoic, fluid-filled structures around the bladder. Occasionally they may contain debris, clot, stones or tumour. They may be mistaken for ovarian cysts, bladder duplication and loculated ascites or urachal remnants. Paraureteric diverticula may distort the vesicoureteric junction and cause reflex.

4.1.48 VESICAL DOME MASSES

Urachal neoplasm

These tumours make up less than 0.34 per cent of bladder cancers, 95 per cent are mucin-secreting adenocarcinomas, whilst 5 per cent are transitional, squamous and anaplastic. The site of origin is the juxtavesical or intravesical part in 90 per cent, the middle of the urachus in 6 per cent and near the umbilicus in 4 per cent. The tumour most commonly involves the anterior bladder dome and grows outwards. The tumour affects the 40 to 70 year age group, the majority present with haematuria. Sonography reveals a midline or slightly off midline, solid, complex or cystic tumour. The tumour calcifies in 50 to 70 per cent of cases.

Urachal cysts

See p. 376.

Vesical, ovarian, gastrointestinal tract, prostatic and cervical cancers

These tumours may involve the vesical dome by direct spread. However this is a late occurrence in the course of disease and the primary site has often been determined by other means.

4.1.49 PERFORATION OF THE UTERUS

This is a rare complication of dilatation and curettage, that may result in an inflammatory mass mimicking a carcinoma. A history of recent surgical intervention will usually be forthcoming.

4.1.50 PELVIC LIPOMATOSIS

Marked increase in the deposition of fat in the pelvis usually affects obese middle-aged men. This results in bladder compression increasing its craniocaudal length and narrowing it from side to side. The fat is seen as echogenic material filling the pelvis around the bladder. The majority of other diseases which result in bladder compression give rise to hypoechoic masses.

Hypoechoic masses causing lateral compression of the bladder

Venous collaterals in inferior vena cava thrombosis.
Bilateral iliac artery aneurysms.
Lymphadenopathy.
Pelvic tumours.
Haematoma.
Lymphocoele.

4.1.51 CYSTITIS

There are many causes of inflammation of the bladder wall including infection, radiation, drugs (for example cyclophosphamide) and trauma (for example indwelling catheter or surgery). The bladder appears sonographically normal in the majority of cases but may show thickening of its wall because of oedema. The bladder mucosa is normally less than 2 mm thick measured at full distension.

4.1.52 BLADDER TUMOURS

Tumours of the bladder wall are seen as echogenic masses protruding into the bladder lumen from their wall attachment. Uncommonly bladder tumours can be benign, for example fibroma, endmetrioma and rarely a pheochromocytoma. Malignant bladder tumours are transitional cell carcinomas in 90 per cent of patients, squamous carcinomas in 6 to 8 per cent and adenocarcinomas in 2 per cent of patients. Clinical staging is inaccurate in 45 per cent of patients whilst CT has an accuracy of 90 per cent.

Jewett Marshal staging system of bladder carcinoma

O – tumour is confined to the mucosa.
A – spread to submucosa.
B – spread to muscle layers.
C – perivesical disease.
D – spread to adjacent organs, nodes or distant sites.

Transurethral scanning using a 12.5 or 20 MHz transducer in a 6.2-F catheter has been used as means of staging bladder tumours. This is a promising technique but not practical at the moment. The same technique has been used in staging renal pelvic and ureteric tumours. Superficial non-invasive tumours have a well-defined base without bladder wall deformity or fixation. Tumours spreading into the bladder wall are seen as hypoechoic areas within the wall causing loss of continuity of normal wall echoes. More extensive tumour spread is seen as hypoechoic tumour extending into the perivesical fat.

4.1.53 BLADDER CALCULI

Bladder calculi are usually secondary to chronic incomplete bladder emptying and stasis. Calculi are seen as echogenic masses within the bladder lumen, that are usually mobile and cause distal shadowing. A similar appearance occurs with blood clot, foreign bodies and tumours encrusted with calcium salts. Sonography is particularly good at picking up lucent calculi which may not be visualised on plain abdominal radiographs.

Bladder calculi may be mimicked by sub-ureteric teflon injection, which gives rise to echogenic mounds that may shadow.

4.1.54 BLADDER WALL CALCIFICATION

Tuberculosis.
Schistosomiasis.
Bladder tumours.
Post-irradiation cystitis.

4.1.55 BLADDER WALL HAEMATOMA

Bladder wall haematomas are not uncommon if the bladder is examined sonographically immediately after instrumentation. Lesions may appear solid or cystic depending upon the nature of the blood. Focal oedema may also give rise to focal masses. Any such anomalies found after cystoscopy should be followed up to ensure resolution.

4.1.56 NEUROPATHIC BLADDER

The bladder should be routinely scanned before and after micturition. Loss of normal neurological control of bladder function may affect bladder volume and appearance. Posterior nerve root lesions usually give rise to a spastic bladder which is trabeculated and may have multiple diverticula. In long-standing cases the bladder volume may be markedly reduced.

4.1.57 BLADDER INJURY

The bladder is much more prone to injury in a child than in an adult owing to its abdominal position. Blunt abdominal trauma, penetrating injury or pelvic fractures may injure it. The latter may cause urethral injury.

Types of bladder injury

- Bladder contusion (the most common injury).
- Interstitial bladder injury (rare).
- Bladder rupture:
  extraperitoneal 80 per cent
  intraperitoneal 20 per cent (higher in children)
  combined intraperitoneal and extraperitoneal (rare).

Sonography

Sonography may show the 'bladder-within-a-bladder sign' (bladder surrounded by free fluid) with extraperitoneal rupture. With intraperitoneal rupture, which usually occurs at the bladder dome, one may expect to see urinary ascites.

4.1.58 PERIVESICAL FLUID COLLECTIONS

Pelvic ascites.
Haematoma.
Abscess or pus.
Urinoma.
Lymphocoele.
Post-ovulation fluid.
Contrast – post-hysterosalpingography.
Ultrasound contrast – post-sonohysterosalpingography.
Uterine rupture.
Ovarian cyst rupture.
Ectopic pregnancy.

4.1.59 INTRALUMINAL BLADDER MASSES (*Including bladder wall lesions bulging into the lumen*)

Malignant bladder tumours – transitional cell carcinoma, squamous cell carcinoma, adenocarcinoma, rhabdomyosarcoma (usually children), leiomyosarcoma, lymphoma.
Bladder tumours metastatic – melanoma, stomach carcinoma, breast carcinoma, renal cell carcinoma, bronchial carcinoma.
Benign prostatic hyperplasia.
Prostatic malignancy.
Blood clot.
Calculi.
Foreign body.
Bladder trabeculation.
Localised haemorrhage or bladder wall oedema.
Ureterocoele.
Extension of an adjacent malignancy – prostate, rectum, colon, uterus, ovary or cervix.
Abscess spreading to the bladder wall.
Endometriosis.
Polyp.
Fungus ball.

Granuloma (tuberculosis, schistosomiasis).
Benign bladder wall tumours – leiomyoma, neurofibroma, haemangioma, phaeo-
chromocytoma, rhabdomyoma, nephrogenic adenoma.
Cystitis (inflammatory polyps).
Leukoplakia.
Cystitis cystica.
Malakoplakia.
Prolapsing urethral polyp.

4.1.60 BLADDER-WALL THICKENING

Thickness of the normal wall is

- less than 5 mm for a non-distended bladder
- less than 3 mm for a distended bladder.

Causes of bladder-wall thickening

Increased muscle thickness (urethral valves, prostatic hypertrophy).
Neurogenic bladder.
Cystitis.
Bladder malignancy.

4.1.61 MASSES COMPRESSING THE BLADDER

Uterus – pregnancy, fibroid.
Ovarian masses.
Ectopic kidney.
Prostatic hypertrophy (cancer).
Lymph nodes.
Sacrum or coccyx bone tumour.
Hip arthroplasty.
Meningomyelocoele.
Pelvic lipomatosis.

4.1.62 THE URETHRA

The urethra is not usually seen during bladder sonography although urethral diverticula have been diagnosed sonographically. Bladder outflow
obstruction by urethral valves causes distension of the posterior urethra
which may then be visualised. This is the commonest form of lower urinary
tract obstruction in boys; it is very rare in girls.

Urethral valves

Classification

Type 1 – exaggeration of plicae colliculi which extend from the verumontanum and attach to the anterolateral walls of the urethra.

Type 2 – folds arising from the verumontanum, that pass proximally to the bladder base (this may not be a true cause of obstruction).

Type 3 – diaphragm with a small central perforation, situated proximal or distal to the verumontanum but not actually attached to it.

The posterior urethra is dilated and visible in only 50 per cent of causes of posterior urethral valves if the bladder is scanned at rest. Dilatation is more obvious if scanning is undertaken during micturition. Posterior urethral dilatation is better seen with transperineal scanning. A dilated utricle may also be observed with perineal scanning. Other evidence of bladder outflow obstruction includes bladder wall thickening and upper tract dilatation due to reflux or retrograde transmission of increased bladder pressure. An over-distended bladder is seen in 30 per cent of children. As posterior urethral valves may be detected antenatally, the child may be born with hypoplastic or multicystic dysplastic kidneys. Dilated renal pelvis may be absent in a newborn if the bladder has ruptured antenatally or in association with renal dysplasia or pelviuretral atresia.

Female urethral sphincter

The female urethral sphincter (the external rhabdosphincter of the bladder) is regularly observed on routine scanning of the female bladder. This sphincter which has been dubbed as the 'female pseudo-prostate', is seen as a rounded or oval midline structure measuring $1.30 \times 1.33 \times 0.96$ cm in longitudinal, transverse and anteroposterior dimensions at the bladder base. The structure is fairly well defined and rounded. This is a normal anatomical structure and should not be confused with a pathological polyp or mass.

Transperineal sonography in children

Transperineal sonography is an effective technique for revealing the morphology of the urethra, periurethral soft tissues, anterior rectum and the vagina and distal genital tract in girls. A linear 5 to 7.5 MHz transducer covered with gel and a plastic wrap is applied to the perineum in a lithotomy position.

4.1.63 ACQUIRED URETHRAL DIVERTICULA IN THE FEMALE

Acquired urethral diverticula are thought to occur in 3 per cent of asymptomatic women. However they may be an overlooked cause of persistent urinary symptoms on the face of normal routine urological investigations. Symptoms are often mistaken for cystitis, stress incontinence, infected periurethral glands or endometriosis. The standard technique for investigating suspected urethral diverticula is retrograde urethrography or voiding cystourethrography. Sonography is useful in women with suspected urethral diverticula. Several approaches have been used including perineal, transrectal, endovaginal and transurethral sonography. Endoscopic urethral ultrasound appears particularly good and provides information on the extent and location of the diverticular neck both of which are important in surgical excision. The technique also provides information on lesions not connected to the urethra. The diverticula appear as echopoor masses with a debris level.

Differential diagnosis of female urethral diverticula

Urethral diverticula.
Gartner's duct cysts.
Endometrioma.
Ectopic ureterocoeles.
Vaginal inclusion cysts.
Skene gland abscesses.
Haematoma.
Accessory phallic urethra with obstructed and dilated dorsal urethra.

4.1.64 DIFFERENTIAL DIAGNOSIS OF A CYSTIC URETHRAL MASS IN A MALE

Posterior urethral valves.
Congenital urethral diverticulosis – lacuna magna-diverticula in the urethral roof, narrow-mouthed saccular, wide-mouthed saccular, scaphoid megalourethra (floor of anterior urethra, rare), fusiform megalourethra (involves the entire urethra, rare).
Accessory ventral urethra with cystic dilatation.
Cowper's syringocoele.
Stenosed or occluded Cowper's duct.
Periurethral abscess.
False passage (following instrumentation).
Traumatic diverticula.

Haematoma.
Patulous urethra in neuromuscular disorders affecting the bladder.
Perineal diverticula.

4.1.65 PERINEAL DIVERTICULA

These diverticula are typically located in the membranous urethra and occur after bilateral ischiectomy as a result of which there is severance of the attachment of the triangular ligament inferior to the pubic ramus. With loss of the triangular ligament the unprotected bulbous urethra becomes subject to direct weight bearing.

4.1.66 COWPER'S SYRINGOCOELE

The bulbous urethral glands (Cowper's) are paired dorsal structures where their ducts (bulbourethral ducts) drain into the bulbous spongiosum, proximal to the bulbous urethra. Cystic dilatation of the bulbourethral ducts may occur because of either stenosis or occlusion of the duct ostia because of stasis and pressure changes. Patients present with recurrent urinary tract infections, urethral discharge and urinary obstructive symptoms. Four types of syringocoeles have been described

1. simple – minimal dilatation of the distal bulbourethral duct allowing reflux from the urethra
2. perforate – dilated distal duct communicating with the urethra via a patulous orifice
3. imperforate – complete obstruction of the duct orifice resulting in a cyst that does not communicate with the urethra
4. ruptured – a thin frail membrane remains within the bulbous urethra following rupture of the syringocoele.

Perforated syringocoeles are readily seen on urethrography as a diverticulum communicating with the urethra whilst the imperforate variety gives an appearance of an extrinsic mass impressing on the urethra, usually with smooth margins.

On transperineal sonography a cystic structure is seen in relation to the bulbous urethra with septations or internal echoes. Ultrasound would rule out lesions such as urethral tumours.

Differential diagnosis of imperforate syringocoeles

Imperforate syringocoele.
Periurethral abscess.
Periurethral haematoma.

False passage following instrumentation.
Benign tumours of the bulbourethral glands.
Adenocarcinoma of the bulbourethral glands.

4.1.67 BARTHOLIN GLAND ABSCESS

Bartholin glands are paired vulvovaginal mucus-secreting epithelial-lined glands. These glands drain via ducts (approximately 2.5 cm) at the junction of the hymen and labia minora on the posterolateral aspect of the vagina. Lined by transitional epithelium these ducts are particularly prone to obstruction at their ostia. Accumulation of secretions within these ducts gives rise to cystic dilatation, which may become secondarily infected and inflamed. Treatment is usually surgical; this is particularly the case in women over the age of 40 years because of the risk of a Bartholin gland carcinoma. Sonography reveals a hypoechoic mass with a small anechoic component concentrically surrounded by multilayered echogenic structures. A guide aspiration may help in arriving at a diagnosis and aid in the placement of a Word catheter for drainage.

4.1.68 URETHRAL TUMOURS

Urethral tumours in the male

Benign mesenchymal tumours – fibrous polyp (children), haemangioma (extremely rare), myoblastic (extremely rare).
Benign epithelial tumours – transitional cell papilloma (elderly), adenomatous tumour of the prostatic urethra, adenomatous metaplasia, papillary urethritis (polypoid urethritis).
Malignant tumours – transitional cell carcinoma, squamous cell carcinoma, metastases (kidney, bladder, prostate, colon, spermatic cord, testis).

Urethral tumours in the female

Benign tumours – polyp, papilloma, adenoma (these three types of tumour have a *recorded association with malignancy*).
Malignant tumours – transitional cell carcinoma (proximal urethra), squamous cell carcinoma (distal urethra).

4.1.69 DETRUSOR SPHINCTER DYSSYNERGIA

Detrusor sphincter dyssynergia refers to the inability of the bladder neck to open when the bladder contracts (spinal cord lesion or trauma above the sacral outflow), that can be detected on ultrasonography. By an intravenous delivery of 5 to 10 mg of phentolamine (an alpha-adrenergic blocker) it is possible to demonstrate the opening of the neck within 5 minutes of the injection, confirming the diagnosis of detrusor-sphincter dyssynergia. A further refinement is to use a combination of ultrasound and electromyography to establish the diagnosis. An electromyography needle is placed into the periurethral striated sphincter using transrectal ultrasound for guidance. Diagnosis is confirmed when increased electromyographic activity of the periurethral striated sphincter is observed during bladder contraction, whilst the distal half of the prostatic urethra remains narrow as observed by sonography, associated with an increased prominence of the verumontanum.

4.2 ADRENAL GLANDS

The adrenal glands each weigh approximately 5 grams and measure $4 \times 2 \times 0.4$ cm in size. The right gland is triangular or pyramidal in shape and lies in front of the right crus of the diaphragm behind the inferior vena cava and bare area of the liver at the upper pole of the right kidney. The right crus of the diaphragm may be mistaken for the adrenal surrounded by perirenal fat. The left adrenal gland is prerenal in position extending from the upper pole of the left kidney almost down to the left renal hilum. It lies in front of the left crus of the diaphragm behind the splenic vessels and pancreas and is crescentic or semilunar in shape.

Sonography

Although the adrenal glands may be seen as slightly echogenic bands, it is fat around the adrenal gland that is more frequently visualised. The adrenals appear hypoechoic relative to the surrounding fat but they are frequently only visualised when enlarged or calcified. They may appear normal despite clinically proven disease, for example sonographic changes are only present in 50 per cent of proven cases of bilateral adrenal hyperplasia. In the neonate on the other hand it has been shown that 97 per cent of the normal right adrenal and 83 per cent of the normal left adrenal glands can be identified. The reasons for the improved visualisation of the normal neonatal adrenals include the larger size of the neonatal adrenal glands relative to other intra-abdominal organs, the smaller size of the patient and less retroperitoneal fat. The left adrenal gland has to be distinguished from a pancreatic mass, splenic artery aneurysm and accessory spleen.

4.2.1 ADRENAL MASSES

Small adrenal masses can frequently be visualised, as they tend to be hypo-echoic and are outlined by adjacent fat. However ultrasound has difficulty in showing masses less than 1.3 cm in size and has an accuracy of 70 per cent as compared to an accuracy of 90 per cent with CT. Small adrenal masses lie anteromedial to the kidney whilst larger masses lie more anteri-orly and may appear hepatic or renal in origin. Hepatic, renal, splenic and pancreatic cysts need to be distinguished from adrenal cysts. Ultrasound is superior to conventional CT in this respect because of its multiplaner capa-bility. Adrenal calcification is not uncommon and gives rise to echogenic foci within the gland, that may shadow. Bowel loops may be mistaken for adrenal masses but they are inconsistent when the patient's position is changed, par-ticularly if the patient is scanned erect. The most common adrenal tumours are adenoma, phaeochromocytoma, adrenocortical carcinoma and metastases.

Causes of neonatal adrenal calcification

Adrenal haemorrhage.
Neuroblastoma.
Virus simplex infection (calcification is also found in the liver).
Wolman's disease (abnormal leukocyte acid lipase).

Adrenal calcification in older children and adults

Solid tumours – neuroblastoma, phaeochromocytoma, adenoma, carcinoma, dermoid, metastases, melanoma (metastatic or primary), haemangioma (rare), ganglio-neuroma, angiosarcoma (extremely rare), myelolipoma (rare), osteoma (rare).
Adrenal haemorrhage – overwhelming bacterial infections, neonatal adrenal haem-orrhage, anticoagulant therapy, pseudocyst (secondary to haemorrhage).
Infections – *Echinococcus granulosis* cyst, tuberculosis, histoplasmosis, virus simplex infection, meningococcal septicaemia.
Miscellaneous – Addison's disease, Wolman's disease.

Neonatal adrenal masses

Haemorrhage.
Neuroblastoma.
Adrenal carcinoma.

Bilateral adrenal masses

Metastases.
Adrenal hyperplasia.

Lymphoma.
Haemorrhage.
Tuberculosis.
Histoplasmosis.
Phaeochromocytoma.
Haemangioma (very rare).

Adrenal tumours

Functioning tumours of the adrenal gland may be quite small but may have profound systemic effects, for example Conn's adenomas. Benign tumours usually have a solid appearance with well-defined margins. Adrenal hyperplasia is difficult to identify and is easily mistaken for an adenoma if hyperplasia is nodular. Metastases are the commonest malignant adrenal lesions, they are usually hypoechoic but may be echogenic and are frequently bilateral. Haemorrhage and necrosis give rise to a heterogenous appearance.

Differential diagnosis of adrenal masses

Benign non-functioning masses – lipoma, fibroma, cysts, leiomyoma, haemangioma, myelolipoma, collision tumour (partly functioning), osteoma, neurofibroma.
Functioning cortical tumours – adenoma, carcinoma, adrenal hyperplasia.
Functioning medullary tumours – phaeochromocytoma, neurogenic tumours.
Non-functioning medullary tumours – neuroblastoma, ganglioneuroma (benign), primary malignant melanoma.
Non-functioning malignant tumours – metastases: (breast, lung, ovary, gastrointestinal tract, melanoma and kidney), angiosarcoma (extremely rare), leiomyosarcoma (rare), fibrosarcoma (extremely rare).

Neuroblastoma

Neuroblastoma is relatively common in children and is the commonest abdominal mass in a young child. Thirty per cent occur in the first year of life whilst 85 per cent occur in children less than 5 years of age. The prognosis is age dependent and is most favourable in the neonate. Neuroblastoma is a malignant neoplasm derived from the sympathetic neuroblast tissue, 70 per cent arise within the abdomen though only 37 per cent arise primarily in the adrenal glands. Neuroblastoma is usually a solid tumour which is often large at presentation. They have a more heterogeneous echopattern than Wilms' tumour and calcific foci are frequently seen in both the primary tumour and metastases. The tumour may spread directly to the liver via the blood stream. Cases of neuroblastoma frequently present with evidence of metastases (up to 60 per cent) before the primary tumour is evident. In these cases ultrasonography is invaluable at demonstrating adrenal pathology.

Differential diagnosis of a neuroblastoma

Tuberculoma – presents in an older age group, it is unusual in Europe and the US.

Exophytic Wilms' tumour – this involves the kidney.

Adrenal haemorrhage – this has a changing echopattern over time and is bilateral.

Retroperitoneal teratoma – more often has cystic components.

Ganglioneuroma – affects an older age group.

Ganglioneuroblastoma is indistinguishable from a neuroblastoma.

Multicystic dysplastic kidney – the normal renal architecture is replaced.

Mesoblastic nephroma – this is a multiloculated renal mass.

Haemangioma – extremely rare and affects older patients.

Inflammatory pseudo-tumour.

Adrenal carcinoma

Adrenal carcinoma is a rare adrenal cortical malignancy which has a poor prognosis with no survivors at 5 years. Adrenal carcinomas make up 0.3 to 0.4 per cent of all childhood malignancies and presentation in neonates has been described. Adrenal carcinomas are usually large at diagnosis even when the tumour is functioning (carcinomas demonstrate less endocrine function than adenomas relative to their size). Of the functioning carcinomas 36 per cent present with Cushing's syndrome, 20 per cent with a combination of Cushing's and virilism, 6 per cent with feminisation and 1 per cent with mineralocorticoids and other hormones. Twenty per cent of adrenal carcinomas secrete no functioning hormones.

Sonography

A heterogeneous mass is the commonest appearance though haemorrhage and necrosis may give rise to a more complex mass with cystic areas, with irregular walls. The mass is generally hypoechoic as compared to normal adrenal tissue. The tumour may invade the renal vein and inferior vena cava and metastases may spread to the regional lymph nodes, lungs, diaphragm, bone and brain. The tumour may occasionally calcify. Calcification and large size suggest malignancy on imaging. A needle biopsy is fraught with problems as a well-differentiated carcinoma may be misinterpreted as an adenoma.

Adrenal adenoma

Non-functioning adenomas

These masses are found incidentally on CT or ultrasound. The levels of adrenal hormones are normal with clinical features of hyperfunction. They are found in 0.6 to 1.5 per cent of CT examinations, whilst the exact incidence on ultrasound is unknown. They are found in 3 to 9 per cent of individuals at autopsy series. When found in the presence of a primary tumour such as a lung carcinoma, it is difficult to differentiate an adenoma from a metastatic deposit on imaging. Surveillance with CT or ultrasound will confirm a lack of growth. In case of doubt a fine-needle aspiration biopsy is usually recommended. They represent well-defined solid masses which are uniformly hypoechoic to the normal adrenal gland.

Functioning adenomas

Conn's syndrome hypersecretion of aldosterone causing hypertension. These tumours are quite small at presentation and are not usually visible on ultrasound. When seen these tumours are less than 1 centimetre, hypoechoic and well defined. Conn's syndrome may also result from adrenal hyperplasia.

Cushing's syndrome hypersecretion of corticosteroids. These tumours make up 10 per cent of adenomas.

Virilising adenomas hypersecretion of testosterone. These tumours cause virilising characteristics in boys and girls.

Feminising adenomas oestrogen producing tumours.

Functioning adenomas are usually less than 5 cm with an average size of 2.0 to 2.5 cm. They are well-defined tumours hypo- to hyperechoic depending upon fat content. These are usually no areas of necrosis in the average-sized tumours.

Phaeochromocytoma

This is a neuroectodermal tumour arising from the adrenal medulla (90 per cent) or the sympathetic chain. Phaeochromocytomas produce catecholamines and thus patients present with hypertension which may be intermittent. Most are benign but 10 per cent are malignant, 10 per cent bilateral and 10 per cent are extra-adrenal. Approximately 40 per cent of extra-adrenal phaeochromocytomas are missed, of which 5 per cent are multiple. Most of the extra-adrenal phaeochromocytomas lie in the abdomen or pelvis. Phaeochromocytoma can occur as a familial disorder. The tumour has a known association with multiple endocrine neoplasia type IIa and IIb (type III) and neuroectodermal disorders.

Sonography

Sonographic appearances are those of a well-defined homogeneous hypo-echoic mass in approximately 50 per cent of patients. However the mass may be complex or even cystic (16 per cent) and hyperechoic to the renal parenchyma (approximately 20 per cent). Most phaeochromocytomas are 5 to 6 cm in size at presentation.

Ganglioneuroma

This is a benign neural crest tumour closely related to ganglioneuroblastoma and neuroblastoma. The retroperitoneum is the commonest site of occurrence, while 20 per cent occur in the adrenal gland. Most cases of ganglioneuroma occur in patients over the age of 40 years (60 per cent). A minority are functioning, producing hypertension, virilisation, myasthenia gravis, diarrhoea and sweating depending upon the dominant hormone produced.

Sonography

The sonographic appearances are those of a solid heterogeneous tumour. The tumour has a tendency to surround blood vessels with no compromise to the vessel or compromise is minimal. Calcification has been recorded in 8 to 27 per cent of cases. The differential diagnosis is from a neuroblastoma when in the adrenal, and from a neurofibroma and schwannoma when in the retroperitoneum.

Ganglioneuroblastoma

This is a rare neural crest tumour that is intermediate in cellular maturity between a ganglioneuroma and a neuroblastoma. The tumours usually present in early childhood, most involve the sympathetic ganglia with extension into the epidural space through neural foramina. The exact incidence of adrenal location is unknown but it is rare. The sonographic appearances may be indistinguishable from a ganglioneuroma or neuroblastoma. A cystic appearance has been described in adrenal tumour.

Myelolipoma

Myelolipoma is a rare benign tumour which contains mature fat tissue and proliferating haematopoietic cells. Its prevalence at autopsy series is estimated at 0.08 to 0.4 per cent. Most are asymptomatic but some may produce pain from a mass effect. Endocrine dysfunction has been reported but this is probably related to a coexisting adrenal adenoma. Calcification is rare but punctate when it occurs.

Sonography

Sonographically these tumours are well defined and hyperechoic. Computed tomography may suggest the diagnosis as fat content may be demonstrated; CT values are higher than those of retroperitoneal fat, as myelolipomas contain bone marrow cells. Tissue diagnosis has been achieved by fine-needle aspiration. The differential diagnosis includes lipoma, retroperitoneal liposarcoma and upper pole angiomyolipoma of the kidney.

Haemangioma

Adrenal haemangiomas are extremely rare with fewer than 20 cases reported in the world literature. The age group affected is between 50 and 70 years. The tumour is twice as common in women and bilateral involvement has been reported. A giant cavernous haemangioma of the adrenal gland 25 cm in diameter has been reported. Most haemangiomas are cavernous and rarely capillary.

Sonography

The sonographic appearances are those of a hypoechoic, hyperechoic or a mixed echogenicity mass. Sixty four per cent of tumours have calcification demonstrated on plain radiographs. Haemorrhage within the tumour may occur. The most helpful signs on CT are demonstration of phleboliths and contrast enhancement of peripheral lakes. However similar CT features have been described with haemangioblastoma.

Sarcoma

Malignant mesenchymal tumours of the adrenal gland are extremely rare. Only a few cases of soft tissue sarcomas including leiomyosarcoma and angiosarcoma have been reported. There is usually diagnostic difficulty in differentiating these tumours from metastases.

Adrenal lymphoma

Adrenal lymphomatous infiltration is not uncommon. At autopsy series 25 per cent of lymphoma patients have adrenal involvement due mainly to direct spread from the retroperitoneum. However primary lymphoma of the adrenal gland occurs. Forty-six per cent of adrenal lymphomas are bilateral. The most common type of lymphoma to involve the adrenal is non-Hodgkin's lymphoma. Adrenal lymphoma is said to respond the same way to chemotherapy as other systemic or lymph node disease. Thus if presumed lymphoma involvement of the adrenal gland does not respond to treatment as do other sites, the diagnosis of adrenal lymphoma should be reconsidered.

Sonography

Sonographically these tumours, in common with other sites of lymphoma involvement, are echopoor, however areas of echogenicity may occur because of haemorrhage or infarction. The appearances may closely resemble metastases.

Adrenal metastases

The adrenal gland is a common site for metastases and is said to be the fourth most common site after the lungs, liver and bone. The commonest tumours to metastasise to the adrenal gland are the breast, lung, melanoma and kidney and as many as 53 per cent of breast, and 38 per cent of lung, carcinomas have adrenal metastases at autopsy. Theoretically any malignant tumour can metastasise to the adrenal gland.

Sonography

On sonography adrenal metastases appear homogeneously hypoechoic, however the echogenicity varies with the occurrence of haemorrhage and necrosis. Usually by the time adrenal metastases are seen on imaging the primary site is already known. However non-functioning adrenal adenomas do cause confusion from time to time, in which instance CT or ultrasound surveillance for growth or a fine-needle aspirate is recommended. Magnetic resonance imaging can differentiate non-functioning adrenal adenoma from metastases, adrenal carcinoma and phaeochromocytoma in 70 per cent of cases.

Adrenal haemorrhage

Adrenal haemorrhage can occur in two settings: in the neonate where the majority of cases occur and in the adult. The clinical implications differ considerably in the two groups. In the neonate adrenal haemorrhage usually occurs between the second and seventh day of life. The aetiologic factors include birth trauma, hypoxia, infants of diabetic mothers, septicaemia and haemorrhagic diathesis. The right adrenal appears to be more commonly affected as compared to the left, whilst 10 per cent are bilateral. The latter carries more serious clinical implications of adrenal hypofunction. In the adult population adrenal haemorrhage has been associated with anticoagulant therapy, septicaemia, neoplasia, blunt abdominal trauma, liver transplantation and adrenal venous sampling.

Sonography

On sonography the haematoma may have a solid or cystic appearance depending upon the stage of haematoma formation or liquefaction. In the neonate adrenal haemorrhage has to be differentiated from an adrenal carcinoma and neuroblastoma. Colour-coded Doppler sonography and power Doppler has shown vessels within the neuroblastoma whilst no flow was shown in an adrenal haemorrhage. However colour Doppler or power Doppler has been shown not to be helpful in differentiating benign from malignant adrenal masses in the adult. Long-standing cases may calcify giving a densely echogenic appearance with shadowing. In the neonate calcification may be present as early as 10 days after haemorrhage. Adrenal haemorrhage may occur *in utero* and bilateral adrenal calcification may be present at birth.

Adrenal cysts

Adrenal cysts are classified into four groups.

Endothelial cysts (45 per cent)

Lymphangiomatous cysts (93 per cent) – endothelial-lined multiloculated cysts which may result from obstructed lymphatic channels.

Angiomatous cysts – probably a result of recurrent haemorrhage within a haemangioma.

Hamartomatous cysts.

Pseudocysts (39 to 42 per cent)

Pseudocysts lack a true lining

Haemorrhage into a normal adrenal gland.

Haemorrhage into a benign or malignant tumour.

Epithelial cysts (9 per cent)

Unusual cystic adenomas.

Glandular or retention cysts.

Cystic transformation of embryonic cell rests.

Parasitic cysts (7 per cent)

These are usually due to *Echinococcus granulosus* and associated with disseminated hydatid disease although solitary adrenal disease may occur.

Anechoic suprarenal masses

Adrenal haemorrhage.

Cyst – adrenal, renal, hepatic, pancreatic or mesenteric.

Hydronephrosis of the upper moiety of a duplex kidney.

Abscess.

Necrotic tumour – adrenal or renal.

Multiloculated adrenal cysts

Lymphangiomatous cyst.
Pseudocyst.
Hydatid cyst.
Necrotic tumour (thick-walled septa).

Endothelial adrenal cysts

The majority of these cysts are lymphangiomatous (93 per cent). These cysts are usually an incidental finding although rarely they may be become symptomatic because of a local mass effect. A few cases with associated hypertension have been reported, these cases were cured after resection of the cysts. Fifteen per cent are thought to calcify. Most are purely cystic and multiloculate although rarely a hypoechoic or hyperechoic pattern may occur because of haemorrhage. Haemorrhage may also cause a pseudo-nodular appearance. A debris level may be seen on sonography. Doppler ultrasound shows no flow in the cyst or nodules. In atypical cases an aspiration biopsy is recommended.

Adrenal pseudocysts

These make up 39 to 42 per cent of the adrenal cysts. They do not have a true lining but do develop a fibrotic capsule. They form as a result of intraglandular haemorrhage or infarction. Rarely cystic degeneration or infarction of a primary adrenal tumour may cause adrenal pseudocysts. About 15 per cent of pseudocysts display calcification. In uncomplicated pseudocysts sonography may show well-defined cystic lesions with good through transmission, indistinguishable from upper pole paracortical renal cysts. However with complications internal septa and debris may be seen. Calcification may appear as echogenic foci or a curvilinear echogenic surface with shadowing.

Hydatid cyst of the adrenal gland

Hydatid cysts of the adrenal gland are rare and represent 7 per cent of all adrenal cysts whilst the adrenal gland is involved in 0.5 per cent of all *Echinococcus granulosis* infections. The ultrasound features depend upon the stage of evolution of disease. Early lesions appear purely cystic and unilocular, indistinguishable from other benign cysts. Eventually the capsule become fibrotic and some may calcify. The discharge of daughter cysts from the wall gives it a multilocular appearance.

Adrenal pseudo-tumours

Adrenal pseudo-tumours represent either a normal anatomical structure adjacent to the adrenal gland or pathology in adjacent organs that mimic adrenal pathology.

Fluid-filled gastric fundus.
Renal upper pole cyst or tumour.
Tortuous splenic vessels.
Varices.
Splenic lobulation.
Accessory spleen.
Hepatic tumour.
Nodules or variation of the diaphragm.
Hepatic flexure or splenic flexure colonic masses.
Pancreatic masses.
Loculated ascites.
Retroperitoneal tumours.
Retroperitoneal lymphadenopathy.

4.3 FURTHER READING

Abulafia O, Sherer DM: Bartholin gland abscess: sonographic findings. J Clin Ultrasound 25:47-49, 1997.

al-Murrani B et al.: Echogenic rings: an ultrasound sign of early nephrocalcinosis. Clin Radiol 44:49-51, 1991.

Amin R: Primary non-Hodgkin's lymphoma of the bladder. Br J Radiol 68:1257-1260, 1995.

Avni EF et al.: Ultrasound demonstration of pyelitis and ureteritis in children. Pediatr Radiol 18:134-139, 1988.

Avni EF et al.: Can careful ultrasound examination of the urinary tract exclude vesicoureteric reflux in a neonate? Br J Radiol 70:977-982, 1997.

Baxter GM, Morley P, Dall B: Acute renal vein thrombosis in renal allografts: new Doppler ultrasonic findings. Clin Radiol 43:125-127, 1991.

Belli AM, Joseph AEA: The renal rind sign: a new ultrasound indication of inflammatory disease in the abdomen. Br J Radiol 61:806-810, 1988.

Blane CE et al.: Renal sonography is not a reliable screening examination for vesicoureteral reflux. J Urol 150:752-755, 1993.

Borgstein RL, Moran B, Davison LM: Characteristic ultrasonographic appearance of a large renal oncocytoma. Clin Radiol 43:426-428, 1991.

Bosio M: Cystosonography with echocontrast: a new imaging modality to detect vesicoureteric reflux in children. Pediatr Radiol 28:250-255, 1998.

Brandt TD et al.: Ultrasound assessment of normal renal dimensions. J Ultrasound Med 1:49-52, 1982.

Bruno MA et al.: Bile nephrosis in a neonate: sonographic findings of rapid kidney enlargement and increased echogenicity. Am J Roentgenol 159:628-630, 1992.

Butler H, Bick R, Morrison S: Unsuspected adrenal masses in the neonate: adrenal cortical carcinoma and neuroblastoma. Pediatr Radiol *18*:237–239, 1988.

Chan H: Non-invasive bladder volume measurement. J Neurosci Nurs *25*:309, 1993.

Chancellor MB *et al.*: Intraoperative endo-luminal ultrasound evaluation of urethral diverticula. J Urol *153*:72–75, 1995.

Chen JH, Lee SK: Renal leiomyosarcoma mimicking transitional cell carcinoma. Am J Roentgenol *169*:312–313, 1997.

Chippindale AJ, Bisset RAL, Mamtora H: Two patients with symptomatic renal metastases. Clin Radiol *40*:95–97, 1989.

Chuung Y-F, Tsai T-C: Sonographic findings in familial juvenile nephronophthisis-medullary cystic disease complex. J Clin Ultrasound *26*:203–206, 1998.

Clautice-Eagle T, Jeffrey RB: Renal hypoperfusion: value of power Doppler imaging. Am J Roentgenol *168*:1227–1231, 1997.

Cremin BJ, Davey H, Oleszczuk-Raszke: Neonatal renal venous thrombosis: sequential ultrasonic appearances. Clin Radiol *44*:52–55, 1991.

Dacher JN *et al.*: Power Doppler sonographic pattern of acute pyelonephritis in children: comparison with CT. Am J Roentgenol *166*:1451–1455, 1996.

Darge K *et al.*: Reflux in young patients: comparison of voiding ultrasound of the bladder and retrovesical space with echo enhancement versus voiding cytourethrography for diagnosis. Radiology *10*:201–207, 1999.

Deeg KH, Bettendorf U, Hofmann V: Differential diagnosis of neonatal adrenal haemorrhage and congenital neuroblastoma by color Doppler sonography and power Doppler sonography. Eur J Pediatr *157*:294–297, 1998.

Diament MJ: Is ultrasound screening for urinary tract infection 'cost effective'? Pediatr Radiol *18*:157–159, 1988.

Domjan JM, Dewbury KC: Multiple highly reflective foci in the renal parenchyma are not specific for pseudoxanthoma elasticum. Br J Radiol *69*:871–872, 1996.

Duncan AW, Charles AK, Berry PJ: Cysts within septa: an ultrasound feature distinguishing neoplastic from non-neoplastic renal lesions in children? Pediatr Radiol.

Emamian SA *et al.*: Kidney dimensions at sonography: correlation with age, sex and habitus in 665 adult volunteers. Am J Roentgenol *160*:83–86, 1993.

Felson B, Moskowitz A: Renal pseudotumours: The regenerative nodule and other lumps. Bumps and dromedary lumps. Am J Roentgenol *107*:720–729, 1969.

Fernbach SK, Feinstein KA: Renal tumours in children. Semin Roentgenol vol. XXX *2*:200–217, 1995.

Fernbach SK *et al.*: Fatty Wilm's tumour simulating teratoma: occurrence in a child with horseshoe kidney. Pediatr Radiol *38*:424–426, 1988.

Fredericks BJ *et al.*: Glomerulocystic renal disease: Ultrasound appearances. Pediatr Radiol *19*:184–186, 1989.

Friedman EP, De Bruyn R, Mathew S: Pseudotumoral cystitis in children: a review of ultrasound features in four cases. Br J Radiol *60*:605–608, 1993.

Fung Y, Yeh HC: Renal aspergilloma mimicking a tumour on ultrasonography. J Ultrasound Med *16*:555–557, 1997.

Galli L, Gaboardi F: Adrenal myelolipoma: report of diagnosis by fine needle aspiration. J Urol *136*:655–657, 1986.

Gilbert TJ, Parker BR: Juvenile xanthogranuloma of the kidney. Pediatr Radiol *18*: 169–171, 1988.

Gold RP, Thayaparase R, Romes N: Myxomatous degeneration of renal capsular leiomyoma. Am J Roentgenol *161*:978, 1993.

Goldman I *et al.*: Infected urachal cysts: a review of 10 cases. J Urol *140*:375–378, 1988.

Gorg C, Weida R, Schwerk WB: Unusual perirenal sonographic pattern in malignant lymphoma of the kidney. Clin Radiol 50:720-724, 1995.

Goyal M et al.: Congenital anterior urethral diverticulum: sonographic diagnosis. J Clin Ultrasound 24:543-544, 1996.

Guber SJ, de Bruyn R: Laurence Moon-Biedl syndrome: renal ultrasound in the neonate. Br J Radiol 64:631-633, 1991.

Habboub HK et al.: Accuracy of color Doppler sonography in assessing venous thrombus extension in renal cell carcinoma. Am J Roentgenol 168:267-271, 1997.

Haberlik A: Detection of low-grade vesicoureteral reflux in children by color Doppler imaging mode. Pediatr Surg Int 12:38-43, 1997.

Hauser M, Krestin GP, Hagspiel KD: Bilateral solid multifocal intrarenal and perirenal lesions. Differentiation with ultrasonography, computed tomography and magnetic resonance imaging. Clin Radiol 50:288-294, 1995.

Hirai T et al.: Usefulness of color Doppler flow imaging in differential diagnosis of multilocular cystic lesions of the kidney. J Ultrasound Med 14:771-776, 1995.

Hisham AN, Samad SA, Sharifah NA: Huge adrenal haemangioma. Australas Radiol 42:250-251, 1998.

Jackson DMA, Collins CD, Cosgrove DO: Diffuse fatty infiltration of the renal parenchyma secondary to bilateral angiomyolipoma: features on ultrasound and computed tomography. Br J Radiol 68:318-320, 1995.

Jain M et al.: High-resolution ultrasonography in the differential diagnosis of cystic diseases of the kidney in infancy and childhood: preliminary experience. J Ultrasound Med 16:235-240, 1997.

Jequier S, Kaplan BS: Echogenic renal pyramids in children. J Clin Ultrasound 19:85-92, 1991.

Kay CJ: Renal diseases in patients with AIDS: sonographic findings. Am J Roentgenol 159:551-554, 1992.

Keane MAR, Finlayson C, Joseph AEA: A historical basis for the sonographic snowstorm in opportunistic infection of the liver and spleen. Clin Radiol 50:220-222, 1995.

Kedar RP, Collins CD, Cosgrove DO: Cachexia of the kidney: a cause of pseudohydronephrosis. Br J Radiol 67:596-598, 1994.

Keesling CA et al.: Sonographic appearance of the bladder after endoscopic incision of uretrocoeles. Am J Roentgenol 170:759-763, 1998.

Kenny IJ: Renal sonography in long-standing Lesch-Nyhan syndrome. Clin Radiol 43:39-41, 1991.

Kenny PJ: Imaging of chronic renal infections. Am J Roentgenol 155:485-494, 1990.

Kim SH et al.: Duplex Doppler ultrasound in patients with medical renal disease: resistive index vs serum creatinine level. Clin Radiol 45:85-87, 1992.

Kincaid W, Edwards R: Intra-renal varices mimicking hydronephrosis. Br J Radiol 65:1038-1039, 1992.

Kodama K et al.: New sonographic finding in renal infarction. Br J Radiol 67:499-500, 1994.

Kronthal AJ et al.: Uterine perforation, simulating urachal carcinoma: CT diagnosis. Am J Roentgenol 154:741-743, 1990.

Lavocat MP et al.: Imaging of pyelonephritis. Pediatr Radiol 27:159-165, 1997.

Lee HJ et al.: Doppler sonographic resistive index in obstructed kidneys. J Ultrasound Med 15:613-618, 1996.

Leonor de Gonzalez E et al.: The appearances on ultrasound of the female urethral sphincter. Br J Radiol 61:687-690, 1988.

Levine E: Renal cell carcinoma: clinical aspects, imaging, diagnosis and staging. Semin Roentgenol (1995) vol. XXX 2:128-148, 1995.

Levitin A, Becker JA: Tumour like conditions of the kidney. Semin Roentgenol vol. XXX 2:185-199, 1995.

Liu JB *et al.*: Endoluminal sonographic evaluation of ureteral and renal pelvic neoplasms. J Ultrasound Med 16:515-521, 1997.

Lopez Rasines G *et al.*: Female urethra diverticula: value of transrectal sonography. J Clin Ultrasound 24:90-92, 1996.

Lorigan JG *et al.*: Macroglobulinaemic lymphoma presenting with perirenal masses. Br J Radiol 61:1077-1078, 1988.

Lowe LH *et al.*: The role of imaging in complex infections of the urinary tract. Am J Roentgenol 163:363-365, 1994.

Manns RA *et al.*: Acquired cystic disease of the kidney: ultrasound as the primary screening procedure. Clin Radiol 41:248-249, 1990.

Martin KW, McAlister WH, Shackelford GD: Acute renal infarction: diagnosis by Doppler ultrasound. Pediatr Radiol 18:373-376, 1988.

Meilstrup JW *et al.*: Other renal tumours. Semin Roentgenol vol. XXX 2:168-194, 1995.

Mellins HZ: Cystic dilatations of the upper urinary tract: a radiologist's developmental model. Radiology 153:291-301, 1984.

Merchant SA, Amonkar PP, Patel JA: Imperforate syringocoele of the bulbourethral duct: appearances on urethrography, sonography and CT. Am J Roentgenol 169:823-824, 1997.

Miletic D *et al.*: Sonographic measurement of absolute and relative renal length in adults. J Clin Ultrasound 26:185-189, 1998.

Modesto A *et al.*: Renal complications of intravesical bacillus Calmette-Guerin therapy. Am J Nephrol 11:501-504, 1991.

Morrison ID, Reznek RH, Webb JAW: Renal adenocarcinoma with ultrasonographic appearance suggestive of angiomyolipoma. Clin Radiol 50:659-661, 1995.

Morrison SC, Comisky E, Fletcher BD: Calcification in the adrenal glands associated with disseminated herpes simplex infection. Pediatr Radiol 18:240-241, 1988.

Narla LD *et al.*: The renal lesions of tuberosclerosis (cysts and angiomyolipoma): screening with sonography and computerised tomography. Pediatr Radiol 18:205-209, 1988.

Neumyer MM, Healy DA, Thiele BL: Ultrasound assessment of mesenteric and renal ischemia. Ultrasound Quarterly 12:89-103, 1994.

Oak SN, Kulkarni B, Chaubal N: Color flow Doppler sonography: a reliable alternative to voiding cystourethrogram in the diagnosis of vesicoureteral reflux in children. Urology 53:1211-1214, 1999.

Otal P *et al.*: Imaging features of uncommon adrenal masses with histopathologic correlation. Radiographics 19:569-581, 1999.

Paivansalo MJ *et al.*: Hyperechogenic 'rings' in the periphery of renal medullary pyramids as a sign of renal disease. J Clin Ultrasound 19:283-287, 1991.

Pastor-Pons E *et al.*: Isolated renal mucormycosis in two patients with AIDS. 166:1282-1286, 1996.

Patel U, Hartley L, Kellet MJ: Sonographic features of renal obstruction mimicked by perinephric cysts. Clin Radiol 49:481-484, 1994.

Pearlstein G: Renal system complications in HIV infection. Crit Care Nurs Clin North Am 2:79-87, 1990.

Perale R *et al.*: Late ultrasonographic pattern in congenital nephrotic syndrome of Finnish type. Pediatr Radiol 18:71, 1988.

Platt JF *et al.*: The inability to detect kidney disease on the basis of echogenicity. Am J Roentgenol 151:317-319, 1988.

Radin DR *et al.*: Visceral and nodal calcification in patients with AIDS-related *Pneumocystis carinii* infections. Am J Roentgenol *154*:27–31, 1990.

Ramachandani P, Pollack HM: Tumours of the uroepithelium. Semin Roentgenol vol. XXX No 149–167, 1995.

Rees JIS, Evans C: Imaging of renal transplantation. Clin Radiol *43*:4–7, 1991.

Reuter KL, Young SB, Colby J: Transperineal sonography in the assessment of a urethral diverticulum. J Clin Ultrasound *20*:221–223, 1992.

Riccabona M *et al.*: In vivo three-dimensional sonographic measurement of organ volume: validation in the urinary bladder. J Ultrasound Med *15*:627–632, 1996.

Roger SD *et al.*: What is the value of measuring renal parenchymal thickness before renal biopsy? Clin Radiol *49*:45–49, 1994.

Rotterberg GT, De Bruyn R, Gordon I: Sonographic standards for a single functioning kidney in children. Am J Roentgenol *167*:1255–1259, 1996.

Rosenfield AT, Siegel NJ: Renal parenchymal disease: histopathologic–sonographic correlation. Am J Roentgenol *137*:793, 1981.

Salih M *et al.*: Color flow Doppler sonography in the diagnosis of vesicoureteric reflux. Eur Urol *26*:93–97, 1994.

Sarnaik AP, Sanfilippo DJ, Slovis TL: Ultrasound diagnosis of adrenal hemorrhage in meningococcemia. Pediatr Radiol *18*:427–428, 1988.

Schifter T, Heller RM: Bilateral multicystic dysplastic kidneys. Pediatr Radiol *18*: 242–244, 1988.

Schulze S, Holm-Nielsen A, Mogensen P: Transurethral ultrasound scanning in the evaluation of invasive bladder cancer. Scand J Urol Nephrol *25*:215–217, 1991.

Scott DJ, Wallace WIIB, Hendry GMA: With advances in medical imaging can the radiologist reliably diagnose Wilms' tumour? Clin Radiol *54*:321–327, 1999.

Sharma AK: Tumefactive extramedullary hematopoisis of the kidney in a patient with idiopathic thrombocytopenic purpura. Am J Roentgenol *167*:795–796, 1996.

Siegel CL *et al.*: Sonography of the female urethra. Am J Roentgenol *170*:1269–1274, 1998.

Sponge AR *et al.*: Extrapulmonary *Pneumocystis carinii* in a patient with AIDS: sonographic findings. Am J Roentgenol *155*:76–78, 1990.

Sy M *et al.*: Renal pseudotumour recurrence after partial nephrectomy. Br J Radiol *69*:359–62, 1996.

Teele RL, Shase JC: Transperineal sonography in children. Am J Roentgenol *168*: 1263–1267, 1997.

Trigaux JP, Pauls C, Van Beers B: Atypical renal hamartomas: ultrasonography, computed tomography and angiographic findings. J Clin Ultrasound *21*:41–44, 1993.

Vargas-Serrano B *et al.*: Transrectal ultrasonography in the diagnosis of urethral diverticula in women. J Clin Ultrasound *25*:21–28, 1997.

Vergesslich KA *et al.*: Acute renal transplant rejection in children: assessment by duplex Doppler sonography. Pediatr Radiol *18*:474–478, 1988.

Weinberg B, Yeung N: Sonographic sign of intermittent dilatation of the renal collecting system in 10 patients with vesicoureteral reflux. J Clin Ultrasound *6*: 65–68, 1998.

Worthington JL *et al.*: Sonographically detectable cysts in polycystic kidney disease in newborn and young infants. Pediatr Radiol *18*:287–293, 1988.

5

Male genital tract

5.1 THE PENIS

The penis is made up of the radix, which is attached to the perineum, and the free body or corpus. The corpus of the penis is formed by three elongated erectile masses – two dorsal corpora cavernosa overlying a single corpus spongiosum – capable of enlargement when engorged with blood during erection. Each corpus is individually covered by a fibrous membrane (the tunica albuginea) while all three corpora are covered together by two facial coverings. The tunica albuginea does not provide a complete separation allowing vascular communication through distal fenestrations. Penile erection occurs mainly as result of engorgement of the corpora cavernosa. Distally the corpora cavernosa expands to form the glans penis, which does not participate in the erectile function but the erect shaft of the penis is thought to interfere with blood drainage from the glans resulting in some engorgement of the glans.

The arterial supply to the penis is derived from internal pudendal arteries via three sources

1. the paired cavernosal artery to the corpora cavernosa
2. the dorsal penile artery supplying the corpus spongiosum
3. the urethral artery.

Each corpora cavernosa is supplied by an individual artery, which enters it at the base of the penis, traversing it centrally and slightly medially throughout its entire length giving off helicine arteries which terminate in single sinusoids. Venules drain the sinusoids. These draining venules communicate with emissary veins that penetrate through the tunica albuginea before terminating in the dorsal vein of the penis. The dorsal vein of the penis is the main route of penile blood drainage in most men. However, in a minority of males some blood drains via the cavernous and crural veins at the base of the penis. Variation of both penile arterial supply and venous drainage is common, occurring in almost 50 per cent of males. The most common variation is the origin of both cavernous arteries arising from a single pudendal artery and an absent dorsal artery of the penis. Variation in the venous anatomy includes drainage via the veins of the glans and the corpus spongiosum.

The sensory somatic nerve supply of the penis comes via the internal pudendal nerves arising from the sacral plexus (S2, S3 and S4). The somatic nerves are a source of sensory supply and innervation of the penile musculature. The autonomic nerves supply the smooth muscle of the cavernous arteries and cavernosal sinusoids.

5.1.1 PHYSIOLOGY OF PENILE ERECTION

Penile erection is primarily a haemodynamic process resulting from engorgement and enlargement subsequent to blood entrapment, secondary to cyclical changes between arterial inflow and venous outflow. Although haemodynamic change provides the main physiological mechanism of erection, there are other factors at play such as psychological, endocrine and metabolic states and general well being.

Six phases of penile activity have been described from the flaccid state to latent tumescence, to full erection, to detumescence. The haemodynamic parameters are dependent on the phase of penile erection. Peak flow velocity, arterial dilatation and vessel pulsation are the most important indicators of penile arterial disease.

5.1.2 SONOGRAPHY OF THE PENIS

High frequency transducers (7.5 MHz) aided by colour Doppler is used to scan the penis in both longitudinal and transverse sections. The corpora cavernosa and spongiosum are both homogeneously hypoechoic; the tunica is usually seen as a thin echogenic linear structure, less than 2 mm thick in the flaccid state and less than 0.5 mm thick when the penis is erect. Calcification of the tunica or cavernosa is regarded as pathological. Age has no influence on the cavernosa echogenicity. The venous sinusoids are recognised in the engorged state as echopoor cystic spaces whilst the penile arteries are seen as linear structures with echogenic walls identified both in the flaccid and the erect state. Image-directed Doppler sonography of the penile arteries provide quantifiable and reproducible assessment of penile artery flow.

Ultrasound assessment of the penile urethra

A 7.5 MHz linear transducer is ideal for the assessment of the penile urethra. The ventral surface of the perineum, penis and scrotum is scanned after instillation of saline into the urethra via a catheter or syringe. Urethral strictures and other urethral pathology is readily identified. However difficulty is encountered in accurately measuring the depth of spongiofibrosis.

Ultrasound assessment of impotence

Vascular disease constitutes the commonest and most important treatable cause of impotence. Precise diagnosis is vital to identify surgically treatable disease such as segmental arterial occlusion or a venous leak in the presence of normal arteries. Image-directed Doppler sonography assisted by pharmacological erection forms the cornerstone of investigation of impotence. The investigation is carried out using a high-resolution duplex transducer with the facility of real time grey scale scanning in conjunction with a simultaneous display of pulsed-range gated Doppler to analyse blood flow. The high-resolution transducer allows imaging of individual cavernous arteries with simultaneous display of Doppler flow analysis. The colour-coded Doppler facility allows display of flow direction and detection of arterial and venous communications. An initial base-line ultrasound of the flaccid penis is performed identifying each individual corpus and the tunica albuginea. Echogenic foci within these structures are identified and recorded. These echogenic foci may represent pathology that is relevant to the aetiology of impotence, and that may influence the type of therapy. The diameter of the identified cavernous arteries is recorded.

The examination is then repeated 5 minutes after a pharmacological erection has been achieved by means of vasodilators such as papaverine (15 to 30 mg) or alprostadil (10 µg). Images are taken using grey scale and colour Doppler. Aberrant arterial blood supply is recorded. The latter is important as it may contribute to, or be the only blood supply involved in, the process of erection. Once an aberrant arterial supply has been recorded or excluded, the presence of an asymmetric response of the cavernous arteries during erection, or the absence of arterial dilatation, is an indication of significant vascular disease. The effect of pharmacological agents to achieve erection may be influenced by sympathetic activity such as needle phobia, anxiety or embarrassment. These patients may respond to self-stimulation. A second injection of the vasodilator may be required to achieve sustained erection.

Flow parameters measured in the investigation of impotence

Arterial dilatation   The cavernous arterial diameter varies from 0.3 to 1.0 mm. During pharmacological erection the diameter should be more than 0.7 mm. Patients with arterial disease will show minimal or no dilatation after an intracavernous injection of a vasodilator.

Peak-flow velocity   The increased blood flow to the erect penis is not only maintained by arterial dilatation, but also by increased blood flow velocity. The peak systolic velocity within the cavernous arteries should be greater than 25 cm/s within 5 minutes of pharmacological stimulation.

Penile blood flow index   This index can be calculated as the percentage increase in the diameter of the right cavernous artery plus the percentage increase in the diameter of the left cavernous artery.

Total peak flow velocity   When the value of total peak flow velocity of both arteries is <285 impotence is likely to be of vascular origin. This index has a sensitivity of 97 per cent and specificity of 77 per cent in the diagnosis of vascular impotence.

Blood flow acceleration = peak systolic velocity ÷ systolic time rise   The systolic time rise is the time from the start of the systolic curve to its maximum value. Proximal arterial disease produces dampening of velocity waveforms with prolongation of systolic rise time. A systolic rise time greater than 110 m/s is said to have a predictive value of 92 per cent for arteriogenic impotence.

Echogenic foci within the penis

Sinusoidal disease – calcification.
Peyronie's disease.
Penile fibrosis.
Arterial calcification – vascular disease.
Fatty tumours – lipoma and lipofibroma.
Fibrous tumours – usually hypoechoic but may be hyperechoic.
Ulcerated penile carcinoma – air within the ulcer.

5.1.3 PEYRONIE'S DISEASE

Focal areas of fibrosis of the tunica albuginea cause Peyronie's disease. The aetiology is unknown. The severity of the disease varies between patients from completely asymptomatic with abnormalities only detected at palpation, to severely symptomatic with a painful and curved erection. The pain may be responsible for the impotence but there may be a contribution from vascular malfunction. On ultrasound fibrotic nodules of the tunica are seen as echogenic foci, some calcified, that may shadow. The tunica appears diffusely thickened to between 2 to 10 mm with ill-defined margins. Fifty per cent of the patients have a venous leak or arteriogenic impotence.

5.1.4 PENILE FIBROSIS

Cavernosal fibrosis is a separate entity from Peyronie's disease. The aetiology is unknown although trauma may play a role. Sonographically cavernosal fibrosis is shown as echogenic foci within the normally hypoechoic cavernosa.

5.1.5 VENOGENIC IMPOTENCE

In patients with a weak erection but who have a normal arterial flow a venous leak can be surmised. With normal erectile response there is little if any flow within the cavernous arteries during the diastolic phase 15 minutes after the intracavernosal injection of a vasodilator. A diastolic flow greater than 10 cm/s is said to correlate well with venous erectile dysfunction. However measurements of end-diastolic velocity, time-averaged velocity, resistive index and pulsatility index in patients with a repeated and unsatisfactory response to intracavernous vasodilator injection are poor predictors of venous leakage. At the present state of knowledge the measurement of these indices cannot replace dynamic pharmacocavernometry or cavernosography.

5.1.6 SUPERFICIAL DORSAL PENILE VEIN THROMBOSIS

Superficial dorsal penile vein thrombosis (penile Mondor's phlebitis) is a rare disease which may occur either as part of a more generalised phlebitis or in isolation. The condition may present as a cord-like induration on the dorsal aspect of the penis or as an acute phlebitis causing pain and systemic symptoms. Trauma, excessive sexual activity, prolonged sexual abstinence, venous occlusion from a distended bladder and pelvic tumours have all been implicated. On ultrasound examination a thrombus may be identified within the superficial dorsal vein of the penis. The vein may be distended and non-compressible and no flow may be seen within the vein on colour flow Doppler.

5.1.7 PRIAPISM

This is defined as a persistent painful erection. The condition is multifactorial but the basic pathophysiology is that of a persistent sinusoidal engorgement as a result of impaired outflow or prolonged raised cavernosal artery inflow. The distinction between the mechanisms is important as management is different. Ultrasound may demonstrate distended sinusoids and thrombosis of the dorsal vein or intracavernosal thrombosis. Prolonged priapism may cause intracavernosal fibrosis which can be identified as increased echogenic foci within the normally hypoechoic cavernosa. In low-flow priapism Doppler ultrasound may demonstrate high-resistance, low-velocity cavernosal artery waveforms. Doppler ultrasound can detect high flow rates with elevated flow rates recorded at 20 to 30 cm/s associated with low-resistance waveforms. Continuous flow in the dorsal vein and arteriovenous shunts have also been demonstrated.

5.1.8 PENILE TUMOURS

Penile tumours are uncommon and generally present with non-specific symptoms. Penile tumours are sub-divided into benign, precancerous, carcinoma *in situ* and malignant tumours. Generally, it is difficult to differentiate malignant from benign tumours on imaging, particularly in the early stages, histological diagnosis can only be offered on biopsy.

Penile cysts

The exact aetiology of penile cysts is unknown. As with cysts elsewhere diagnosis of cysts with ultrasound is straightforward, they are seen as well-defined anechoic lesions with posterior acoustic enhancement and usually with no internal echoes.

Fibrous tumours

These tumours include fibroma, fibromyoma, neurinomas and haemangioma. The tumours appear as well-defined, solid hypoechoic masses.

Intracavernosal fibromatosis

Intracavernosal fibromatosis presents with multiple palpable nodules, usually at the base of the penis. Sonography reveals solid hyperechoic or hypoechoic nodules, with no evidence of vascularity on colour flow Doppler.

Fatty tumours

Lipomas and lipofibromas can occur within the penis. These tumours are hyperechoic depending upon the mix of fatty and other tissue. They may shadow.

Penile carcinoma

Penile carcinoma is uncommon in Europe, USA and Canada and accounts for 0.5 per cent of cancers in men. It appears to be common in central

Africa (10 to 15 per cent) and Puerto Rico (20 per cent). Because the tumour causes no pain presentation is late and may first present with inguinal lymphadenopathy. Despite the late presentation prognosis appears to be favourable with localised surgery even when inguinal lymph node metastases are present. High frequency transducers can show the relationship to the tunica albuginea and Buck's fascia. This relation is an important determinant of the prognosis. With breach of this fascia the prognosis worsens. The tumour is a homogeneous mass within the glans or corpus cavernosa, anechoic foci may be seen because of necrosis. Hypoechoic masses have been described. In large tumours with ulceration hyperechoic foci may be seen because of the presence of air within the ulcers. The normal tunica albuginea is usually seen as a hyperechoic line, when breached by the tumour this line is lost, thus ultrasound allows for accurate local staging (as accurate as MRI). The authors easily identify inguinal lymph nodes with sonography although differentiation between metastases and reactive nodes cannot always be made. Colour flow Doppler plays no role in the diagnosis or staging.

Malignant penile tumours

Bowen's disease*.
Erythroplasia of Queyrat*.
Carcinoma.
Melanoma.
Basalioma.
Sarcoma.
Lymphoma.
Metastases – prostate, urinary bladder, lung and renal.

5.1.9 PENILE TRAUMA

Penile trauma is rare when the penis is in flaccid state. Most traumas occur in the erect state and are caused by an 'accident' of a sexual nature. The most common form of trauma is penile fracture also known as 'Texas trauma' or 'bent nail syndrome' related to prevailing sexual practices.

Ultrasonic features of penile rupture

1. Extravasation of blood under Buck's fascia resulting in unilateral asymmetrical fluid collection, the 'egg plant deformity'. The blood may dissect into the anterior abdominal wall and scrotum. The appearance of the

---

* Carcinoma *in situ*, dermatological diagnosis; sonography usually plays no role.

subcutaneous haematoma depends upon the time interval between the trauma and scanning. In the first few hours after trauma there is thickening of the lining tissue, this is soon replaced by a poorly defined heterogenous predominantly echogenic pattern.

2. The echogenic line of the tunica albuginea is usually lost on one side because of rupture.
3. Traumatic arteriovenous fistulae may give rise to a high-flow priapism. Colour Doppler will detect turbulence within the lacuna with high velocity flow.
4. Superficial dorsal vein thrombosis.

5.2 THE TESTIS AND SCROTUM

5.2.1 THE ADULT TESTIS

The adult testis is an ovoid structure measuring 4 to $5 \times 3 \times 2.5$ cm, the volume ranges from 16 to 20 ml. The testis usually decreases in size with age. It has a smooth homogeneous parenchyma returning mid-amplitude echoes. Before puberty the immature testis has a similar echogenicity to a mature testis, but the longitudinal diameter is always less than 20 to 25 mm. The epididymus lies on the posterolateral aspect of the testes. It has a coarser echopattern than the testis but is of similar echogenicity. It may be differentiated from the testis by two parallel echogenic lines. The head of the epididymus lies superiorly and is slightly more echogenic than the testis. The rete testis may be visualised as a hypoechoic multiloculated mass adjacent to the epididymus in some normal subjects. These anatomical masses are frequently bilateral and often associated with an ipsilateral spermatocoele. No colour flow signals are recorded in a normal rete testis. In normal testes linear hypoechoic bands are seen traversing the testis perpendicular to the mediastinum of the testis repressing normal blood vessels. A flash of colour is displayed in these normal vessels on the application of colour Doppler. The arterial blood to the testis is derived from the testicular arteries, these arise from the abdominal aorta just distal to the renal arteries, which descend in the retroperitoneum to enter the spermatic cord. Two other vessels also enter the spermatic cord

1. the cremaster artery which is a branch of the inferior epigastric artery
2. the deferential artery which is a branch of the vesicular artery.

There is abundant anastamosis between these arteries in the spermatic cord. The testicular artery and its branches are the major blood supply to the testis and typically show a low-resistance flow. The cremaster and deferential arteries supply the high-resistance bed of the epididymus and other extratesticular tissues. Power Doppler readily detects capsular and centripetal testicular arteries in all normal adult testes. Because of the smaller sized arteries in children this display is not usually seen. The venous drainage of the testis takes place through the pampiniform plexus that drains into the cremaster and spermatic vein, finally entering the testicular vein. The left testicular vein drains into the left renal vein whilst the right testicular vein drains into the inferior vena cava directly. The cremasteric plexus, lying behind the pampiniform plexus, drains the extratesticular tissues before draining into the cremasteric vein. The peak systolic velocity of a normal testis is 4 to 19 cm/s, end diastolic velocity is 2 to 8 cm/s with a resistive index of 0.44 to 0.75. The normal values of testicular flow in adults do not apply to prepubertal boys with testicular volumes less than 4 cm^3. However when testicular volumes exceed 4 cm^3 the adult values of resistive index apply to both prepubertal as well as pubertal boys. Power Doppler improves depiction of intratesticular vessels in adults but flow cannot be identified in all prepubertal testes. A small volume of fluid is frequently seen around the testis lying between the parietal and visceral layers of the tunica vaginalis. The wall of the scrotum has a variable thickness which is usually between 3 to 6 mm.

Testicular measurements

- Length   3 to 5 cm.
- Width   2 to 3 cm.
- Depth (anteroposterior)   2 to 3 cm.
- Testicular volume   length × width × anteroposterior depth × 0.53 cm.
- Normal volume   15 to 20 ml.

The accuracy of ultrasound is within 10 per cent of actual volume and is better than physical examination in detecting testicular asymmetry.

5.2.2 THE PAEDIATRIC SCROTUM

Scrotal swelling in the newborn

Torsion.
Orchitis.
Hydrocoele.
Haematocoele.
Testicular oedema.
Scrotal oedema.
Traumatic haematoma.
Testicular tumour.

Inguinal hernia.
Meconium peritonitis.

Types of scrotal haematoma

Bleeding into testicular tissue – trauma.
Blood entering the scrotum from the abdominal cavity.
Blood dissecting along facial planes into the scrotum from the retroperitoneum.

NB Remember the association of intra-abdominal pathology in association with a scrotal swelling.

Acute scrotal pain

Testicular inflammatory disease – epidymitis, epididymo-orchitis.
Testicular trauma or disruption.
Testicular torsion.
Intrascrotal haematoma – traumatic, non-traumatic (Henoch–Schönlein's purpura).
Intratesticular haematoma from vasculitis.
NB 10 to 15 per cent of patients with testicular tumours first seek attention following trauma, therefore scrotal masses found following trauma warrant follow up.

Testicular inflammatory disease

Epididymitis and epididymo-orchitis are the most common infections and the commonest cause of scrotal pain in adults, with by far the majority of patients over the age of 35 years (see pp. 425–426). The infective organisms involved may be bacterial or viral. Infection is usually unilateral. Acute scrotal inflammatory disease in children is uncommon. The main stay of diagnosis is colour flow Doppler. The normal epididymus shows no flow on colour Doppler so the presence of vascularity in the epididymus represents inflammation. In orchitis focal or diffuse hypervascularity is seen on colour Doppler. The presence of pain and hypervascularity of the epididymus allows distinction from testicular tumours. Pulsed Doppler is not essential for diagnosis, but when done it shows an abnormally elevated diastolic flow. A reactive hydrocoele is common, which may become complex or septate with the complication of pyocoele. Testicular ischaemia may develop from pressure on the venous outflow.

Testicular trauma

See pp. 423–424 for a description of testicular trauma. In young patients colour Doppler sonography can be helpful by showing alteration in the extent of testicular perfusion defects. A testicular haematoma appears as a hypoechoic or hyperechoic avascular mass which displaces blood vessels.

Varicocoele

A varicocoele occurs as result of dilatation of the pampiniform plexus usually because of incompetence of the venous valves. Eighty-five per cent of varicocoeles occur on the left. They almost always occur in adolescent boys. When found in younger children a cause such as extrinsic abdominal compression from an abdominal or pelvic mass should be looked for. Sonography shows tubular peritesticular structures on the dorsal aspect of the testis. Colour Doppler displays venous flow augmentation following valsalva or the child assuming an erect posture.

Scrotal oedema

Scrotal oedema is a cause of pain in young children. The normal scrotal skin is quite thin, and is usually less than 3 mm in thickness. The application of colour Doppler to a normal scrotal skin shows no detectable blood flow. With scrotal oedema colour Doppler ultrasound shows hypervascularity within the thickened scrotal skin. The epididymus may also be affected. Cellulitis of the scrotum because of bacterial infection may show similar hypervascularity. In children with idiopathic scrotal oedema the skin is thickened but colour Doppler does not usually show detectable blood flow.

Differential diagnosis of scrotal thickening in children

Henoch–Schönlein purpura (15 per cent).
Cellulitis.
Idiopathic scrotal oedema.
Trauma.
Postorchiectomy (ipsilateral side).

Testicular torsion

This presents an acute surgical emergency because the occlusion of the blood supply to the testis must be restored within 6 hours to prevent necrosis or infarction of the testis. Colour Doppler will show no detectable blood within the testis. Significantly reduced blood flow can sometimes be shown. Over time the testis becomes more hypoechoic with increased paratesticular hypervascularity. If no flow is demonstrated an isotope scan should be performed to verify testicular perfusion.

Testicular tumours

Testicular tumours in children may appear as either hypoechoic or hyperechoic masses, or as a testicular enlargement with normal echogenicity and no discrete mass. Colour Doppler displays disorganised neovascularity either focally or diffusely. Colour Doppler ultrasound shows hypervascularity in 57 per cent of children with testicular tumours with normal echogenicity on grey scale images. This is contrary to adult tumours where colour Doppler contributes little to grey scale images. Rarely both solid and cystic testicular tumours in children may be hypovascular.

5.2.3 MALE INFERTILITY

Scrotal ultrasound

To confirm findings suspected on physical examination – varicocoele, epididymal and parenchymal irregularities.

To measure testicular volume – 64 per cent of men with male factor infertility have an abnormality of testicular size.

Ultrasound can be used to locate malposition of the testis.

Ultrasound examination of the epididymus is useful in confirming an epididymal cyst or a spermatocoele in infertility evaluation.

The presence of a hydrocoele should provoke a search for a testicular tumour.

The ultrasound appearances of most testicular tumours are those of a hypoechoic mass within the homogeneous echopattern of a testis. Most testicular tumours in the age group concerned about fertility are malignant. However some benign lesions such as microlithiasis testicular cysts and old haematomas are occasionally discovered.

Causes of testicular atrophy

Varicocoele.
Crytorchidism.
Inflammations – epididymitis, orchitis, postpubertal mumps.
Trauma.
Following testicular torsion.
Repeated inguinal hernia surgery.
Prostatic surgery.
Klinefelter's syndrome.
Hepatic cirrhosis.
Renal transplantation.
Debility and senility.
Oestrogen therapy.

Hypothyroidism.
Diseases of the hypothalamus and pituitary.

Ultrasound usually shows a small hypoechoic testis with reduced vascularity but normal epididymus.

Transrectal ultrasound

Transrectal ultrasound is an excellent tool in the investigation of male infertility because of the ease of visualisation of the prostate, seminal vesicles and the ejaculatory ducts. The primary use of transrectal ultrasound is in the investigation of hypoplasia, aplasia or obstruction of the seminal vesicles and the ejaculatory ducts. Recently transrectal ultrasound has been combined with seminal vesiculography to diagnose distal ejaculatory duct obstruction, reducing the need for a more invasive vasography.

Ejaculatory duct obstruction

The union of the seminal vesicle and the terminal ampullary part of the vas deferens form the ejaculatory duct. The normal duct measures 4 to 8 mm in diameter with a 2 mm lumen which may be difficult to visualise in the unobstructed state. When obstructed the patient may present with infertility, azoospermia, oligousthenospermia, haematospermia, perineal or testicular pain and pain on ejaculation. Transrectal ultrasound is now regarded as the initial examination of choice, replacing the more invasive procedure of vasography which remains the 'gold standard'. The ejaculatory ducts can be scanned both in transverse and sagittal planes. Obstructed ejaculatory ducts appear as paired oval convoluted tubular cystic structures medial to the seminal vesicles and superior to the prostate. The obstructed dilated ducts are seen to terminate into the urethra at the level of the verumontanum. Ejaculatory duct cysts, dilated ejaculatory ducts, calcification and seminal vesical dilatation are cardinal features of ejaculatory duct obstruction. When dilatation of the ejaculatory duct is evident a search should be made for possible causes.

Causes of ejaculatory duct obstruction in sub-fertile males

Intraprostatic cysts or masses – Müllerian duct cysts, Wolffian duct cysts, prostatic retention cysts, prostatic carcinoma or other tumours.

Previous genital infection or inflammation – pyogenic conditions, viral infections, tuberculosis.

Previous surgery or trauma – bullet or shrapnel wound, pelvic surgery (for example resection of seminal vesicle cyst), bladder extrophy.

Seminal vesicle anomalies – congenital seminal vesicle cyst.

Congenital ejaculatory duct anomalies – ejaculatory duct cysts or diverticula.

5.2.4 SEMINAL VESICLES

Seminal vesicles are paired cystic elongated structures which lie postero-superior to the prostate. They serve as a reservoir for seminal fluid.

Mean dimensions of seminal vesicles

- Length 3.0 ± 0.8 cm.
- Width 1.5 ± 0.4 cm.
- Volume 13.7 ± 3.7 ml.
- Vasal ampulla (mean diameter) 0.4 ± 0.1 cm (this is best visualised in the transverse section, just medial to the seminal vesicle).

There is no significant change in volume following ejaculation. Ninety per cent of men with congenital absence of vas deferens have an underlying ipsilateral aplasia of the seminal vesicle whilst 20 per cent have aplasia of the contralateral seminal vesicle. Eighty-five per cent men with congenital absence of vas deferens have associated upper renal tract anomalies such as ipsilateral renal agenesis, ipsilateral renal ectopia, and crossed fused renal ectopia and horseshoe kidneys. Hypoplasia of the seminal vesicles is said to be present when there is a decrease in size of 30 per cent or more.

Transrectal ultrasound can also be used for guided aspiration of the seminal vesicles and seminal vesiculography can be performed in the diagnostic work up of ejaculatory duct obstruction. Transrectal ultrasound-guided vesiculography has the advantage of lower risk of vasal scarring as compared with operative vesiculography. A perineal approach has also been used to perform contrast vesiculography with transrectal ultrasound guidance.

5.2.5 THE UNDESCENDED TESTIS

The testes arise on the posterior abdominal wall and descend into the scrotum late in foetal life. There is maldescent of the testes in 0.23 to 0.88 per cent of males and it is bilateral in 10 to 25 per cent of cases. At birth 4 per cent of testes have failed to reach the scrotum but the incidence falls to 0.8 per cent by 6 weeks of age. Lack of normal descent increases the risk of trauma, torsion and tumour, and is also associated with decreased fertility. Seventy per cent of the undescended testes lie in the inguinal canal and these may be seen as hypoechoic structures relative to adjacent soft tissues. They are smaller than a normal gonad because of testicular atrophy. Testes lying on the lateral pelvic wall can sometimes be identified but are frequently obscured by bowel gas.

5.2.6 SCROTAL FLUID COLLECTIONS

Hydrocoele – neonatal (frequent, the processus which closes at 18 months is idiopathic (common), still open), inflammatory, tumour, trauma, surgery (bladder, prostate, hernia), torsion, testicular infarction.

Haematocoele – trauma, surgery, anticoagulants (haemorrhagic diathesis), inflammations.

Lymphocoele – following renal transplantation.

Pyocoele – epididymitis or orchitis, secondary infection of hydrocoele.

Varicocoele – extratesticular (common), intratesticular (rare).

Intrascrotal cyst and spermatocoele.

Testicular haematoma.

Testicular abscess.

Testicular cystic neoplasm.

Fluid-filled bowel loop (hernia).

Low-level echoes in hydrocoeles

Inappropriate gain settings.

High protein content – infections (tuberculosis, lymphocoele).

Tunica adenocarcinoma.

Cholesterol crystals – predispose to scrotal calculi.

Blood – trauma, surgery, etc.

Egg masses – filariasis.

5.2.7 CYSTIC SCROTAL MASSES

Hydrocoele

A hydrocoele is the commonest cause of scrotal swelling. It is usually painless but without treatment it may become large. It occurs as a result of abnormal accumulation of fluid in the potential space between the two layers of the tunica vaginalis. The normal scrotum contains only a few millimetres of fluid. The majority of hydrocoeles are idiopathic but they may be secondary to any scrotal pathology such as tumour, trauma, torsion or inflammation. Sonographically the hydrocoele is seen as an anechoic fluid collection around the testicle except posteriorly at the site of attachment of the epididymus. The presence of fluid makes assessment of testicular echogenicity unreliable and the testicle may appear abnormally echogenic relative to the fluid. Long-standing cases may be associated with thickening of the tunica vaginalis and infection or haemorrhage may give rise to internal septae or debris. Sonographic appearances may be identical to paratesticular abscesses or haematocoeles and these must be differentiated on clinical grounds or aspiration. Loculated hydrocoeles may also occur along the course of the processus vaginalis. If the processus vaginalis fails to close the hydrocoele may be seen to extend into the pelvis.

Loculated hydrocoele

Loculated hydrocoeles occur along the processus vaginalis, they can be difficult to differentiate from other scrotal cysts but their cephalad placement may suggest the diagnosis. Their course is benign and usually asymptomatic.

Infected hydrocoele or pyocoele

Infected hydrocoeles have a large amount of fluid and may have a fluid–fluid or fluid–debris level. Besides other organisms, infected hydrocoeles may be tuberculous. In filariasis the fluid may contain fine echoes because of egg masses. In neglected cases, filariasis may be associated with calcification of the tunica and solid masses of varying sizes within the spermatic cord. *Schistosoma haematobium* is also a common cause of hydrocoeles in endemic areas. Both filariasis and schistosomiasis may be associated with scrotal elephantiasis in which instance the scrotal fluid is echofree.

Scrotal masses resulting from urethral complications of catheterisation

Patients with long-term urinary catheterisation may develop complications such as false urethral passages, and patients with paraplegia may acquire urethral diverticula. These can become infected and dissect through fascial planes and present as cystic scrotal swellings. The differential diagnoses of an apparent scrotal swelling in a debilitated catheterised patient must therefore not only include epididymo-orchitis but also urethral abscess, misplaced catheter and urethral diverticulum.

Recurrent and chronic hydrocoele

Recurrent hydrocoele may occur after surgery. These commonly have a multiseptate appearance; chronic hydrocoeles may have a similar appearance. The diagnosis is usually suggested by the history.

Hydrocoele associated with scrotal malignancy

Hydrocoeles associated with underlying malignancy are usually small. Large hydrocoeles are usually of idiopathic or inflammatory aetiology.

Haematocoele

Haematocoeles may follow trauma, surgery or bleeding diathesis such as Henoch–Schönlein purpura. The appearance depends upon the evolution of the blood clot. Initially the blood may be echofree, the blood then clots and becomes echogenic; the blood then reliquefies finally giving rise to a multiseptate appearance before resorption.

Varicocoele

A varicocoele is a common entity described as an abnormal dilatation exceeding 2 mm in diameter of the veins of the pampiniform venous plexus associated with tortuosity. The normal diameter is up to 2.2 mm, which may increase to 2.7 mm during valsalva. Varicocoele is said to occur as a result of absent venous valves, venous compression or pressure gradients. The condition is said to occur in one-third of men undergoing evaluation for infertility. The incidence of sub-clinical varicocoele diagnosed by colour Doppler ultrasound is even higher. The veins forming a varicocoele are usually uniform in size measuring up to 5 mm in diameter. The vessel size increases if the patient is scanned when standing or whilst a valsalva manoeuvre is performed. Colour flow Doppler ultrasound has provided the highest level of confidence by demonstrating flow within a varicocoele. Over 90 per cent of cases occur on the left, the occurrence of a varicocoele on the right should raise suspicion of the possibility of underlying abdominal pathology. A left-sided varicocoele can be secondary to a renal cell carcinoma.

Intratesticular varicocoele

Intratesticular varicocoele is an extremely rare condition characterised by dilated intratesticular veins and associated with ipsilateral varicocoele. The mechanism of causation is the same as extratesticular varicocoele. The dilated intratesticular veins are seen as straight or serpentine hypoechoic tubular structures within the mediastinum testis radiating into the testicular parenchyma. With colour flow Doppler it is demonstrated within the tubular intratesticular structures enhanced during valsalva. The main differential diagnosis is tubular ectasia which displays no flow on colour Doppler ultrasound.

Scrotal arteriovenous malformation

These may be difficult to differentiate from varicocoele on real time sonography, but colour Doppler shows a high passive flow unlike that of a varicocoele. The venous spectral Doppler shows high flow with pulsatility.

Pulsatility does not occur in the normal pampiniform plexus or varicocoele. High diastolic arterial flow indicating a low peripheral resistance is characteristic of an arteriovenous malformation.

Spermatocoele

Spermatocoeles represent a cystic collection of seminal fluid, usually within an efferent duct near the head of the epididymus. This is secondary to efferent duct obstruction as a result of inflammation, trauma or vasectomy. Small spermatocoeles may resemble epididymal cysts. Larger spermatocoeles may be septate, and may have either low-level echoes within or a fluid–fluid level. Larger cysts may displace the testis anteriorly. Colour Doppler ultrasound shows no flow within the cysts or within the walls of the cysts. Aspiration of these cysts yields sperm-like fluid. Guided aspiration and sclerotherapy with ethanolamine oleate is said to have a cure rate of over 80 per cent.

Epididymal cyst

Epididymal cysts are common and are said to occur in 40 per cent of males, they may be associated with tubular ectasia. These sonolucent fluid collections tend to occur in the body of the epididymus. They vary in size from a few millimetres to very large so as to mimic a hydrocoele, but unlike a hydrocoele there is no fluid collection anterior to the testis. The appearance may be indistinguishable from a spermatocoele or cystic degeneration of the epididymus secondary to inflammation.

Cysts of tunica albuginea

Several tissue layers envelop the testes. The tunica albuginea overlies the capsule of the testis and mediastinum testis is a reflection of this capsule. Above is the tunica vaginalis (peritoneum) with two layers (visceral and parietal). External to these layers is the dortos muscle lying below the scrotal skin. These layers cannot be differentiated by the current generation of ultrasound machines. Tunica albuginea cysts are uncommon. They affect patients in their fifth and sixth decades. They are 2 to 5 mm in size, single or multiple, unilocular or septate, and are placed in the upper anterior or lateral zone of the testis. They may be large and indistinguishable from tunica vaginalis cysts. They may rarely appear as intratesticular and complex lesions.

Dilated rete testis

Dilated rete testes are related to ectasia of the seminiferous tubules, producing a 1 to 3 cm area of hypoechoic tubular structures near the mediastinum. The condition is frequently bilateral and tends to occur in an older age group than testicular tumours. The multiple internal coarse echoes blend in with the testicular echoes at the margin of the lesion, resulting in an ill-defined lesion. No pulsed or colour Doppler is detected within these tubular structures.

Scrotal hernia

Scrotal hernia may contain omentum, bowel or a combination of the two. Bowel loops may reach the scrotum and may be recognised sonographically when fluid filled, as they will show peristalsis on prolonged examination, although peristalsis is not always present. When filled with air or omental fat they will appear echogenic and may shadow. Another clue that the mass has descended from the peritoneal cavity is a 'tail' that points towards the abdomen along the line of the spermatic cord.

Epidermoid cyst of the testicle

These represent rare benign tumours affecting the 20 to 40 year age group although they have been reported from 3 years to the age of 70 years. They are usually asymptomatic and discovered on routine examination. Although described as cysts the ultrasonic appearances are variable but usually seen as a sharply circumscribed lesion which may be hypoechoic, hyperechoic or of mixed echogenicity. A target or onion-like pattern has been described. Occasionally a sharply marginated mass because of rim calcification may be seen which may shadow.

Ruptured ovarian follicle

Ruptured ovarian follicle in ovotestis in a true hermaphrodite may give rise to an expanding hypoechoic testicular mass, leading to a multiseptate mass with posterior enhancement.

Papillary cystadenoma of the epididymus

See p. 434.

Testicular trauma

Clinical examination is an unreliable means of assessing testicular integrity, particularly if the testicle is surrounded by a haematoma. Scrotal trauma may produce testicular rupture, intratesticular haematoma, infarction haemato-coele, and lacerations of the scrotum and traumatic epididymitis. Ultrasonography allows visualisation of the testicle despite the presence of a haematoma, though rupture may still be difficult to identify unless the testicle is fragmented or extrusion of testicular material is shown. Haemorrhage within the testicle may be seen as anechoic blood or echogenic clot. Infarction may be identical. An established haematoma may give a bizarre complex mass appearance. Without a history of trauma the appearances are similar to those of infarction, abscess and tumour, and haemorrhage is more likely to occur if the testicle is already diseased. Sonography of traumatic epididymitis shows enlargement of the epididymus and hypervascularity of the epididymus on colour flow Doppler. Colour flow Doppler ultrasound shows findings indistinguishable from infective epididymitis. Generally, of course, the clinical presentation should be sufficient to distinguish the two.

Haemo-epididymus

This may follow trauma, giving rise to a multiloculated mass representing blood within the epididymus.

Cystic testicular tumours

It is said that 24 per cent of testicular tumours have a cystic element although they usually occur in combination with more solid components and may form a complex mass.

Testicular prosthesis and postorchiectomy appearance

Following orchiectomy the scrotal sac on the ipsilateral side forms a potential space which is occupied by a small amount of fluid, the fluid eventually resolves leaving behind a few echoes in an empty scrotum. Haematomas, which are more common after the inguinal approach, should resolve within 6 weeks. Testicular prostheses are made up of silicone rubber. On sonography they appear echofree. They cannot be compressed and the scotal sac appears full and distended.

5.2.8 SOLID TESTICULAR MASSES

Torsion of the testis

Testicular torsion usually presents with acute pain and swelling but may present as a painless scrotal swelling particularly in young children (see p. 415). Surgery must be performed within 6 hours of the onset of symptoms if function is to be preserved. In the early stages the testis appears normal. It then becomes swollen and may appear of increased or decreased echogenicity. Six hours after the onset of symptoms the testis is normally hypoechoic and a normal scan at this time makes torsion unlikely. Colour Doppler ultrasound may show decreased or absent blood flow to the testis. The testis may also appear rather high in the scrotum and may be noted to have a rather horizontal axis.

If testicular torsion is not treated surgically in the acute phase the hypoechoic testicle becomes enlarged and a hydrocoele may develop. The testis then atrophies making the epididymus appear relatively large and echogenic in comparison. The main differential diagnosis of testicular torsion in clinical practice is that of epididymo-orchitis. Colour Doppler is said to be 91 per cent sensitive and 100 per cent specific for epididymo-orchitis (see below). Radionuclide scanning has a true positive rate of 99 per cent for epididymo-orchitis.

Ischaemic orchitis

Ischaemic orchitis occurs as result of testicular infarction following a testicular torsion or scrotal surgery where extensive dissection of the spermatic cord to mobilise the testis is carried out. Overuse of diathermy to control bleeding from the dissected spermatic cord may also result in damage to the spermatic artery or pampiniform plexus, leading to testicular infarction or ischaemic orchitis. Testicular atrophy complicates 0.03 to 0.5 per cent of primary inguinal repairs and 0.8 to 5.0 per cent of recurrent hernia surgery. Testicular infarction can also result from trauma, bacterial endocarditis, polyarteritis nodosa and Henoch–Schönlein purpura. Rarely testicular infarction may occur spontaneously. Presentation is with pain, tenderness and swelling of the testis and spermatic cord. Pyrexia may precede local manifestation. Sonography shows a hypoechoic small testis, ill-defined hypoechoic lesions may be seen in focal infarction. There is no spectral or colour Doppler signal.

Epididymitis and epididymo-orchitis

Epididymo-orchitis is the commonest intrascrotal inflammation. Sonographic appearances are variable depending upon the stage and severity of the disease. The epididymus is usually enlarged and hypoechoic, but it may be intensely echogenic. In uncomplicated cases of epididymitis the testicle is usually not involved though there may be hypoechoic foci in the testicular parenchyma adjacent to the epididymus. Colour Doppler imaging shows hypervascularity within the epididymus. Orchitis gives rise to hypoechoic foci and in severe cases results in an enlarged hypoechoic testicle with secondary hydrocoele formation. Focal or diffuse hypervascularity may be seen on colour flow Doppler. In chronic epididymitis the epididymus becomes echogenic. In tuberculous epididymitis the epididymus may become heterogeneous and hypoechoic associated with concomitant hypoechoic lesions in the testis and a discharging sinus. The testis may become stony hard associated with extratesticular calcification.

Testicular tumours

Testicular tumours occur most frequently in the 20 to 40 year age group and make up 1 to 2 per cent of all cancers in males and 1.5 per cent of all childhood malignancies. Their incidence is increased 5 to 100 times in undescended testicles and orchidopexy after the age of 6 years does not appear to reduce this risk. There is an increased risk of testicular cancer in Caucasians, Jews and patients with a family history or previous testicular cancer. Fifteen per cent of testicular tumours present with a hydrocoele whilst others present with a testicular mass or distant metastases. Ten per cent of patients present with acute pain due to intratesticular haemorrhage. Metastases may be present at presentation in 4 to 14 per cent of patients to lung, liver, bones, brain and lymph nodes. Tumours are usually classified by germ cell (for example seminoma and teratoma) and non-germ cell origin. Seminoma is the commonest in children. Over the age of 50 years 50 per cent of testicular neoplasms are lymphomas. Over 90 per cent of testicular neoplasms are completely or predominantly hypoechoic. Infarction and inflammation may also give rise to focal hypoechoic areas and thus a hypoechoic focus does not necessarily indicate malignancy. High-frequency sonography is a very accurate means of demonstrating testicular parenchyma and a normal scan is almost 100 per cent accurate at excluding testicular malignancy. Colour Doppler sonography show little vascularity in tumours less than 1.5 cm in size but tumours larger than 1.6 cm consistently display hypervascularity and distortion of blood vessels.

Germ cell tumours

Seminoma

This tumour accounts for 50 per cent of primary testicular neoplasms and is the most common tumour in the undescended testis. The age group affected is between 30 and 40 years. The tumours may be multifocal. A quarter already show metastases at presentation usually to the lungs. Tumour activity can be monitored by beta-human chorionic gonadotrophin (β-hCG), which is elevated in 10 to 15 per cent patients. The serum alpha fetoprotein is usually normal. The ultrasound appearances are those of a uniformly hypoechoic lesion.

Embryonal cell tumour

These make up approximately a quarter of testicular tumours and are the most common component of mixed testicular tumours. They usually affect patients in their second and third decades and children under the age of 2 years. These tumours are the most aggressive testicular neoplasms that predispose to visceral metastases. The commonest ultrasound appearance is that of a hypoechoic mass with irregular borders, that may show echogenic foci because of areas of calcification and cystic areas because of haemorrhage and necrosis.

Teratoma

Teratoma accounts for less than 10 per cent of primary testicular tumours but is the second most common testicular tumour in young boys. The tumour may be benign in children but may transform into malignancy. The alpha fetoprotein may be elevated. The tumour may appear primarily solid, cystic or complex. The presence of cartilage and bony elements may give rise to echogenic areas with shadowing.

Choriocarcinoma

The incidence of this tumour is 1 to 3 per cent with a peak age incidence of 20 to 30 years. Pulmonary metastases occur in 81 per cent of cases, metastases may occur without evidence of a primary neoplasm. The prognosis is poor and is rapidly fatal. The serum β-hCG is invariably elevated which may cause gynaecomastia. Choriocarcinoma usually gives rise to a complex mass with cystic areas because of haemorrhage and necrosis and may also have echogenic foci caused by calcification.

Yolk sac tumour

This is a rare tumour which is considered equivalent to the endodermal sinus tumour of the ovary. Yolk cell tumour elements are said to be present in 38 per cent of other adult germ cell tumours except a seminoma. The yolk sac tumour (endodermal sinus tumour) is therefore not regarded as a distinctive tumour of the infant's testis, but a germ cell neoplasm differentiating in the direction of yolk sac vitelline structures, and occurring in the testis, ovary and extragonadal sites in common with other germ cell neoplasms. The tumour primarily affects children under 3 years of age. The serum alpha fetoprotein is invariably elevated. The tumours frequently metastasise to the lung. Specific ultrasound appearances have not been described.

Testicular lymphoma

Non-Hodgkin's, especially B-cell lymphoma, represents the most common secondary neoplasm of the testis and the most common testicular malignancy in men over the age of 60 years. The testis is usually the first site of recurrence after initial response to chemotherapy in the setting of diffuse disease. The presentation is that of a painless testicular mass, bilateral in 40 per cent of cases. The ultrasound appearances are those of a focal homogeneous hypoechoic mass without a definable capsule, similar to a seminoma. The testis may be diffusely involved resulting in a global reduction of the echogenicity. The tumour may extend into the epididymus and spermatic cord but invasion of the tunica albuginea is usually rare.

Testicular leukaemia

The testis may be a 'sanctuary organ' for haematological malignancies such as acute lymphocytic leukaemia and lymphoma because of the lack of accumulation of chemotherapeutic agents in the testes. Testicular leukaemia is described in chronic as well as in acute myelogenous leukaemia (chloroma), but most testicular involvement is due to acute lymphocytic leukaemia which occurs in 8 per cent of children but is said to be rare in adults. Testicular involvement presents with scrotal enlargement, often bilateral, and carries a poor prognosis with a median survival of 9 months. Sonography reveals diffuse or focal nodular decreased echogenicity with preservation of the ovoid testicular shape. Doppler ultrasound shows a strikingly increased vascular flow unrelated to the size or extent of the tumour, unlike that with primary testicular tumours.

Metastases to the testis

Metastases are more common than germ stem tumours in males over the age of 50 years. They are often bilateral and multiple. In adults the common primary sites that metastasise to the testis include the prostate, lungs, kidneys, gastrointestinal tract, bladder, thyroid and melanoma. In children neuroblastoma and Wilms' tumour is often implicated. Sonographically metastases are often hypoechoic but echogenic masses may occur. The sonographic findings may be indistinguishable from lymphomas or primary testicular tumours.

Stromal cell tumours (interstitial cell tumours)

Large-cell calcifying Sertoli cell tumour

These testicular tumours, which arise from the Sertoli cells of the seminiferous tubules, are associated with hormonal abnormalities such as gynaecomastia and precocious puberty. There is a known association with tuberous sclerosis, Peutz–Jeghers syndrome, pituitary tumour with gigantism and Carney complex (endocrine overactivity, cardiac myxomas and spotted pigmented skin lesions). Over 90 per cent of these tumours are benign and usually arise in the first year of life. The sonographic appearances are those of a smooth rounded area, 5 to 10 mm in size, with curvilinear calcification. Calcification within the testis without an associated soft tissue mass is strongly suggestive of this tumour. Doppler ultrasound may display increased blood flow within or adjacent to the lesion. If this diagnosis is made preoperatively local excision may allow preservation of testicular parenchyma.

Leydig cell tumour

These tumours arise from the interstitial cells that form the fibrovascular stroma of the testis. They usually affect children between the ages of 3 and 6 years. As with Sertoli cell tumours they may be hormone secreting, which may be feminising or result in precocious puberty. Over 90 per cent of these tumours are benign. The ultrasonic appearances are those of a hypoechoic mass. Calcification is uncommon.

Gonadoblastoma

These tumours, arising from primitive gonadal stroma, are exceptionally rare. They usually arise on the background of dysgenetic gonads and an abnormal karyotype.

Carney complex

This is a familial neoplastic syndrome (mendelian dominant) associated with pigmented lesions of the skin and a variety of myxomatoid and endocrine tumours, including uterine myxoid tumours and in the male large cell Sertoli calcifying tumours. The tumours are benign therefore recognition is important so testicular-conserving surgery can be carried out. Precocious puberty can occur. Ultrasonography reveals echogenic masses a few millimetres to 2 centimetres in size with chunky calcification associated with shadowing.

Testicular microlithiasis

Testicular microlithiasis is detected by ultrasound as diffuse punctate non-shadowing hyperechoic foci within the testis. The condition is found both in adults and children. It occurs in 6 per cent of adults with a 40 per cent incidence of germ cell testicular neoplasms. Other associations described include cryptorchidism, delayed testicular descent and sub-fertility. Because of this association close clinical follow up with periodic (every 6 to 12 months) scrotal ultrasound is indicated. The time between the detection of microlithiasis and the development of testicular cancer remains unknown.

Testicular sarcoidosis

Sarcoidosis is an immunologically mediated multisystem disease of unknown aetiology with a variable prognosis. Testicular involvement is rare. The race of the patient, presence of systemic sarcoidosis and normal levels of tumour markers should suggest the diagnosis. However we have seen patients in whom scrotal sarcoidosis was the only evidence of disease. The following ultrasound findings have been described

- hypoechoic masses, single or multiple in the testes and epididymus
- a solitary echogenic mass occupying the whole of the epididymus and the cephalad portion of the testis
- homogeneous abnormality of the whole testis
- multifocal hypoechoic lesions with no epididymal involvement
- hypoechoic areas with calcification.

Carcinoid of the testis

Carcinoid of the testis is exceedingly rare, three types have been described

1. primary testicular carcinoid, the most benign type
2. carcinoid associated with a teratoma, even rarer
3. carcinoid metastatic to the testis, this is rare and has a poor prognosis.

Most testicular carcinoids are not clinically functional and therefore diagnosis is not suspected. Sonographically they may show a solid hypoechoic mass with areas of small nodular calcification.

Splenic–gonadal fusion

Splenic–gonadal fusion is a rare congenital anomaly, it is always left sided, most present in childhood and 3 per cent at autopsy. Accessory splenic tissue can be confirmed on a Tc-99m sulphur colloid scan. Ultrasonically it presents as a hypoechoic mass in the left testicle surrounded by normal testicular tissue. There is an association with inguinal hernia and cryptorchidism. The presence of other congenital abnormalities together with a left testicular mass should arouse suspicion of a splenic–gonadal fusion.

Polyorchidism

Polyorchidism usually presents clinically as a painless scrotal mass. On ultrasound supernumerary testes appear similar to the normal testis.

Testicular adrenal rest tumours

Testicular adrenal rest tumours occur in patients who have congenital adrenal hyperplasia and elevated levels of ACTH. If congenital adrenal hyperplasia is not recognised and treated in childhood, isosexual precocious puberty may ensue. On imaging these patients have a moderate to marked symmetrical or asymmetrical adrenal enlargement, which may appear unilateral and mimic an adrenal tumour. In late onset congenital adrenal hyperplasia the presenting feature may be a testicular mass. It is postulated that the sustained elevation of ACTH stimulates adrenal cell rests within the testis to grow and become functionally active adrenal rest tumours. On sonography these tumours appear as hypoechoic eccentrically placed testicular masses, often bilateral, which may have hyperechoic nodules (because of fibrosis) within them that may shadow. Uniformly hyperechoic lesions have been described.

'Burned-out' testicular tumour

Germ cell testicular tumours can undergo spontaneous regression, although metastases to the retroperitoneum, mediastinum, the cervical and axillary chain of lymph nodes, the lungs and liver may be the presenting feature. Within the testis the 'burned-out tumour' may be seen as a highly echogenic focus which may or may not shadow.

Differential diagnosis of echopoor testicular masses

Tumour.
Orchitis.
Torsion.
Infarction.
Abscess.
Haemorrhage.
Granuloma – tuberculosis, sarcoid.
Splenic–gonadal fusion.
Ruptured ovarian follicles – ovotestis in true hermaphrodites.

Differential diagnosis of bilateral testicular masses

Lymphoma.
Leukaemia.
Metastases.
Multiple primary tumours (1.1 to 3 per cent only 9.5–11 per cent present at the same time).
Sarcoidosis.

Carney complex.
Testicular adrenal rest tumours.

Calcification within the testes

Malignant tumours – teratocarcinoma, seminoma, embryonal cell carcinoma, carcinoid metastases to the testis.

Benign tumours – primary testicular carcinoid tumours, adenomatoid tumour, mature teratoma, stromal tumours (Lydia cell and Sertoli cell), Carney complex (Sertoli cell tumours), papillary cystadenoma of the epididymis.

Other causes – tuberculosis, sarcoidosis, trauma, microlithiasis, burned-out germ cell tumour, filariasis, phleboliths.

5.2.9 SOLID EXTRATESTICULAR INTRASCROTAL MASSES

Epididymitis

See pp. 425–426. Epididymitis may be acute or chronic and related to infection or trauma. Focal epididymitis may occasionally present as an asymmetric enlargement of the epididymis with a mass-like appearance. A clinical history consistent with either infection or trauma and relative hyperaemia on colour flow Doppler should suggest the correct diagnosis.

Sperm granuloma

Focal enlargement of the epididymis can also occur with sperm granulomata, which can arise as a complication of vasectomy and appear as a heterogeneous hyperechoic extratesticular mass.

Scrotal hernia

See p. 423.

Torsed appendix testis

In the setting of acute scrotal pain, a torsed appendix testis can appear as a paratesticular hypoechoic nodule with surrounding hyperaemia detected with colour Doppler.

Scrotal calculi

Small nodular paratesticular masses are common findings in physical examinations. Scrotal calculi 3 mm or larger present as mobile dense masses associated with calcification within the tunica vaginalis on ultrasound. There is skin thickening and/or chronic epididymitis (4.3 per cent). They may represent sloughed appendices testis that has undergone dystrophic calcification. They are usually asymptomatic.

Fibrous pseudo-tumour of the epididymus

Paratesticular fibrous pseudo-tumours are benign masses which may be diffuse, multiple or focal. They typically involve the tunica vaginalis but may rarely involve the epididymus. The pseudo-tumour usually presents as a painless scrotal mass or masses discovered incidentally. Histologically these tumours are composed of proliferative fibroblasts and hyalinised collagen, sometimes with inflammatory cells and granulomatous tissue. The importance of these benign tumours is the difficulty in differentiating them from the more common malignant intrascrotal tumours that need orchiectomy. Fibrous pseudo-tumours may need only local resection sparing the testis. Sonographically these masses present as hypoechoic or hyperechoic discrete nodules distinct from the testis.

Fournier's gangrene

This is a rare, potentially lethal, necrotising fasciitis of the scrotum. Diabetes mellitus is a frequent predisposing factor. If treatment is to be successful it has to be initiated early.

Lipoma of the spermatic cord

This is the most common benign tumour of the spermatic cord. It appears homogeneously echogenic, distinct from both the epididymus and testis.

Fibrolipoma of the spermatic cord

These are rare benign tumours presenting with a supratesticular mass of varying size. On sonography the appearances are those of a partially solid mass with a diffuse irregular internal structure.

Benign solid tumours of the epididymus

These tumours are rare. The most common is the benign adenomatoid tumour which accounts for 30 per cent of all extratesticular masses and usually presents as a heterogenous solid mass. It is usually confined to the tail of the epididymus but may occur elsewhere. Other benign tumours of the epididymus include leiomyoma, lipoma, hamartoma, lymphangioma and neurofibroma. Extremely rare tumours of the testicular adnexa include teratoma, melanotic hamartoma and Brenner tumour.

Papillary cystadenoma of the epididymus

Papillary cystadenoma is a rare benign tumour of the epididymus associated with von Hippel–Lindau syndrome in 10 to 26 per cent of cases. When the tumours are bilateral they are virtually pathognomonic of von Hippel-Lindau disease. It is rare in the general population and unilateral when it occurs. The tumours, 1.6 to 5 cm in size are found in young adults and are usually asymptomatic. Sonographically they are solid masses which may occasionally display cystic spaces. Echogenic nodules caused by calcification may be seen that may shadow. The cysts may be so closely spaced that they appear echogenic. Dilated rete testis may be seen with ectatic ductules within the testis. Testicular atrophy may occur but there is no malignant potential.

Paratesticular rhabdomyosarcoma

This is a rare tumour but it accounts for 97 per cent of the malignant neoplasms of the scrotal tunics. The tumour is seen in all ages but usually there is a bimodal age distribution, 5 and 16 years with a mean of 7 years. Clinical presentation is with a painless mass. Metastases usually occur to the para-aortic and paracaval lymph nodes (26 to 71 per cent) and parenchymal metastases (25 per cent) to the lungs and cortical bone. Because of the highly aggressive nature of the tumour early recognition is important. On ultrasound they are usually homogeneously echogenic extratesticular masses. The homogeneous echogenicity does not guarantee a benign lesion. Areas of necrosis may show as hypoechoic areas. A complex mass has been described. There is usually a clear plane of separation from the testis. Ultrasound is 100 per cent accurate in differentiating testicular from extratesticular masses although testicular invasion may occur.

Leiomyosarcoma

Leiomyosarcoma is less common than other testicular tumours. They are also seen in a much older age group and often show slow growth. Following excision local recurrence may occur. Haematogenous spread and local recurrence determines the prognosis. Sonographically they cannot be differentiated from other extratesticular tumours.

Other extratesticular malignant mesenchymal tumours

Fibrosarcoma, liposarcoma and myxochondrosarcoma have been described. With fibrosarcoma a mass with both echogenic and sonolucent components compressing an atrophic testicle has been described. However there are no characteristic features on ultrasound to suggest a diagnosis but sonography is very accurate in differentiating testicular from extratesticular tumours.

Extratesticular germ cell tumours

These have been described in the thorax and retroperitoneum. Exceptionally they may occur in an extratesticular site within the scrotum. Extratesticular seminoma has been shown to have a hypoechoic septate appearance whilst an extratesticular embryonic cell tumour has been shown to present with an inhomogeneous mass caused by haemorrhage and calcification. Although one cannot offer specific diagnoses on ultrasound it is important to know the existence of these entities because of prognostic implications.

Mesothelioma of tunica vaginalis

The tunica vaginalis is an extension of the peritoneum and is formed by a single layer of mesothelial cells. A primary mesothelioma (benign or malignant) analogous to the pleural or peritoneal tumour may affect the tunica vaginalis. The histological appearance of this rare entity may be of three types

1. carcinomatous
2. fibrosarcomatous
3. mixed type

each with a preferential site. Sonography demonstrates a paratesticular mass associated with a complicating hydrocoele. Diagnosis is made at surgery.

Differential diagnosis of mesothelioma of tunica vaginalis
Mesothelial hyperplasia (a) spontaneous (b) secondary to an inflammatory process.
Pseudofibrous tumours.
Metastatic adenocarcinoma (a) distant site (b) adjacent site.
Adenomatoid tumours.

Metastatic tumour of the tunica vaginalis

Metastatic tumour can occur in the epididymus, spermatic cord and/or the tunica vaginalis. The primary sites may be the male breasts, pancreas, kidneys, gastrointestinal tract, melanoma and the prostate gland among other sites. Metastases from a squamous carcinoma of the penis have been recorded. The pancreas and the gastrointestinal tract are the most common sites implicated with metastases to the tunica vaginalis, probably as a result of venous or lymphatic intraperitoneal and retroperitoneal seeding.

Sonography reveals thickening of the sheaths of the testis, as is seen in pachy vaginalitis, related to chronic inflammation of variable often undetectable aetiology associated with hyperaemia on colour flow Doppler.

Hyperechoic uniform scrotal masses – benign

Collagenous scar.
Adenomatoid tumour embedded in the testis.
Focal chronic epididymitis with surrounding fibrosis.
Suture in the capsule of the testis.
Fibrous plaque involving the tunica albuginea.
Spermatic granuloma.
Adenomatoid tumour of the epididymus.

5.2.10 DEEP PELVIC CYSTS IN A MALE

Differential diagnosis of deep pelvic cysts in a male (Fig 5.1)

Congenitally large prostatic utricle.
Müllerian duct cyst.
Seminal vesicle cyst.
Congenital prostatic cyst.
Prostatic retention cyst.
Diverticular prostatis.
Ejaculatory duct diverticulum or cyst.
Prostatic abscess.
Urachal diverticulum or cyst.
Bladder diverticulum.
Seminal vesicle abscess.
Congenital anomalies of the vas deferens.
Cystic prostatic carcinoma.
Cystic degeneration of a hypoplastic nodule.
Ectopic ureter.
Ureterocoele.
Caecoureterocoele.
Pseudoectopic ureterocoele.
Blind ectopic ureterocoele.
Congenital urethral duplication.
Cowper's syringocoele.
Acquired diverticula of the urethra.
Urethral defects following transurethral resection of prostate (TURP)

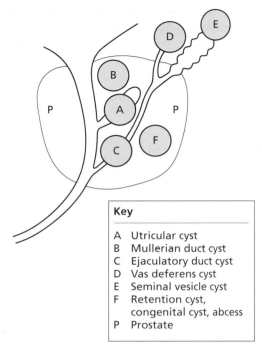

Key

A   Utricular cyst
B   Mullerian duct cyst
C   Ejaculatory duct cyst
D   Vas deferens cyst
E   Seminal vesicle cyst
F   Retention cyst,
    congenital cyst, abcess
P   Prostate

Figure 5.1 Sagittal line diagram of the location of various prostatic cysts

Hydatid cyst.
Pelvic lymphocoele.
Deep pelvic abscess.
Anterior sacral meningocoele.
Plexiform neurofibroma (cystic).
Iliac artery aneurysm.
Pelvic haematoma.
Cystosarcoma phyllodes of the prostate and seminal vesicle.

Congenitally large prostatic utricle

All males have a tiny prostatic utricle (utriculus masculinus) which is not normally visible on sonography. The prostatic utricle may enlarge and become visible as a tubular or pear-shaped cystic structure with underlying anomalies of the lower urinary tract. Enlargement is associated with hypospadias, ambiguous genitalia, undescended testis or a congenital urethral polyp. The utricle normally communicates with the urethra where it inserts into the verumontanum. Presentation is usually in the first or second decades. Complications are rare but occasionally patients may present with epididymitis.

Müllerian duct cysts

Müllerian duct cysts are oval or pear-shaped midline cystic structures lying posterior to the verumontanum and extending cephalad above the prostatic base. Communication with the urethra is rare. They vary in size from a few millimetres to several centimetres. Unlike the prostatic utricle they are not associated with lower urinary tract anomalies and unlike the seminal vesicle they do not contain spermatozoa or fructose. There is an increased incidence of adenocarcinoma and squamous cell carcinoma. Presentation is usually in the third or fourth decades with epididymitis. On sonography they have a variable echogenicity depending upon the type of fluid they contain, i.e. serous, mucoid or purulent. They are the only cysts at this site that may contain calculi.

Seminal vesicle cysts

The seminal vesicles are paired organs which serve as reservoirs of seminal fluid. They are paired, elongated, convoluted, cystic structures lying posterolateral to the prostate. Congenital vesicle cysts usually present between the ages of 15 to 60 years. The symptoms depend upon the cyst's size. Small cysts are usually asymptomatic but larger cysts may be giant and fill the pelvis and they may cause urinary or ejaculatory obstructive symptoms. There is a close association with renal agenesis and dysgenesis. On transabdominal or transrectal sonography these cysts have considerable variation in size and may be unilocular or multilocular. Rarely the cysts may be bilateral. These cysts, if large enough, can be punctured under ultrasound guidance and injected with radiographic or ultrasonic contrast which may outline a seminal-vesicle-shaped structure. The cyst aspirate contains red blood cells, leukocytes, epithelial cells and non-motile spermatozoa.

Congenital prostatic cysts

Cysts of the prostate may be acquired or congenital. Congenital cysts develop as a result of focal dilatation of the prostatic ducts. These cysts are usually small, lie on either side of the midline and may be seen incidentally on transrectal ultrasound. They may come to the attention of the clinician following a digital rectal examination. Paradoxically they are said to feel hard to the finger and mimic prostatic carcinoma. The best way of examining suspected prostatic cysts is by transrectal sonography. These cysts are small appearing well defined, with no internal echoes and are placed on either side of the midline. When large they may be aspirated under ultrasound guidance. The aspirate should contain no spermatozoa.

Ejaculatory duct diverticulum or cyst (the urogenital sinus cyst)

This cyst or diverticulum may be unilateral or bilateral, or both the ejaculatory ducts may open into a single midline cyst. Clinically they are felt as a mass just above the base of the prostate on rectal examination. Presentation is usually with symptoms of acute prostatitis, haemospermia or painful ejaculation. They are best seen on endorectal ultrasound. They may be punctured under ultrasound guidance, injected with radiographic contrast and further evaluated with a radiograph.

Prostatic abscess

A prostatic abscess usually develops as a complication of prostatitis but occasionally haematogenous spread may occur. Predisposing causes include diabetes mellitus immunosuppression, urethral instrumentation and prostatic carcinoma. The symptoms may be those of pelvic pain and systemic symptoms of urinary tract infection such as pyrexia and chills. Endorectal ultrasound is the preferred method of evaluation. Sonographically the abscess may be seen as a hypoechoic mass which may eventually develop thick septae. If the abscess contains gas it may appear hyperechoic. The sonographic appearances are non-specific, none the less when read in conjunction with the clinical presentation a diagnosis can be suggested. Moreover ultrasound guidance allows aspiration for diagnostic and therapeutic purposes.

Urachal diverticulum or cyst

A urachal diverticulum forms when the urachus closes partially, the closure occurring at the umbilicus but not at the bladder end. A urachal cyst forms when the urachus closes both at the umbilical and bladder end, and the cyst forms between the two occluded areas. Both the diverticulum and cyst are asymptomatic and are an incidental finding. They may become symptomatic when complicated by infection or neoplasia. A urachal cyst is seen on abdominal sonography as a well-defined cyst usually with no internal echoes, placed between the umbilicus and the dome of the urinary bladder. The vesicourachal diverticulum appears as a cystic conical area continuous with the bladder dome. There is an increased incidence of carcinoma within the diverticulum after puberty, and also tendency to calculus formation.

Urinary bladder diverticulum

Most bladder diverticula are acquired as a result of bladder outlet obstruction. Congenital diverticula are usually found at the bladder apex or the ureterovesical junction with no associated bladder hypertrophy. They are seen as a cystic pouch-like structure continuous with the bladder lumen. Tumours and calculi can occasionally complicate diverticula.

Seminal vesicle abscess

Seminal vesicle abscess may complicate seminal vesiculitis or congenital mesonephric duct anomalies, the most common being ureteral insertion into the seminal vesicles. An ectopic renal position or renal agenesis may be associated with congenital mesonephric anomalies. The seminal vesicles and their complications are best seen on endorectal sonography. The abscess is seen as a hypoechoic or anechoic, partially fluid-filled structure at the base of the bladder. It may be aspirated under ultrasound guidance through the endorectal probe or through transperineal sonography.

Congenital anomalies of the vas deferens

The commonest cause of congenital absence of the vas deferens is cystic fibrosis. The ejaculatory duct is often absent with an absent vas deferens but the seminal vesicle may become cystic or rudimentary. There are often associated abnormalities of the epididymus where the tail and body, but not the head, are absent. Eighty per cent of absent vas deferens are bilateral. Various types of vaso-ureteral communications associated with an ectopic vas deferens have been described (persisting mesonephric duct: high junction of vas deferens and ureter). These communications may be seen as cystic masses above, or above and behind, the bladder. Associated renal tract anomalies are common.

Cystic prostatic carcinoma

Most prostatic carcinomas are solid tumours, which may be isoechoic, hypoechoic or hyperechoic; most are situated in the peripheral zone under the capsule. Contour anomalies may provide secondary evidence as to the presence of a prostatic tumour. Rarely prostatic carcinomas may be completely cystic, making aspiration biopsy under transrectal ultrasound mandatory in order to differentiate them from other cystic lesions.

Cystic degeneration of hyperplastic prostatic nodules

Hyperplastic benign prostatic nodules are common and may be difficult to differentiate from cancers. They may undergo cystic degeneration with conversion of the nodule into ragged cystic masses. It may not be possible on transrectal ultrasound alone to differentiate these from cystic cancers or prostatic abscesses. Cyst aspiration or biopsy under transrectal ultrasound guidance may be necessary.

Prostatic retention cyst

Prostatic retention cysts develop as a result of dilatation of glandular acini caused by acquired glandular duct obstruction. They may be located in any part of the prostate and generally affect men in the fifth and sixth decades. The cysts are usually 1 to 2 cm in size, unilocular with smooth intraluminal walls.

Diverticular prostatitis

Chronic prostatis may eventually lead to fibrosis, which may constrict or obstruct glandular ducts leading to stasis of glandular secretions, breakdown of intra-acinar septa and cavity formation.

Ectopic ureter

Unilateral ectopic ureters are almost always dilated and may open into the urethra or the genital tract. When one opens into the urethra it invariably does so in its upper third near the verumontanum. Ultrasound will show a tubular cystic structure which extends posterior to the bladder but separate from it. When ectopic ureters are bilateral they rarely open into the genital tract and usually open into the urethra just proximal to the verumontanum. With bilateral ectopic ureters, transverse scans show both ureters as cystic structures symmetrically placed posterior to the bladder, although one ureter may be more dilated. There may be associated renal dysplasia and hydronephrosis.

Ureterocoeles

See p. 375.

Caecoureterocoele

Caecoureterocoeles account for about 5 per cent of ureterocoeles. There is a large orifice opening into the bladder, but the ureterocoele extends into the submucosa of the urethra as a blind pouch or caecum. This pouch or caecum may distend with urine and obstruct the urethra causing bladder neck obstruction.

Pseudoectopic ureterocoele

Pseudoectopic ureterocoeles are rare. They are represented by a dilated distal ureter which forms a submucous mass at the bladder base. The ureter is uniformly dilated and no true ureterocoele exists. The condition has been called a pseudoectopic ureterocoele as the appearance mimics a true ureterocoele on an intravenous pyelogram.

Blind ectopic ureterocoele

Five per cent of ureterocoeles on double ureters are blind ending (there is no ureteral orifice). These may appear as cystic fusiform intravesical structures pointing towards the urethra, and extend into a tubular structure cephalad representing the dilated ureter.

Congenital urethral duplication

Duplication of the urethra is rare. Three types have been described.
Type 1   accessory blind urethra

- type 1A   opening distally onto the dorsal or ventral penile surface but with no proximal connection with bladder or the functioning urethra.
- type 1B   Opening proximally but with no distal connection, this type may mimic a urethral diverticulum.

Type II   complete duplication, patency is maintained at both ends

- type IIA   two functional urethras or two urethras, the second arising from the first and coursing independently
- type IIB   two urethras arising from the bladder joining to form one common urethra distally ending in one meatus.

Type III   duplicated urethra arising from a double or septate urinary bladder.

The accessory urethra may open into the seminal vesicle causing a cystic mass, or an accessory blind duplicated urethra may form a cyst.

Cowper's syringocoele

The Cowper's glands drain into the bulbous urethra. Three types of congenital anomalies affect the Cowper's glands.

1. The gland duct is abnormally dilated (although the opening is wide and unobstructed) and the Cowper's syringocoele develops, appearing as a cystic structure on transrectal ultrasound or perineal ultrasound.
2. The entry of the gland duct enters an ectopic location into the more distal bulbous urethra.
3. A dilated gland duct, caused by meatus stenosis, that may compress the urethra.

Acquired diverticula of the urethra

In contrast to females urethral diverticula are rare in men. They may complicate trauma, infection, surgery or urethral instrumentation. Diverticula in the posterior urethra are most commonly related to the rupture of a prostatic abscess into the urethra whilst anterior urethral diverticula are more likely to be related to instrumentation trauma or infection. Sonographically the diverticula may be single or multiple, unilocular or multilocular, wide or narrow necked with smooth or ragged intraluminal walls.

Urethral defects following TURP

Widening of the prostatic urethra is a common finding after all types of simple prostatectomies. Soon after prostatectomy the prostatic fossa is quite large and takes several weeks to involute, however some residual dilatation remains for years. Following a cryocaustic prostate surgery a 'bottle-brush-like' defect may be seen.

Primary pelvic hydatid cyst

A pelvic hydatid cyst is rare and usually presents with pressure symptoms involving adjacent organs (bladder and rectum). It may present with obstructive uropathy leading to renal failure. Ultrasound appearances are those of a multiloculated cyst.

Pelvic lymphocoele

Lymphocoeles are extraperitoneal lymph collections. They are lined by the parietal peritoneum and have no true lining. They are a recognised complication of abdominal or pelvic surgery, particularly lymphadenectomy for malignant disease. They may occur anywhere in the pelvis but appear to be more common on the pelvic side-wall. They are seen sonographically as multilocular cystic masses but hypoechoic or complex masses may occur. Dependent debris may be seen when a secondary infection supervenes. Calcification within a lymphocoele is rare.

Deep pelvic abscess

Deep pelvic abscess in the male is a known complication of appendicitis, diverticulitis, traumatic injury to bowel, pelvic surgery and Crohn's disease. The abscesses have variable echogenicity, which may be cystic multiseptate, hypoechoic or complex. The walls show intraluminal irregularity. They may be drained percutaneously or transrectally under ultrasound guidance.

Anterior sacral meningocoele

Anterior sacral meningocoele is a herniation of the dural sac through an anterior sacral wall defect. As well as containing arachnoid membrane the sac contains cerebrospinal fluid. The majority of cases present in the third decade with a female preponderance. There is an association with Marfan's syndrome. Sonography reveals a midline cystic structure posterior to the bladder. Computed tomography and MRI may demonstrate the vertebral connections.

Plexiform neurofibroma

Plexiform neurofibromas are associated with neurofibromatosis. Pelvic neurofibromas are usually solid as elsewhere in the body, but cystic neurofibromas have been described.

Iliac artery aneurysm

Pelvic arteriovenous malformations and aneurysms of the iliac arteries present as cystic masses within the pelvis. Aneurysms of the common iliac arteries may displace the bladder anteriorly. Most iliac artery aneurysms are associated with aortic aneurysms. With real time ultrasound there should normally be no difficulty in differentiating vascular cystic spaces from other pelvic cysts. Colour Doppler is diagnostic.

Pelvic haematoma

Haematomas, whether postoperative or traumatic, typically appear anechoic initially and then, as they resolve, they may become complex or multicystic masses. A psoas haematoma may occasionally be difficult to differentiate from other cystic masses.

Cystosarcoma phyllodes of the prostate

Cystosarcoma phyllodes have been given several names including cystic adenoma, cystadenoleiomyofibroma and atypical prostatic hyperplasia.

There is a wide age range of presentation of 22 to 78 years. The tumour may reach quite large proportions and, unlike a prostatic carcinoma, these tumours are soft on digital rectal examination. Patients usually present with urinary obstructive symptoms, haematuria, dysuria or a palpable abdominal mass. The ultrasound appearances reported have been of a complex or cystic mass. The cyst may be very large and multicystic.

5.3 THE PROSTATE

Although the prostate may be visualised on abdominal scanning it is seen most clearly on rectal scanning. The gland may be subdivided into an inner and outer gland. The prostate consists of

1. a heterogenous slightly echogenic central zone surrounding the ejaculatory ducts
2. a more homogeneous slightly hypoechoic peripheral zone.

Glandular tissue makes up 25 per cent of the central zone and 75 per cent of the peripheral zone. The lower echogenicity of the peripheral zone is due to its higher muscle content. This zone comprises the posterior, apical and lateral lobes and is the site of origin of 70 per cent of prostatic carcinomas. The seminal vesicles can often be visualised lying behind and slightly above the prostate. They are hypoechoic relative to adjacent prostatic parenchyma. The normal prostate measures 2.8 (craniocaudal length) × 2.8 (anteroposterior length) × 4.8 (width) cm.

5.3.1 BENIGN PROSTATIC HYPERTROPHY

The size of the prostate increases in middle-aged and elderly males. As it enlarges the prostate becomes asymmetrical and bulges upwards into the bladder. Hypertrophy is usually most prominent in the central zone. The enlarged gland may have a homogeneous echopattern, but it may appear heterogeneous particularly if previously affected by prostatitis or if complicated by areas of infarction, ductal dilatation or stone formation.

5.3.2 PROSTATIC TUMOURS

At post mortem 12 to 46 per cent of men over the age of 50 years have foci of prostatic carcinoma on gland histology. The incidence rises to reach 90 per cent by the age of 90 years. The clinical incidence of prostatic carcinoma is far lower and the natural history of the disease is not fully understood at present. Over 70 per cent of primary prostatic malignancies arise

Table 5.1 Positive predictive value and sensitivity of commonly used tests in the diagnosis of prostatic cancer

Test	Positive predictive value	Yield	Sensitivity
Digital rectal examination	22%	2.4%	45%
Transrectal ultrasound	24–29%	3.3%	89%
Prostatic specific antigen	38%	2.9%	88%

in the peripheral zone of the gland causing loss of normal gland symmetry and echotexture. Prostatic carcinoma does not have a specific sonographic appearance though most tumours are hypoechoic. Calcification may give rise to echogenic foci.

Prostatic cancer: ultrasound sensitivity

1. Eighty per cent of peripheral lesions are benign.
2. Most prostatic carcinomas are peripheral.
3. Prostatic specific antigen is organ specific but not cancer specific.

General appearance of prostatic carcinoma

Although echolucent, isoechoic and hyperechoic carcinomas occur, by far the majority of prostatic carcinomas are echopoor (more than 90 per cent). Transrectal sonography with simultaneous prostatic biopsy via the perineal approach allows accurate tissue diagnosis of prostatic lesions. Ultrasonography is also a valuable means of disease staging since extension of carcinoma through the gland capsule may readily be demonstrated with loss of capsular continuity and gland outline. The majority of predominantly hypoechoic lesions prove to be malignant whilst predominantly hyperechoic areas are rarely malignant. Sonography may follow up these tumours, therapy usually results in an increase in parenchyma echogenicity. Isoechoic tumours may be missed on grey scale ultrasound. In 18 per cent of patients when grey scale sonography is normal colour flow Doppler will reveal a tumour. Conversely 18 per cent of colour flow Doppler is normal when grey scale ultrasound shows an abnormality. Most prostatic carcinomas (75 per cent) will show on ultrasound, the addition of colour flow Doppler can identify another 16 per cent and another 9 per cent are diagnosed on random sexton biopsy. The tumours seen on colour flow Doppler and sexton biopsy have a relatively similar range of Gleeson scores and degree of biopsy core infiltration. The use of colour flow Doppler may obviate excessive biopsies and target the lesions. Hypoechoic lesions containing diffuse stippled echogenicity may be a sonographic sign of comedocarcinoma, which is an aggressive variety of prostatic carcinoma (Gleeson Potters).

5.3.3 PROSTATITIS

Prostatic inflammation gives rise to a tender enlargement of the gland, which has a rather soft consistency of palpation. In acute prostatitis the gland may be of normal size but it is often enlarged and deformed. The capsular margin becomes ill defined and the enlarged gland shows hypoechoic areas. The presence of calculi within the gland gives rise to echogenic foci. With treatment the gland size and contour return to normal but the abnormal echotexture may persist. In chronic prostatitis the gland shows a persistently abnormal echopattern which may be heterogeneously echogenic with evidence of calculi, these calculi usually lie posterior to the urethra and in the gland periphery (calculi tend to occur around the urethra in urethritis).

5.3.4 DIFFERENTIAL DIAGNOSIS OF HYPOECHOIC PROSTATIC MASSES

Prostatic carcinoma.
Comedocarcinoma.
Benign prostatic hyperplasia.
Focal prostatis.
Tuberculosis granuloma.
Tuberculosis.
Prostatic abscess.
Sarcoma.
Focal amyloid deposition.

5.4 FURTHER READING

Ablett MJ *et al.*: A rapidly expanding testicular mass due to ruptured ovarian follicle. Br J Radiol *69*:366–367, 1996.
Al-Otaibi L *et al.*: Fibrous pseudotumour of the epididymus. Am J Roentgenol *168*:1586, 1997.
Ardil RH *et al.*: Epididymitis associated with Mullerian duct cyst and calculus: sonographic diagnosis. Am J Roentgenol *155*:91–92, 1990.
Biyani CS *et al.*: Case report: Fournier's gangrene roentgenographic and sonographic findings. Clin Radiol *50*:728–729, 1995.
Connolly JA *et al.*: Ultrasound evaluation of the penis for assessment of impotence. J Clin Ultrasound *24*:481–486, 1996.

Crone KD, Carroll BA: Scrotal ultrasound. Radiol Clin North Am 25:121, 1985.

Eroso CE et al.: Sonographic findings in testicular sarcoidosis simulating malignant nodule. J Clin Ultrasound 27:81-83, 1999.

Eskey CJ et al.: Malignant lymphoma of the testis. Am J Roentgenol 169:822, 1997.

Flanagan JJ, Flower RL:Testicular infarction mimicking tumours on scrotal ultrasound: a potential pitfall. Clin Radiol 50:49-50, 1995.

Freimanis MG et al.: Ultrasound appearance of extratesticular myosarcoma. J Clin Ultrasound 19:101-104, 1991.

Gierk CL et al.: Large-cell calcifying Sertoli cell tumour of the testis: appearances on sonography. Am J Roentgenol 163:373-375, 1994.

Gooding GAW et al.: Cholesterol crystals in hydrocoeles: sonographic detection and possible significance. Am J Roentgenol 169:527-529, 1997.

Gordon LM et al.:Traumatic epididymitis: evaluation with color Doppler sonography. Am J Roentgenol 166:1323-1325, 1996.

Grimshaw ND, Gopi Chandran TD: Case report. Primary carcinoid tumour of the testis: ultrasound appearances. Clin Radiol 47:290-291, 1993.

Henderson RG et al.: Case report. Splenic-gonadal fusion: the ultrasonic appearances. Clin Radiol 44:117-118, 1991.

Holloway BJ et al.: Scrotal sonography: a valuable tool in the evaluation of complications following inguinal hernia repair. J Clin Ultrasound 26:341-344, 1998.

Kim ED, Lipshultz LI: Role of ultrasound in the assessment of male infertility. J Clin Ultrasound 24:437-453, 1996.

Lavoipierre AM et al.: Prostatic cancer: role of color Doppler imaging in transrectal sonography. Am J Roentgenol 170:205-210, 1998.

Lile R et al.: Prostatic comedocarcinoma: correlation of sonograms with pathologic specimen in three cases. Am J Roentgenol 155:303-306, 1990.

Luker GD, Siegel MJ: Color Doppler sonography of the scrotum in children. Am J Roentgenol 163:649-655, 1994.

Luker GD and Siegel MJ. Scrotal ultrasound in pediatric patients: comparison of power and standard color Doppler ultrasound. Radiology 188:381-385, 1996.

Malvica RP: Epidermoid cyst of the testicle: an unusual sonographic finding. Am J Roentgenol 160:1047-1048, 1993.

Mario A et al.: Ultrasound evaluation of unusual pelvic cystic masses. J Clin Ultrasound 21:651-655, 1993.

Martinez-Berganza M et al.: Cysts of the tunica albuginea: sonographic appearance. Am J Roentgenol 170:183-185, 1998.

Mason BJ and Kier R. Sonographic and MR imaging appearance of paratesticular rhabdomyosarcoma. Am J Roentgenol 171:523-524, 1998.

Miller RL et al.: Testicular microlithiasis: a benign condition with a malignant association. J Clin Ultrasound 24:187-202, 1996.

Monette RJ and Woodward PJ. MR appearances of dilated rete testis. Am J Roentgenol 163:482, 1994.

Morey AF, McAninch JW. Ultrasound evaluation of the male urethra for assessment of urethral stricture. J Clin Ultrasound 24:473-479, 1996.

Nghiem HT et al.: Cystic lesions of the prostate. Radiographics 10:635-650, 1990.

Ozcan H et al.: Color Doppler ultrasonographic findings in intratesticular varicocoele. 25:325-329, 1997.

Parvey HR et al.: Urethral complications of urinary catheterisation presenting as primary scrotal masses: sonographic diagnosis. J Clin Ultrasound 26:261-264, 1998.

Pattiel HJ et al.: Maturational changes in arterial impedance of the normal testis in boys: Doppler sonographic study. Am J Roentgenol 163:1189-1193, 1994.

Pavlica P, Barozzi L: Ultrasound of penile tumours and trauma. Ultrasound Quarterly *14*:95–109, 1998.

Rowling SE *et al.*: Intrascrotal vasculitis simulating a testicular neoplasm. J Ultrasound Med *15*:161–163, 1996.

Seenu V *et al.*: Primary pelvic hydatid cyst presenting with obstructive uropathy and renal failure. Postgrad Med J *70*:930–932, 1994.

Shapiro RS *et al.*: Superficial dorsal penile vein thrombosis (penile Mondor's phlebitis): ultrasound diagnosis. J Clin Ultrasound *24*:272–274, 1996.

Shawker TH *et al.*: Intratesticular masses associated with abnormally functioning adrenal glands. J Clin Ultrasound *2*:51–58, 1992.

Tartar VM *et al.*: Tubular ectasia of the testicle: sonographic and MR imaging appearance. Am J Roentgenol *160*:539–542, 1993.

Tesler FN *et al.*: Ultrasound assessment of testicular and paratesticular masses. J Clin Ultrasound *24*:423–436, 1996.

Torres GM *et al.*: Bacille Calmetti-Guerin vaccine induced granulomatosis prostatis: another hypoechoic non-neoplastic lesion. Am J Roentgenol *155*:195–196, 1990.

Tumeh SS *et al.*: Acute diseases of the scrotum. Semin Ultrasound CT MR *12*:115, 1991.

Tweed CS, Peck RJ: A sonographic appearance of testicular lymphoma. Clin Radiol *43*:341–342, 1991.

Vilana R *et al.*: Cystic prostatic carcinoma. Am J Roentgenol *162*:1502, 1994.

Wachsberg RH *et al.*: Posterior urethral diverticulum presenting as a midline prostatic cyst: sonographic and MRI appearances. Abdom Imaging *20*:70–71, 1995.

Yang WT *et al.*: Neonatal adrenal haemorrhage presenting as an acute right scrotal swelling (haematoma) – value of ultrasound. Clin Radiol *50*:127–129, 1995.

6

Female genital tract

6.1.1 OVARIES

The ovaries can be identified in the majority of children. Their relationship to the uterus varies because of the mobility of the ligamentous attachments. They may be located cephalad, lateral or posterior to the uterine body. There is considerable variability in the ovarian shape although most are ovoid. The ovary shows a heterogeneous echopattern at all ages. Small follicles less than 1 cm are not uncommon at all ages whilst follicles larger than 1 cm are seen in the majority of postpubertal women.

Ovarian size

Ovarian size at birth $1.5 \times 0.3 \times 0.25$ cm.
Ovarian size after puberty $2.4\text{-}4.1 \times 1.5\text{-}2.4 \times 0.85\text{-}1.9$ cm.
Ovarian volume   length $\times$ width $\times$ depth $\times 0.52$ ml (assuming that the ovary is elliptical in shape)

ovarian volume in a child	1 ml
ovarian volume in an adult	7-7.5 ml
postmenopausal ovarian volume	1.5-10 ml.

Before the menopause the ovarian volume depends upon the number and size of developing follicles.

Neonatal ovarian cysts

Ovarian cysts are found in the majority of neonatal and infant ovaries. Maternal hormones are responsible for follicular growth *in utero*. The neonatal ovary is usually of heterogeneous echopattern with cysts. In children 1 day to 3 months old cysts smaller than 9 mm are found in 82 per cent and cysts larger than 9 mm in 20 per cent of individuals. Cysts may reach enormous proportions and may fill the entire abdomen. It may sometimes be impossible to differentiate ovarian cysts from mesenteric or enteric cysts. Neonatal ovarian cysts may undergo haemorrhage, torsion and amputation. The sonographic appearance therefore depends on whether the cyst is uncomplicated or complicated. Uncomplicated cysts are anechoic with an imperceptible wall. A complicated cyst may contain a fluid–debris level, septa and retracting clot, or it may have a solid appearance because of multiple echoes. The walls of the cyst may become echogenic because of calcification. A fluid–debris level and retracting clot has been suggested as specific signs of cyst torsion that had occurred antenatally. Complex cysts may be impossible to differentiate from ovarian neoplasms which fortunately are extremely rare.

Differential diagnosis of neonatal ovarian cysts

Mesenteric cysts.
Enteric cysts.
Hydrometrocolpos.
Cloacal malformation mass – frequently present in duplication of uterus and vagina resulting in a multicystic mass.
Cystic meconium peritonitis.
Urachal cyst.
Bowel atresia or obstruction.
Renal cyst.
Anterior meningocoele.
Ovarian neoplasms – cystic teratoma, cystadenoma and granulosa cell tumour.

6.1.2 PREPUBERTAL UTERUS

The foetus is subject to the influence of maternal hormones and thus at birth the neonatal uterus has the same configuration as the postpubertal uterus. The uterus involutes over the next few weeks. Intracavitary fluid is a common finding. The uterus can be identified in the majority of children with adequate bladder distension. The uterus may be anteverted or retroverted. The prepubertal uterus is tubular in configuration with similar anteroposterior measurements to the fundus and cervix. After the early neonatal period the uterine size regresses and remains unchanged until the age of 7 years. At about 7 years of age the uterus shows signs of growth. Although there is a general increase in uterine size the growth is much more pronounced in the fundus, which gives the uterus a pear-shaped configuration. The myometrium appears hypoechoic and the endometrium is isoechoic to the myometrium in prepubertal girls. Following the onset of menstruation the endometrium becomes more echogenic and acquires differing echogenicity during the menstrual cycle.

Uterine measurements

Average size of the neonatal uterus   length 3.4 cm, width 1.25 cm.

NB   the foetus is subject to the influence of maternal hormones and thus the uterus has a similar configuration to the postpubertal uterus.

Average size of the prepubertal uterus   length 2–3.3 cm, width 0.5–1 cm.

NB   at this stage the body and cervix are of a similar length, giving a body to cervix ratio of 1:1. After puberty the ratio increases to 2:1.

Average size of the uterus at puberty   length 5–8 cm, width 1.6–3 cm.
Uterine volume   approximately 1.5 × length × width × breadth
   prepubertal uterine volume is less than 2 ml
   at puberty uterine volume is 25 ml.
Pregnancy   during pregnancy the uterus increases up to 30 times by muscle hypertrophy. After pregnancy it involutes but usually remains larger than before.
Uterine hypoplasia   this is not usually evident until puberty. Causes include lack of oestrogens, chromosomal anomalies and *in utero* exposure to diethylstilbestrol.

Intersex

Ambiguity of the genitalia at birth poses an urgent clinical problem, as the sex of the child needs to be settled to enable the parents to bring up the child appropriately. Sonography can be useful because demonstration of the presence of a uterus and ovaries suggests a virilised female whereas their absence suggests male pseudohermaphrodism. True hermaphrodism may occur but is exceptionally rare. In this condition both ovarian and testicular tissues are present.

Female pseudohermaphrodism
- Congenital adrenal hyperplasia
- Exposure of female foetus to excessive androgens

Male pseudohermaphrodism
- Defects in testicular differentiation
- Defects in testicular hormones
- Defect in androgen action

Uterine malformations

Congenital maformations of the uterus are found in 0.1–0.5 per cent of women, these may be associated with anomalies of the urinary tract because of their similar embryological origins. These anomalies may be visualised sonographically and the diagnosis is confirmed by hysterosalpingography. They are usually asymptomatic although there is an increased incidence of spontaneous abortion.

Non-obstructive genital anomalies
Uterine agenesis.

Mayer–Rokitansky–Kuster–Hauser syndrome – dysplasia of the Müllerian ducts with resultant absence of the uterus and vagina.

Uterine hypoplasia – a small uterine cavity is noted usually associated with hormonal dysfunction. Hypoplasia is not clinically evident until puberty. Causes include lack of oestrogens, chromosomal anomalies and *in utero* exposure to diethylstilbestrol.

Uterus didelphys – complete duplication (two uterine horns, two cervices, and two vaginas).

Uterus bicornis bicollis – complete division of the uterus down to the internal os (one vagina, two cervices and two uterine bodies).

Uterus bicornis unicollis – partial division of the uterus (one vagina, one cervix and two uterine horns).

Uterus unicornis unicollis with a rudimentary remnant.

Septate uterus – partial or non-resorption of the uterine septum.

Uterus unicornis unicolis – unilateral arrested development.

Obstructive genital anomalies
Imperforate hymen.

Transverse vaginal septum.

Vaginal atresia.

NB In the above anomalies mucous secretions accumulate resulting in cystic dilatation of the vagina (hydrocolpos).

Urogenital sinus or cloacal malformation – there is a single exit chamber for the bladder and vagina, while in cloacal malformation there is a single chamber for bladder, vagina and rectum. This may result in hydrocolpos or hydrometrocolpos.

Sonography Sonography is the modality of choice in the diagnosis of obstructive genital anomalies (hydrocolpos and hydrometrocolpos). The vagina is a distensible organ and with distal obstruction a large pelvic, usually cystic, mass with scattered internal echoes may result. A fluid–debris level may be seen. Occasionally the vaginal mass may be hypoechoic. The cystic vagina should not be confused with a distended urinary bladder. The identification of the uterus capping the vaginal mass is important for the diagnosis of vaginal obstruction, but this may not always be easy to demonstrate because of difficulty in identifying the less distensible uterus and its displacement into the abdomen. The vaginal mass may also cause hydronephrosis because of ureteric obstruction. Hydronephrosis can also occur from bladder obstruction because of the narrow urogenital sinus or cloaca. There is an association with renal dysplasia and renal agenesis.

Uterine obstructive lesions at menarche

Most obstructive lesions are diagnosed at menarche as a result of accumulation of menstrual blood in the vagina (haematocolpos), uterus (haematometra) or vagina and uterus (haematometrocolpos).

Causes of obstructive genital lesions at menarche

Imperforate hymen.
Transverse vaginal septum.
Congenital absence of the vagina and cervix (uterus present).
Congenital absence of the vagina (cervix and uterus present).
Mayer–Rokitansky–Kuster–Hauser syndrome associated with an active rudimentary uterine cavity with functional endometrium thus resulting in unilateral haematometra.
Uterine didelphys with obstructed hemivagina – this presents with dysmenorrhea and lower abdominal pain.
Unicornuate uterus with an obstructed rudimentary uterine horn – this typically presents with dysmenorrhea and lower abdominal pain.

6.1.3 PRECOCIOUS PUBERTY

The development of secondary sexual characteristics before the age of 9 years in a female child is considered to be precocious puberty.

True precocious puberty

This is usually secondary to early activation of the hypothalamus–pituitary–gonadal axis. No cause is found in 80 per cent of children. Twenty per cent of children have intracranial neoplasm, hydrocephalus or post-encephalitic or post-traumatic scars.

Pelvic sonography reveals ovarian and uterine enlargement with a pear-shaped adult uterine configuration.

Precocious pseudopuberty

Development of secondary sexual characteristics without activation of the hypothalamus–pituitary-gonadal axis is classified as precocious pseudo-puberty. The causes include ovarian neoplasms, ovarian cysts, oestrogen-secreting adrenal neoplasms and exogenous oestrogens.

Sonography reveals a small uterus and ovaries. The cause of precocious pseudopuberty such as ovarian neoplasm, ovarian cysts or an adrenal tumour may be identified on abdominal scanning.

6.1.4 DELAYED DEVELOPMENT OF PUBERTY

Delayed puberty is said to occur when there is an absence of breast development or menstruation by the age of 15 years. Most cases are said to be familial or caused by constitutional delay.

Causes of delayed development of puberty

Familial.
Constitutional.
Infections.
Neoplasms affecting the hypothalamus–pituitary–gonadal axis.
End-organ sensitivity to gonadotrophins.
Gonadal dysgenesis – Turner's syndrome, Noonan's syndrome, Perrault's syndrome, Kallman's syndrome, Swyer's syndrome, pure gonadal dysgenesis.
Ovarian failure (with no chromosomal anomalies) – ataxia-telengiectasia, galactos-aemia, type 1 autoimmune polyendocrinopathy, girls receiving cytotoxic drugs, pelvic irradiation.
Sonography may reveal streak ovaries or ovaries with no follicles visible. The uterus is small, tubular and of prepubertal type.

6.1.5 POLYCYSTIC OVARIAN DISEASE

Polycystic ovarian disease or Stein–Leventhal syndrome classically presents with obesity, hirsutism and secondary amenorrhea. However this triad is not always present. This hormonal dysfunction involving the hypothalamus-pituitary–ovarian axis usually manifests itself with menstrual irregularities and infertility. Presentation is usually at puberty or shortly thereafter. The diagnosis is usually based on hormonal criteria rather than imaging. Sonographic appearances are variable. The ovaries are enlarged in the majority of patients. Ovarian echogenicity is compared to the uterus where the echopattern of the ovaries may be the same as the uterus or echoes within the ovaries may be less than the uterus (hypoechoic). Discrete cysts within the ovaries are seen in a minority of patients. The ovaries may show an increased number of follicles at varying stages of maturation and atresia.

6.1.6 OVARIAN CYSTS

Ovarian cysts are common in females of all ages. By far the majority of ovarian cysts are either follicular or corpus luteal. A corpus luteal cyst arises when the corpus luteum does not involute, follicular cysts result when the mature follicles do not ovulate. Follicular cysts are usually anechoic whereas corpus luteal cysts often have internal echo because of haemorrhage. Functional ovarian cysts may become large and palpable and may present with pain due to haemorrhage, torsion or rupture. Most functional cysts resolve within weeks. The ultrasonic appearances depend upon haemorrhagic and other complications. They may acquire a multiseptate appearance with fluid–debris levels. Occasionally they may appear as hyperechoic. See p. 452 for neonatal cysts.

6.1.7 OVARIAN TORSION

Ovarian torsion occurs as a result of rotation of the ovarian pedicle resulting in vascular compromise. The risk of torsion increases with ovarian size particularly with cysts and tumours over 5 cm in diameter. Torsion of a normal ovary is rare except in young girls before menarche. There is increased mobility of the adnexa in young girls. The sonographic appearance of ovarian torsion is variable. The ovary may be solid, cystic or complex, hypoechoic or hyperechoic and multiple follicles may be noted around the periphery of the ovary. A fluid–debris level associated with a septate appearance and retracting clot may be seen in a torsed ovarian cyst. Because flow on Doppler ultrasound cannot always be demonstrated in a normal ovary, the absence of flow on colour Doppler does not diagnose torsion. However if normal flow is seen in the ovary on colour flow Doppler, torsion is excluded. Weeks after ovarian torsion the walls of the ovarian mass may become echogenic because of calcification.

6.1.8 OVARIAN TUMOURS

Germ-cell tumours and teratodermoids make up most ovarian tumours in children. The sonographic appearance of a mature teratoma depends upon its constitution and may be purely cystic, solid or complex. The most characteristic appearance is said to be a hypoechoic or cystic mass with mural nodules. Highly echogenic foci within the mass may represent teeth, bone or fat. Other benign tumours such as fibroma and cystadenoma are rare in children (see p. 452).

Tumours arising from primitive germ cells of the embryonal gonads make up the majority of malignant ovarian tumours in children. These tumours include dysgerminoma (associated with XY gonadal dysgenesis), immature teratoma (elevation of alpha fetoprotein), endodermal sinus tumour (elevation of alpha fetoprotein and human chorionic gonadotrophins), choriocarcinoma and malignant mixed germ-cell tumour.

Sonographic appearances are those of a large solid or complex mass. Calcification may occur in dysgerminoma and immature teratoma. The existence of a cystic mature teratoma does not exclude a co-existent malignant neoplasm.

Malignant stromal tumours are rare and include granulosa-theca-cell, Sertoli–Leydig cell tumours and arrhenoblastoma, whilst some sex cord tumours defy characterisation. These are functioning tumours which may precipitate precocious puberty or cause virilisation depending upon the predominant hormone secreted. These tumours are large at presentation and may appear solid or complex.

Ovaries are a sanctuary site for leukaemia and may also be involved in lymphoma. Both the ovaries are usually involved often with asymmetrical enlargement. The ovaries appear solid and hypoechoic.

6.1.9 UTERINE TUMOURS

The most common uterine tumour in children is a rhabdomyosarcoma. Other uterine tumours are exceptionally rare in children, they include leiomyoma, adenocarcinoma, and cervical intraepithelial tumours and mixed mesodermal tumours. Clear-cell adenocarcinoma of the cervix and vagina are, again, a rare neoplasm typically seen in adolescents exposed to diethylstilbestrol. These patients usually present with vaginal bleeding.

6.1.10 VAGINAL TUMOURS

The vagina is seen in the majority of children as a midline tubular structure behind the bladder. The collapsed mucosa is seen as an echogenic stripe. The walls of the vagina are hypoechoic measuring less than 1 cm in thickness. The most common vaginal tumour in children is a rhabdomyosarcoma. The common site of origin is the anterior vaginal wall often involving the adjacent cervix and possibly extending into the bladder neck and base. The sonographic appearances are those of a solid heterogeneous mass, which may have hypoechoic or cystic foci because of haemorrhage and necrosis.

6.1.11 PELVIC INFLAMMATORY DISEASE

See p. 492.

6.1.12 ECTOPIC PREGNANCY

Over the past 25 years there has been a sharp rise in the incidence of teenage ectopic pregnancy. The clinical presentation and sonographic appearance is no different to adult ectopic pregnancy. See pp. 494–496.

6.1.13 EFFECTS OF EXPOSURE TO DIETHYLSTILBESTROL

Increased incidence of vaginal carcinoma.
Increased incidence of genital anomalies – abnormal vaginal mucosa 56 per cent, vaginal adenosis 35 per cent, vaginal fibrous ridges 22 per cent, small T-shaped uterus.

6.1.14 PELVIC MASSES IN CHILDREN

Ultrasound patterns of pelvic masses in children

Cystic adnexal masses – simple ovarian cyst, cystadenoma, cystadenofibroma, teratoma, hydrosalpinx.
Complex adnexal masses – cyst, teratoma, tubo-ovarian abscess, haemorrhagic cyst.
Solid adnexal masses – haemorrhagic cyst, teratoma, dysgerminoma, fibroma.

Uterine and vaginal masses in children

Cystic masses – hydrocolpos, haematometrocolpos.
Complex masses – pregnancy, infection.
Solid masses – rhabdomyosarcoma, hydatidiform mole.

Non-gynaecologic pelvic masses in children

Cystic masses – abscess (appendicitis, Crohn's disease), lymphocoele, enteric duplication, ureteral dilatation, cysts of urachus, bladder diverticulum.
Complex masses – sacrococcygeal teratoma, abscess, haematoma.
Solid masses – haematoma, neuroblastoma.

6.2 FERTILE AND POSTMENOPAUSAL WOMEN

6.2.1 OVARIES

Ovarian size has been discussed on p. 451. The ovaries are fairly mobile structures because of their loose attachment to the pelvic wall and uterus via the broad and other ligaments. Whilst the ovaries can be visualised in the majority of children and fertile females, only 64 to 78 per cent can be visualised in postmenopausal women, the longer the interval after menopause the lower the chances of identifying the ovaries. Following hysterectomy only 43 per cent of normal ovaries can be identified. Doppler signals in the non-functioning ovary are those of a high-impedance waveform. In a functioning ovary the Doppler signals vary and depend upon the ovarian cycle. The understanding of the ovarian cycle is important to understand the development of follicles and physiological cysts. The ovarian cycle occurs as follows.

1. The follicular phase lasts from 1 to 14 days when primordial follicles begin to mature in response to follicle-stimulating hormone. The ovary at this stage will have multiple small cysts. By the fourth day two to three follicles on each side show enlargement to approximately 1 centimetre. The graafian or dominant follicle appears in one ovary by the tenth day and grows to 20 to 25 mm in size by the fourteenth day of the menstrual cycle. Doppler sonography may show a progressively increasing diastolic flow in the ovary bearing the dominant follicle. From day 1 to day 6 there is a high-impedance waveform with a resistive index close to 1.0. From day 7 to day 22 there is continuous diastolic flow with a resistive index close to 0.5.
2. The ovulatory phase begins on the fourteenth day, this is when mid-cycle pain, 'mittelschmerz', just prior to the release of the ovum occurs. There is usually a sudden decrease in the follicular size on the release of the ovum.
3. The luteal phase lasts 15 to 28 days and gives rise to a 16 to 24 mm corpus luteum cyst which is almost isoechoic with ill-defined margins and internal echoes due to haemorrhage. Before involution the corpus luteum cyst may grow to 3 to 4 cm in size because of further haemorrhage. Finally before the end of the menstrual cycle the corpus luteum cyst undergoes considerable atrophy by approximately the twenty-fourth day. Doppler waveforms from day 23 to day 28 show a high-impedance waveform with a resistive index close to 1.0.

Signs of ovulation

The graafian follicle varies in size from 17 to 29 mm, it grows by 3 mm a day until 24 hours before ovulation when there may be a sudden increase in size.

The appearance of the 'cumulus', which represent a 1 millimetre echogenic focus projecting into the follicle, is followed by ovulation within 36 hours.

Solid echoes develop within the graafian follicle following ovulation.

A decrease in diameter or sudden collapse of the graafian follicle indicates that ovulation has occurred.

The appearance of a ring structure within the uterine fundus.

The appearance of fluid or blood in the pouch of Douglas.

Non-visualisation of the ovary

Normal ovary obscured by gas – this is more common on the left side because of the sigmoid colon

Bladder is overdistended or underdistended.

Previous oophorectomy.

Displaced ovary (anteversion or retroversion), uterine masses, leiomyoma.

Ectopic ovary – in the inguinal canal, failure of descent, low ovary.

Children – most ovaries are seen by modern scanners.

Postmenopausal small ovaries.

Atrophic ovaries – radiotherapy.

Developmentally small ovaries – Turners syndrome.

Müllerian dysgenesis.

Distorted pelvic anatomy – previous surgery or radiotherapy.

Ultrasound mimics of ovaries and ovarian masses

Low-lying caecum

This may mimic an ovarian dermoid as faeces and gas in the caecum and the adjacent omental fat may appear as an echogenic mass. It is particularly likely to be confused with an ovarian tumour if the caecum is low lying or pelvic in location. A repeat examination after an interval may reveal the true nature of the caecum.

Fluid or faeces-filled bowel

A fluid-filled bowel in the vicinity of the adnexa may mimic an ovary or ovarian cyst. Reverberation echoes from gas can be mistaken for the margins of a mass. Scanning over a period of time would demonstrate peristalsis and a changing 'pseudo-mass'.

Bladder duplication artefact

This happens particularly with an over-distended bladder, the pseudo-mass effect may resolve with partial voiding.

Ectopic pregnancy

The incidence of ectopic pregnancy is rising for a variety of reasons and now accounts for 1 per cent of pregnancies. The most common presentation is with an adnexal mass (see p. 494).

Hydrosalpinx and pyosalpinx

These may present cystic, solid or complex masses in relation to the adnexa.

Vascular aneurysms and malformations

These show characteristic flow on pulsed or colour Doppler.

Pelvic varices and ovarian varicocoele

Varicose veins in the broad ligaments may cause ill-defined pelvic pain associated with enlargement of the uterus and adnexa, pelvic congestion, congested breasts and varicosities of legs (Taylor's syndrome). Because of the congestion and enlargement of the adnexa a 'real' adnexal mass may be mimicked. Sonography shows a cystic or complex adnexal mass. Duplex Doppler with colour flow shows normal ovaries and the cystic spaces would demonstrate blood flow.

Uterine masses

Uterine masses, particularly exophytic fibroids, may mimic ovarian masses. In most instances ultrasound should be able to differentiate the uterus from the mass.

Paraovarian cysts

Separate from the ovary these cysts represent vestigial remnants of the wolffian duct in the mesosalpinx, they account for 10 per cent of pelvic masses.

Massive ovarian oedema

This is a tumour-like condition due to oedema and marked enlargement of one or both ovaries. It is probably related to intermittent torsion resulting in occluded venous and lymphatic drainage. The presentation may be with intermittent lower abdominal pain over a few weeks. Masculinisation may occur in the chronic phase. The ultrasound appearances are those of an enlarged ovary or ovaries and occasionally a multicystic ovarian mass may be seen.

Pelvic kidney
These kidneys usually maintain a reniform shape and recognisable parenchymal structure. Pelvic kidneys may become hydronephrotic.

Pseudomyxoma peritonei
The gelatinous ascites in pseudomyxoma peritonei may implant on serosal surfaces. When implantation occurs in the region of the broad ligament an ovarian mass may be mimicked.

Pelvic fat and connective tissue
Any of these structures may be confused with the ovaries. Confusion is less likely with endovaginal sonography.

Pelvic muscles
The ovaries are located between the iliopsoas muscles and the uterus. On cross section the iliopsoas muscles may be mistaken for ovaries. The iliopsoas muscles can be scanned by positioning the transducer along the midline, immediately above the pubis with the transducer angled away from the midline.

Presacral masses
Masses such as sacrococcygeal teratomas and presacral meningocoele may at times be confused with adnexal masses. Computed tomography or MRI may identify their dorsal location.

Lymphocoele and haematoma
These usually follow surgery and may resemble adnexal cysts, they may be difficult to differentiate from gynaecological masses. They are usually multiseptate and ill defined and may be placed at a distance from the uterus.

Colonic carcinoma
Carcinoma of a low-lying caecum and the sigmoid may mimic adnexal masses but these masses on careful inspection may be seen to present a typical or atypical target sign. However, recurrent carcinoma after surgery may be difficult to differentiate from adnexal masses.

Diverticular abscess or mass
Ultrasound may reveal bowel wall thickening or fluid surrounding a 'target lesion'.

Markedly constipated bowel
Constipated bowel may mimic a dermoid. Rectal examination may identify the cause.

Matted omentum

Polypoid fatty masses may mimic adnexal masses. With endovaginal sonography confusion is less likely.

Obturator internus

The obturator internus muscle lies along the posterior pelvic side wall. This muscle can occasionally be confused with an ovary.

Peritoneal inclusion cysts

Patients with peritoneal inclusion cysts usually give a history of previous surgery. Ultrasound findings are those of an anechoic septate mass surrounding the ovary. Doppler sonography shows low resistive flow in the septations.

Endosalpingiosis

This condition, akin to endometriosis, is said to be implantation of ectopic oviduct epithelium involving the peritoneum or pelvic or para-aortic lymph nodes. The condition is usually asymptomatic and affects women of child-bearing age. These deposits are usually incidentally seen as multiple peripheral echogenic foci involving the ovaries. These foci are of calcific density on plain abdominal radiographs and CT.

Structures mistaken for ovarian follicles

Ovarian cysts.
Iliac vessels.
Ovarian vessels.
Uterine vessels.
Hydrosalpinx.
Pyosalpinx.

Palpable pelvic masses not seen on ultrasound

No true mass present.
Mass resolved spontaneously.
Mass hidden by bowel loops.
Bowel loops or soft tissues mistaken for a mass.
Mass displaced into the abdomen (the position of a mass may vary depending upon the degree of bladder distension).
Large ovarian masses may mimic the bladder or ascites
A dermoid or calcified mass giving rise to an echogenic anterior surface with distal shadowing may not give the appearance of a mass (need plain abdominal radiograph), the 'tip-of-the-iceberg sign'.

Bilateral ovarian enlargement

Polycystic ovary syndrome.
Cystic disease.
Ovarian tumours – primary and secondary.
McCune–Albright syndrome.
Haemorrhage.

6.2.2 OVARIAN AND ADNEXAL MASSES

Cystic ovarian masses

Malignant cysts
Malignancy is suggested by thick-walled cysts, excrescences, thick septa (particularly if they are complete), intramural nodules, a low pulsatility index less than 1 and a resistive index less than 0.4 (elevated diastolic flow). A unilocular cyst which appears well defined with good through transmission and a diameter less than 5 cm is nearly always benign. The presence of ascites is not a discriminating factor as it may accompany both benign and malignant cystic tumours. The presence of colour flow on Doppler in the regular wall or septa does not indicate malignancy. Therefore the addition of colour flow Doppler to conventional ultrasound in the diagnosis of cystic tumours adds little to the diagnostic work up.

Follicular cysts
These are functional ovarian cysts, usually due to an unruptured follicle or failure to ovulate and are regarded as a sign of an anovulatory cycle. They are particularly common during puberty and menopause. They are generally small cysts (1 to 2.5 cm), single or multiple, unilocular and thin walled. Internal echoes, septa and fluid–debris levels may be seen as a result of haemorrhage. As they can elaborate oestrogen, their persistence can cause endometrial hyperplasia with associated prominent endometrial echo complex.

Corpus luteum cysts
Corpus luteum cysts occur during the luteal phase of the ovarian cycle (15 to 28 days). They vary in size from 16 to 40 mm, are usually smooth walled and vary in echogenicity from almost isoechoic through anechoic to hypoechoic. They may give rise to a complex adnexal mass due to internal haemorrhage. Rupture may occur resulting in free pelvic fluid. By approximately the twenty-fourth day involution and atrophy of the corpus luteum cyst occurs (corpus luteum atreticum).

Theca lutein cysts

These cysts are often bilateral, thick walled, well defined and septate, they may grow up to 10 centimetres in diameter. Theca lutein cysts are usually secondary to an underlying functional disorder such as hydatidiform mole, choriocarcinoma or ovulation induction therapy.

Haemorrhagic ovarian cysts

Haemorrhage may complicate both benign and malignant cysts. The sonographic appearances are variable depending upon the state of blood within the cyst. The cyst may appear anechoic, solid, complex or septate and a fluid–debris level may be seen.

Polycystic ovaries

Large ovaries in 35 to 40 per cent with five or more cysts of 5 to 8 mm in each ovary, 30 per cent normal sized ovaries. Serial examinations show failure of the follicles to change size or configuration. 25 per cent – hypo-echoic ovary with no discrete individual cysts, 5 per cent – enlarged ovaries isoechoic with uterus. There is a 5 to 17 per cent risk of ovarian neoplasm and increased incidence of endometrial carcinoma. A normal ultrasound appearance does not exclude polycystic ovary syndrome.

Ovarian remnant syndrome

Occasionally adnexal cystic masses may occur after partial oophorectomy. The small amount of ovarian tissue may be hormonally stimulated and produce a haemorrhagic functional cyst. Sonographically an echogenic mass, which can be quite large, may be identified.

Paraovarian cysts

These represent vestigial remnants of the wolffian duct in the mesosalpinx, they account for 10 per cent of all adnexal masses. They are usually sited in the broad ligament separate from the ovary. They do not regress on serial scanning. Haemorrhage, torsion and rupture may complicate the cyst. A specific diagnosis can only be made if normal ovary separate from the mass can be identified on the ipsilateral side.

Endometrioma

Endometriosis is a common condition resulting from encysted functional end endometrial epithelium in an ectopic location outside the uterus. It has been found in 8 to 20 per cent of women undergoing pelvic surgery. A more localised form of disease consists of discrete masses called endmetriomas or 'chocolate cysts'. These are fairly well-defined, thick-walled cysts with low-level internal echoes. Recurrent bleeding may give rise to cystic areas with variable internal echoes, that may mimic solid masses. Endometriosis may occur internally within the uterine wall or in several external locations including the ovary, broad ligament, pouch of Douglas and many other non-gynaecological locations.

Ovarian torsion

Torsion of the ovary occurs as a result of rotation of the ovary on its axis producing compromise of the vascular pedicle. The risk of torsion increases with ovarian enlargement, ovarian mass lesion and hypermobility of the adnexa which is more frequent in children and during pregnancy. Ultra-sonography may show a unilaterally enlarged hypo- or hyperechoic mass with multiple peripheral cysts 8 to 10 mm in diameter. An associated cystic or solid mass may be seen. Engorged vessels may appear as small multiple cystic structures of uniform size at the periphery of the torsed ovary. Free fluid is detected in the cul-de-sac in 32 per cent of patients. Doppler sonography may show absence of flow but this is not a reliable sign.

Ovarian hyperstimulation syndrome

Ovarian hyperstimulation may result during assisted conception (human chorionic gonadotrophin and clomifene), hydatidiform mole, chorioepithe-lioma and occasionally from multiple pregnancies. It is diagnosed when the ovary measures over 5 cm in the longest diameter and contains multiple follicles. Ovarian cysts over 10 cm in size are found in almost all cases. There are marked constitutional symptoms such as abdominal pain, nausea, vomiting and dyspnoea. Ascites, pleural effusions and hydroureters may occur. Electrolyte imbalance and venous thrombosis are complications. In severe cases death may result from intra-abdominal haemorrhage or a thrombo-embolic episode.

Serous cystadenoma

This is the second most common benign tumour of the ovary (20 per cent of all benign tumours). The initial appearance is indistinguishable from a simple cyst, but the cysts are large at presentation and may be up to 20 cm in diameter. They may be bilateral and can undergo malignant transformation to a cystadenocarcinoma. The malignant tumour usually affects patients in an older age group (40–50 years). They are usually unilocular but may contain thin-walled septa with occasional papillary projections. Ascites may rarely occur.

Serous cystadenocarcinomas

These represent 60 to 80 per cent of all ovarian carcinomas. The tumours are quite large and over half are over 15 cm in size. They are often multiloculated with thick septa, with numerous papillary projections and echogenic material within the locules. The tumours are bilateral in 50 to 60 per cent of cases, and ascites due to surface implantation is also common. Associated lymphadenopathy due to metastases may be seen on ultrasound. These tumours may calcify.

Mucinous cystadenomas

These tumours represent 20 per cent of all benign ovarian tumours affecting the 30 to 50 year age group. They are usually unilateral with prominent septations. The locules frequently have a high protein content (mucin) presenting as low-level echoes on sonography. Rupture of the tumour leads to pseudomyxoma peritonei.

Mucinous cystadenocarcinoma

These are rare tumours and generally difficult to differentiate from their benign counterpart, serous cystadenocarcinoma. The tumour is not purely cystic and contains thick septa and other solid components within the locules. They may be bilateral in 20 per cent of patients. Metastases from a mucinous cystadenocarcinoma or rupture of the tumour may lead to pseudomyxoma peritonei.

Endometroid carcinoma

These account for 15 per cent of all malignant ovarian tumours. An association with endometrial hyperplasia and endometrial carcinoma has been described in 20 to 30 per cent of patients. Sonographic appearances are varied and may range from cystic, with papillary projections, to solid, to complex solid areas with necrosis and haemorrhage.

Brenner's tumour

See p. 469.

Clear cell carcinoma of the ovary

See below.

Other cystic masses

Ectopic pregnancy, pelvic inflammatory disease, pyosalpinx, and tubo-ovarian abscesses may be indistinguishable from other adnexal masses on sonography alone. Clinical history is frequently of primary importance in achieving a diagnosis. The masses may be cystic, solid or complex, and are often associated with fluid in the cul-de-sac.

Solid or complex ovarian masses

Clear cell carcinoma

This is thought to arise from the müllerian ducts, is almost always invasive and makes up 5 to 10 per cent of all malignant ovarian tumours. The sonographic appearances are non-specific and frequently seen as solid or complex masses. However a unilocular cystic appearance with mural nodules may be seen.

Brenner's tumour

This is a rare epithelial benign tumour which may occur at any age but has a peak incidence between the ages of 40 and 70 years. They may have oestrogenic activity. Sonographic appearances are those of a 1 to 2 cm well-defined hypoechoic solid mass although larger tumours up to 30 cm in diameter have occasionally been observed. Extensive calcification has been recorded. Cystic lesions have been described.

Undifferentiated ovarian carcinoma

Undifferentiated ovarian cancers are rare accounting for less than 5 per cent of malignant ovarian tumours. Sonographically these tumours are solid and hypoechoic but may have a complex appearance with areas of cystic necrosis. Prognosis is usually poor.

Germ-cell tumours: teratomas and dermoids

These are common tumours in adolescents and young women but they may also occur in the elderly. Malignant teratomas are rare. Between 10 to 15 per cent of dermoids are bilateral. Cystic teratomas can exhibit a wide range of sonographic appearances reflecting their varied composition of sebum, teeth, hair, etc. Despite the varied appearance of a teratoma, its sonographic features can be distinctive. One such distinctive finding is that of a highly echogenic nodule or 'dermoid plug' within an adnexal mass. A conglomerate of fatty tissue or sebum, hair, teeth and calcification produces the dermoid plug. The size of a dermoid plug varies from a few millimetres to that occupying the entire mass. Another feature of a teratoma is a highly echogenic focus within the mass due to teeth or calcification that may shadow. Hair may float on top of fatty material giving the 'tip of iceberg sign'. A fat–fluid level may be seen.

Mimics of a 'dermoid plug' sign

Acute haemorrhage within a pelvic mass – ovarian cyst, endmetrioma.
Exophytic lipomatous uterine mass.
Uterus obstructed by endometrial carcinoma.
Perforated appendicitis with an appendolith.
Pyometra or haematometra – in elderly patients.
Ovarian neoplasm with echogenic mural nodules.

Unrecognised dermoid plug

Cystic teratoma confused with bladder.
Bowel gas and faecal material.

May be missed on transvaginal ultrasound because of the limited field of view.

The rare feature of fat–fluid level may go unrecognised.

No true recognition with discovery in a misleading clinical context – a teratoma may be an incidental finding.

Ovarian stromal tumours

Stromal tumours are uncommon. They may affect all age groups although ovarian fibroma and fibrothecoma usually present in menopausal and post-menopausal women. Several cell types have been described including granulosa cell tumours, fibroma and fibrosarcoma and Sertoli–Leydig tumours. They are functioning tumours and therefore may present early. Sonographically they appear solid. They may be bilateral. Ovarian thecoma, fibroma or Brenner's tumour may be associated with Meigs' syndrome which represents a clinical triad of pleural effusions, benign ascites and an ovarian tumour.

Krukenberg's tumours

These tumours represent ovarian metastases of which 50 per cent are of gastrointestinal origin including stomach, colon, pancreas and the biliary tree. Two per cent of women with carcinoma of the stomach are said to develop ovarian metastases. In 20 per cent of cases they may antedate the discovery of the primary tumour. The most common appearance is of a pelvic mass, usually showing homogeneous low-level echoes. Appearances identical to cystadenocarcinoma may occur. Echogenic masses containing variable anechoic spaces have been described. Eighty per cent are bilateral.

Lymphoma

The ovaries are a 'sanctuary' organ for lymphoma. Lymphoma of the ovary is usually part of a more extensive disease elsewhere and often results from dissemination from other sites such as lymph nodes; ovarian lymphoma deposits are solid but echopoor. Often bilateral ovarian enlargement is usual.

Other ovarian tumours

Other tumours of the ovary not described above are rare and include dysgerminoma, choriocarcinoma, embryonal carcinoma and polyembryoma mixed cell tumour. Sonographically these are seen as solid or complex masses, diagnosis is seldom possible preoperatively.

Solid non-neoplastic masses

Ectopic pregnancy, pelvic inflammatory disease and salpingitis may all present as solid adnexal masses indistinguishable from ovarian masses on sonography alone.

Doppler sonography of ovarian and adnexal masses

Adding colour Doppler to conventional ultrasound produces a specificity and positive predictive value higher than that achieved with conventional ultrasound alone. Specificity is said to increase from 82 to 97 per cent ($P <$ 0.001) and a positive predictive value to increase from 63 to 91 per cent. Although colour flow and pulsed Doppler may help differentiate between malignant and benign lesions, there appears to be an overlap between malignant and benign pathology, with inflammatory masses and functioning benign tumours mimicking malignant lesions. Corpus luteum flow cannot be differentiated from flow to malignant lesions. In purely cystic masses the presence of colour flow in the wall or septa does not indicate malignancy. In cystic tumours readily diagnosed by conventional ultrasound, colour flow Doppler does not add any helpful information.

Serpentine tubular anechoic pelvic structures in a female
Fluid-filled bowel loops.

Multiloculated ovarian cysts.

Hydatid cysts.

Hydrosalpinx.

Uterine arteriovenous malformation – colour Doppler is an excellent tool for diagnosis.

Ovarian cancer risk

Nulliparity or low parity increases the risk of ovarian cancer, the risk decreases with increasing parity.

The use of oral contraceptives is said to be associated with a low risk.

The risk increases when two or more primary relatives are affected.

The risk increases with advancing age (80 per cent occur in patients over 50 years old).

It takes 2 to 3 years after menopause for the ovary to atrophy to $2 \times 1.5 \times 0.5$ cm. An ovary larger than this after menopause is considered abnormal.

Eighty to ninety per cent of ovarian cancers have a cystic component.

Even in experienced hands 25 to 40 per cent of ovaries are not visualised in postmenopausal women both on transabdominal or transvaginal ultrasound.

Benign ovarian cysts occur in 1 to 14 per cent of postmenopausal women, cysts less than 5 cm in diameter are considered low risk and can be monitored.

Neither transabdominal nor transvaginal ultrasound have shown acceptable sensitivity or specificity for ovarian cancer screening, although specificity is improved with pelvic examination and tumour marker levels (CA 125).

CA 125 is a highly non-specific marker with a tremendous degree of overlap between benign and malignant gynaecological disease – a positive CA 125 may bias an ultrasound examination!

CA 125 is elevated in 1 per cent of healthy women, the first trimester of pregnancy, cirrhosis, endometriosis and in 40 per cent of intra-abdominal non-ovarian malignancies.

CA 125 is elevated in only 50 per cent of patients with stage 1 disease, thus half the patients with potentially curable disease will not be detected.

There is considerable overlap of Doppler indices between benign and malignant disease and therefore reliability cannot be placed on these studies. The demonstration of flow on colour Doppler in the walls or septa of a cystic ovarian mass does not indicate malignancy.

Predominantly solid adnexal masses

Solid teratoma.
Dermoid cysts.
Krukenberg's tumours.
Lymphoma of ovaries.
Fibroma and fibrothecoma.
Arrhenoblastoma.
Granulosa cell tumour.

Differential diagnosis of cystic ovarian masses

Follicular cysts.
Corpus luteum cysts.
Theca lutein cysts.
Polycystic ovary.
Endometriosis (chocolate cysts).
Ectopic pregnancy.
Tubo-ovarian abscess and pelvic inflammatory disease.
Hydrosalpinx.
Paraovarian cysts.
Haematoma.
Adrenal torsion.
Cystic ovarian tumours.
Peritoneal and mesenteric cysts.
Lymphocoele.
Bowel loops.
Bladder diverticula.
Loculated ascites.
Appendix, diverticular, Crohn's abscesses.
Postoperative abscesses.
Dermoid cysts.

Degenerated fibroids.
Vascular aneurysms.

Adnexal calcification

Tumours – dermoid, Brenner's tumour, fibroma ovary, thecoma ovary, mucinous cystadenomas.
Miscellaneous – leiomyoma, previous abscess, calcified haematoma.

Echogenic pelvic masses

Benign cystic teratoma
See p. 469.

Malignant change in cystic teratoma
One to two per cent of teratomas may undergo a malignant change. Most malignant teratomas are found in postmenopausal women and usually represent incidental microscopic squamous cell carcinoma in a benign-looking tumour. However local invasion and distant metastases may occur. The appearances of a prominent solid echogenic tissue within a cyst or contiguous with it may suggest a malignancy. A contrast-enhanced CT may supplement the examination.

Non-teratomatous fatty ovarian tumours
These tumours are exceptionally rare and only a few cases of ovarian lipomas and lipoleiomyomas have been reported. The sonographic appearance of a lipoleiomyoma has been described as a 20 cm hypoechoic solid mass containing 1 to 3 cm hyperechoic nodules.

Fatty uterine tumours
These are rare tumours and only 100 cases have been reported in the world literature. They represent lipomas, lipoleiomyomas and fibromyolipomas. These tumours may be exophytic or endophytic. When exophytic they may be difficult to differentiate from tumours of ovarian origin. The identification of fat within these tumours on sonography (hyperechoic) CT or MRI is virtually diagnostic.

Pelvic lipomas
Lipomas in the retroperitoneum and pelvis are not uncommon. Sonographically they are well defined and hyperechoic, they produce a mass effect and no evidence of invasion. A CT scan may confirm their fat content.

Liposarcoma

These fairly aggressive tumours affect patients in their fifth to seventh decades with no gender predilection. Three histological types have been described

1. lipogenic
2. myxoid
3. pleomorphic.

The lipogenic variety has the most fat content and appears to have the least potential for malignancy. The pleomorphic type is the most invasive and has minimal fat content. The myxoid type is the commonest liposarcoma and is usually a well-circumscribed inhomogeneous mass that contains a variable amount of fat, it often occurs concomitantly with a lipogenic component. The sonographic appearances depend upon the fat content of the tumour. They may be well-defined to ill-defined, hyperechoic to complex, solid masses. Similarly the CT appearance also depends upon the histologic type and the amount of fat content.

Focal calcification in ovaries

- Calcification in a normal ovary is idiopathic, there is no change over time, laparoscopically the ovary appears normal.
- Dermoid shows punctate calcification.
- Adenofibroma shows multiple punctate calcification.
- Mucinous cystadenoma shows curvilinear calcification.
- Previous tubo-ovarian abscess shows punctate calcification.
- Previous ovarian torsion.

NB   Although calcification in benign tumours tends to be punctate it is possible that curvilinear calcification may be the earliest manifestation of malignancy.

Echogenic ovarian tumours

- Adenocarcinoma without serous or mucous collection.
- Teratoma.
- Brenner's tumour.
- Fibrothecoma.
- Granulosa cell tumour.
- Krukenberg's tumour.

Intrauterine contraceptive device

These cause high-amplitude echoes within the uterine cavity, which remain at low gain setting. The majority of intrauterine contraceptive devices shadow (90 per cent). Entrance and exit echoes giving parallel line appearances are seen in 65 per cent of cases. Type specific morphology is seen in 94 per cent.

Air in the uterine cavity

Air within the uterine cavity may be seen following the passage of sound or dilatation and curettage. Air is seen as high-amplitude echoes which may cause reverberation artefact and which may also shadow.

6.2.3 UTERUS

The uterine size in children and postpubertal women has been described (see p. 453). The postmenopausal uterus measures 3.5–6.5 cm (length) × 1.2–1.8 cm (width) × 2 cm (depth). The length of the postmenopausal cervix is one-third of the uterine length. The thickness of the various uterine layers depends upon the phase of the menstrual cycle in premenopausal women and the effect of hormonal medication in pre- and postmenopausal women. The endometrial thickness refers to anteroposterior measurements of the opposing layers of the endometrium across the endometrial cavity, excluding intrauterine fluid.

Endometrial thickness

Menstrual phase 1–5 days   Thickness 1–3 mm. The central interface is represented by a thin interrupted echogenic line.

Proliferative phase 4–6 days   Thickness 4–6 mm. A hyperechoic line represents the endometrial interface, the endometrium itself is a thickened hypoechoic band. The outer myometrium is slightly more echogenic.

Secretory phase 15–28 days   Thickness 7–14 mm. The central echo is bright associated with an echogenic thickened endometrium and a thin hypoechoic myometrium.

Postmenopausal uterus   The endometrial thickness is less than 8 mm in the majority of women (80 per cent) but the thickness may increase to 15 mm with hormone replacement therapy. Endometrial thickness of less than 5 mm is said to be associated with an atrophic hormonally inactive state as judged by histology.

Causes of increased endometrial thickness

Early intrauterine pregnancy (decimal reaction).
Hormonal excess – endogenous or exogenous.
Decidual reaction with ectopic pregnancy.
Retained products of conception.
Anovulatory cycles.

Gestational trophoblastic disease.
Endometrial carcinoma.
Endometrial polyp.
Haematometra.
Tamoxifen therapy.
Pyometra.
Cervical pregnancy.
Adenomyosis.
Endometrial hyperplasia.
Hormone replacement therapy.

Prominent endometrial echo complex

Decidual reaction

This is a normal response to intrauterine pregnancy and is sonographically depicted as echogenic thickened endometrium. An ectopic pregnancy may also cause a decidual reaction in 20–50 per cent of cases.

Secretory phase of the menstrual cycle

This refers to days 15 to 28 of the menstrual cycle. The endometrial thickness varies from 7 to 14 mm and is associated with a central echogenic line and thin hypoechoic myometrium.

Stimulated endometrium

The endometrium in postmenopausal women is thin and no more than 5 mm which is consistently associated with histologic evidence of atrophy. Hormone replacement therapy alters the physiology of the endometrium and causes increased thickness.

Endometrial carcinoma

See p. 480.

Endometrial hyperplasia

This is the most common cause of uterine bleeding and is related to proliferation of the endometrium because of prolonged oestrogenic stimulation. It affects both fertile and postmenopausal women. Classified into simple, complex and atypical hyperplasia, the incidence of subsequent malignancy is as high as 25 to 50 per cent in the atypical variety.

Endometrial polyp

See p. 481.

Pedunculated endometrial leiomyomas
See p. 480.

Endometritis
Endometritis is a bacterial infection of the endometrium, that may occur postpartum, following abortion, instrumentation or subsequent to placement of an intrauterine contraceptive device. The uterus may appear normal or it may be enlarged, with a wide echogenic cavity which may contain air or fluid.

Retained products of conception
The appearances of the 'endometrial complex' depend upon the stage of pregnancy at which abortion occurred and the type of tissue retained, for example osseous tissue.

Persistent corpus luteum cysts
After fertilisation of the ovum the follicle persists, producing hormones necessary to maintain the early pregnancy. The follicle may rupture causing severe lower abdominal pain and serious intra-abdominal haemorrhage in early pregnancy. This complication may mimic ectopic pregnancy. These cysts, when persistent, elaborate progesterone which sustains secretory endometrium.

Intrauterine contraceptive device with progesterone stimulation
This combination gives rise to an echogenic and thickened endometrium. However it is uncertain as to the role of each individual factor.

Haematometra
Several causes of haematometra have been described. The presence of blood in the endometrial cavity alters its echogenicity depending upon the stage of resolution of the blood or clot.

Malignant mixed müllerian tumour
This is a rare tumour but in common with other endometrial neoplasms there is enhancement of endometrial echoes.

Cervical pregnancy
The sonographic criteria for cervical pregnancy include uterine enlargement, diffuse echogenic intrauterine echoes, enlarged cervix and absent intrauterine pregnancy.

Gestational trophoblastic disease

See pp. 496–498.

Adenomyosis

This is the result of diffuse benign invasion of the myometrium by the endometrium. Characteristically there is uterine enlargement and contour anomaly with a normal central echo, although rarely the central echo complex may be prominent.

Tamoxifen therapy

Tamoxifen is widely used in the treatment of carcinoma of the breast. Several abnormalities of uterine endometrium have been described including

1. endometrium thickness is greater than 4 mm
2. the endometrium may be hypoechoic, homogeneous or hyperechoic with multiple small cysts
3. endometrial polyps with cysts within them
4. endometrial carcinoma.

Asherman's syndrome

Asherman's syndrome is an association of complete or incomplete synechiae with menstrual dysfunction and infertility. It may follow caesarean section, myomectomy, trauma, endometritis, curettage, manual removal of the placenta and septic abortion. Over 70 per cent of cases give a history of instrumentation of the endometrial cavity. Sonography reveals thickening of the endometrial cavity. Other features such as solitary or multiple endometrial filling defects, bands of tissues traversing the endometrial cavity and irregularity of the uterine cavity are much more likely to be seen on hysterosalpingography.

Differential diagnosis of prominent endometrial complex

Physiological causes – at the time of menses, normal gestation sac, decidual reaction in a contralateral bicornuate uterus, in neonates due to maternal hormonal stimulation.

Complicated pregnancy – blighted ovum and missed abortion, pseudogestational sac of ectopic pregnancy, incomplete abortion, retained products of conception

Inflammation or infection – endometriosis, endometritis, salpingitis, pelvic inflammatory disease, twisted ovarian cyst.

Haemorrhage – normal or dysfunctional, after dilatation and curettage, ruptured corpus luteum cyst.

Neoplasia – cervical carcinoma, degenerating fibroids, hydatidiform mole, choriocarcinoma, uterine sarcoma, benign cystic teratoma.

Genital tract obstruction (*Causing hydrometra, haematometra or pyometra*) – cervical obstruction whatever the cause, cervical stenosis, cervical carcinoma, endometrial carcinoma, imperforate hymen, previous cervical surgery.

Iatrogenic or traumatic – after dilatation and curettage, uterine perforation, drainage of free peritoneal fluid via the genital tract.

Echogenic foci within the uterine cavity

Intrauterine contraceptive devices
Women with an intrauterine contraceptive device who become pregnant are at a higher risk of an ectopic pregnancy. There is also a higher risk of actinomycosis.

Calcification
This is commonly associated with myomas which may appear intrauterine with the submucous variety.

Retained products of conception
Bright echoes may be demonstrated within the uterus, particularly if osseous parts are retained.

Radiation therapy implants
These may cause high-intensity echoes within the uterine cavity, that may shadow. History of the implant insertion may be obtained.

Air within the uterine cavity
This usually follows dilatation and curettage or culdocentesis.

Cerclage sutures
They may mimic an intrauterine contraceptive device, an obvious history may be obtained.

Intrauterine osseous metaplasia
This may be the result of a previous pregnancy or an inflammation.

Fluid in the cul-de-sac

Blood
Normal ovulation, ruptured ovarian cyst, ruptured ectopic pregnancy, endometriosis, trauma and postoperative causes.

Transudate

Part of generalised ascites, for example heart failure.

Exudate

Pelvic inflammatory disease, part of generalised exudative ascites, for example malignancy.

Encapsulated collections

Bowel, ovarian cyst, endometrioma, abscess, urinoma and lymphocoele.

6.2.4 UTERINE NEOPLASMS AND MASSES

Leiomyomas (fibroids)

These are common smooth muscle tumours found in 20 per cent of women over 35 years old. Classically they appear as hypoechoic, homogeneous masses. They may distort the shape of the uterus and undergo extensive cystic degeneration. Calcification presents as high-level echoes with shadowing. Fat deposition may also cause high-level echoes and may simulate uterine malignancy. Subserosal fibroids may simulate adnexal or ovarian masses. They are more common in Afro-Caribbean people.

Endometrial carcinoma

Endometrial carcinoma is the most common malignant neoplasm of the female genital tract. Over 70 per cent of endometrial carcinomas occur in individuals over the age of 50 years with a peak incidence at the age of 62 years. The prognosis is related to myometrial invasion. Sonographic diagnosis remains difficult because early lesions may be confined to the corpus (stage I) or extend into the cervix (stage II) and may not alter the uterine echopattern. The presence of a prominent endometrial echo complex greater than 4 mm in a woman with postmenopausal bleeding and irregularity or loss of the normal endometrial–myometrial junction is suggestive of this diagnosis. Endometrial thickness over 8 mm in a postmenopausal woman requires a biopsy and/or dilatation and curettage. Doppler waveforms with a resistive index less than 0.7 is said to be suggestive of malignancy. Endometrial carcinomas may obstruct the uterine cavity causing hydrometra, pyometra or haematometra. A fluid–debris level may be identified. Occasionally, spread to other organs in the pelvis may be identified on ultrasound.

Endoluminal ultrasound in endometrial carcinoma

This is performed with an intrauterine 2-mm radial 15 MHz probe. The scan range is limited to 25 mm. The scan is performed while distending the endometrial cavity with fluid. It may be useful in assessing myometrial invasion which is an important prognostic indicator.

Endometrial polyps

These may occur at all ages but are more common at menopause. Sonography may reveal discrete mass(es) within the uterine cavity, enlargement of the uterus and a prominent endometrial echo complex.

Adenomyosis

Adenomyosis characteristically affects porous women over the age of 40 years. It is related to a diffuse or focal invasion of the myometrium by nests of endometrial tissue causing uterine enlargement. The myometrial echopattern, central echo complex and uterine contour may be normal. Focal infiltration is more easily seen as poorly defined hypoechoic heterogeneous areas within the myometrium. A honeycomb or 'Swiss cheese' appearance, caused by the presence of small 1 to 3 mm myometrial cysts, is seen in 50 per cent of patients. There may be thickening of the anterior and posterior myometrial wall. Pelvic endometriosis and adenomyosis may coexist in 30 per cent of patients.

Cervical carcinoma

Cervical carcinoma is the sixth most common cause of death from cancer in women. The peak age incidence is 45 to 55 years. The majority are squamous cell carcinomas (95 per cent), adenocarcinomas make up the rest. A clear cell carcinoma occurs in women exposed to diethylstilbestrol *in utero*. The majority of cervical carcinomas are staged clinically and by MRI. The role of transabdominal ultrasound is limited in the evaluation of cervical cancer. It is used mostly to evaluate obstruction of the urinary tract in patients with advanced disease. Transvaginal and transrectal ultrasound has received attention for evaluating tumour size and local invasion. In evaluation of tumour size opinions range from enthusiastic advocates of endoluminal ultrasound to results that show that endoluminal ultrasound is no more informative than clinical examination. The main drawback of ultrasound is its poor contrast resolution and its difficulty in direct visualisation of the tumour. With large tumours ultrasound may be able to visualise gross invasion of the parametric, pelvic side wall and bladder base. Parametric invasion is seen as irregular tumour margins, vascular encasement or both. The parametrial thickening or soft tissue mass may extend to the pelvic lateral wall, encasement of the iliac vessels may be seen. Bladder base invasion may show as a contiguous tumour invasion associated with lack of mobility of the bladder wall. Concomitant benign uterine and pelvic abnormalities cannot be reliably differentiated from cervical cancer spread. Lymph node metastases are also difficult to evaluate. Sonography therefore is not the sole recommended technique for staging invasive cervical carcinoma.

Uterine sarcoma

Uterine sarcomas are rare tumours making up 3 per cent of all uterine tumours. Individuals of all ages are affected but the majority are approximately 60 years of age. Leiomyosarcomas are believed to arise from pre-existing leiomyomas. Uterine sarcomas may be indistinguishable from large leiomyomas. Commonly, large tumours present with areas of haemorrhage and/or necrosis, with bizarre areas of high-intensity echoes, invasion into the other pelvic organs may be seen as an extrauterine mass. Metastases to the liver suggest leiomyosarcoma. A malignant mixed müllerian tumour often presents as a bulky uterus with polypoid tumours filling the endometrial cavity and protruding from the cervical os.

Uterine arteriovenous malformations

Uterine arteriovenous malformations are rare. They are an even rarer cause of vaginal bleeding affecting women from 18 to 72 years of age. They can be congenital or acquired, an isolated anomaly or they can occur with arteriovenous malformations at other sites. When vaginal bleeding occurs a significant blood loss may ensue needing transfusion in 30 per cent of patients. Rarely cardiac failure can result. Acquired arteriovenous malformations can result from previous surgery, curettage, pelvic trauma, previous pregnancy, gestational trophoblastic disease, exposure to diethylstilbestrol and endometrial and cervical cancer. Sonography reveals tubular cystic structures associated with a mixed arteriovenous pattern on colour flow Doppler. Duplex Doppler reveals swirling pattern of combined arterial and venous flow in an anechoic mass. On transvaginal ultrasound enlarged asymmetric uterine radial vessels are observed in place of symmetrical vessels in size 1 to 2 mm.

6.2.5 INDICATIONS FOR INTRAOPERATIVE GYNAECOLOGIC ULTRASOUND

Sonography is performed operatively by either a transabdominal or transvaginal approach, or via a laparoscope. Intraoperative sonography may be useful in the evaluation of the following.

Difficult dilatation and curettage.
Placement of intracavity radiation applications.

Termination of pregnancy.

Removal of embedded intrauterine devices.

Asherman's disease.

Colour Doppler evaluation of a twisted ovary.

6.2.6 ENDOMETRIOSIS

Endometriosis is the presence of endometrial tissue outside the endometrial lining of the uterus. Endometrial tissue is found within the myometrium in 10 to 50 per cent of menstruating females at post mortem. In only 19 per cent of cases is the ectopic endometrium capable of undergoing cyclical bleeding. At pelvic surgery 8 to 20 per cent of women have evidence of endometriosis. Endometriosis is thus a very common condition but the majority of deposits are small and unlikely to cause symptoms, they are not detectable on sonography.

Sonography

Endometriosis may be focal or diffuse.

Focal form

Recurrent bleeding may give rise to cystic areas with variable internal echoes, which may mimic solid masses.

Irregular cystic spaces, chocolate cyst, thick-walled discrete masses with irregular borders and low-level echoes, which may give a solid or complex appearance. These may occur distant to the uterus.

Cysts may contain echogenic material because of blood.

Hypoechoic enlargement of the uterine wall.

Contour anomaly of the uterus.

Thickening of the posterior myometrium may be mistaken for fibroids.

Distortion of the endometrial cavity.

Diffuse form

The scans may appear normal as the lesions are small and scattered and are not detectable.

Multiple cysts may be detectable bilaterally.

There may be loss of definition of pelvic organs.

Differential diagnosis of endometriosis

Uterine fibroids.

Nabothian cysts – small fluid-filled spaces in the myometrium near the cervix due to retention cysts of cervical glands.

Cystic or solid ovarian tumours.
Tubo-ovarian abscesses.
Uterine tumours.
Pelvic inflammatory disease.
Ectopic pregnancy.
Haemorrhagic cysts.

6.2.7 THE FALLOPIAN TUBES

The fallopian tubes cannot be usually differentiated from other pelvic soft tissue unless affected by disease or outlined by ascites within the pelvis. Salpingography may be performed sonographically by injecting saline or one of the many commercially available galactose-based ultrasound contrast agents. This allows assessment of tubal patency without the use of ionising radiation. The pelvis is scanned as a baseline. A vaginal examination is performed and 20 millilitres of saline or ultrasonic contrast with the dose determined by the manufacturer is injected into the uterine cavity. Tubal patency is demonstrated by the accumulation of fluid or ultrasonic contrast within the pelvis.

Salpingitis

In the acute phase of a first attack of salpingitis pelvic sonography is usually normal and the diagnosis is made clinically. Local spread of infection may give rise to an abscess formation which may be demonstrable sonographically, but ultrasonic findings are more frequent in recurrent or chronic cases. There may be a non-specific appearance of loss of normal tissue planes with or without the presence of hydro- or pyosalpinx, which is seen as a fluid collection in or around the uterine tubes. Abscesses vary from very small to large complex masses. Fluid may be seen in the pelvis and the combination of fluid collections with tissue inflammation and thickening may give rise to complex masses.

6.2.8 THE VAGINA

Provided the urinary bladder is adequately filled the vagina is virtually always visible. The anterior and posterior walls are usually in apposition giving a slit-like appearance in transverse section. In longitudinal section the walls are seen as parallel hypoechoic bands separated by a central echogenic band representing the mucosa and lumen.

True absence of the vagina is rare; this clinical appearance is usually caused by labial or vaginal adhesions. Congenital vaginal obstruction may occur due to the presence of a membrane just proximal to the hymen.

Rarely a membrane may occur at the junction of the upper and middle thirds of the vagina, at the point of fusion of the müllerian duct and sinus derivatives. Vaginal obstruction by a membrane may cause haematocolpos in the newborn or haematometrocolpos in menstruating girls. Sonography may show the area of obstruction and dilatation of the proximal vagina and uterus.

6.2.9 VAGINAL MASSES

Differential diagnosis of vaginal masses

Cystic vaginal masses

Haematocolpos See p. 455.

Gartner's duct cysts These are usually proximal to the vagina in the adnexa or along the anterolateral aspect of the vaginal wall. Arising from the mesonephric duct remnants, they are the most common cystic vaginal masses. They are usually incidental findings.

Vaginal inclusion cysts These are related to the inclusion of the vaginal epithelium during surgery and usually found as cystic masses in the posterior or lateral wall of the vagina.

Mucinous cysts These are related to a developmental anomaly due to remnants of the incomplete separation of the rectum and urogenital sinus by the urachal fold.

Endometriosis Aberrant endometrial tissue rests may occur in the vagina, the most common site being in the posterior fornix. It may be entirely cystic or may appear as a complex mass. The mass may be subject to cyclical change.

Urethral diverticula See p. 386.

Ureterocoeles In about 40 per cent of ureterocoeles, the orifice opens outside the bladder, proximal or distal to the external sphincter. These cystic swellings may project into the vagina and can be recognised on sonography.

Cystocels This is a form of vaginal prolapse of the bladder and urethra. Sonography may reveal a midline cystic swelling in the vagina in communication with the bladder.

Solid vaginal masses

Foreign body A foreign body, for example a tampon (the appearance is variable), may be seen as an echogenic mass with shadowing, but when soaked with fluid the texture of the material may be discernible on ultrasound. The possibility of a foreign body should always be remembered in children who may give no history of insertion of the article which may have been present for some time.

Leiomyoma Pedunculated leiomyomas may prolapse through the cervix into the vagina and be seen as hypoechoic masses.

Leiomyoma of the urethra This has been described as a well-defined, hypoechoic mass in the region of the urethra, in relation to the anterior vagina or vulva on transvaginal sonography.

Vaginal polyp These may be single or multiple finger-like projections that are either echogenic or of low reflectivity on ultrasound.

Neoplasms True vaginal neoplasms are rare in children and uncommon in adults. Clear cell carcinoma may be associated with diethylstilbestrol exposure *in utero*. Primary and secondary tumours are usually seen as solid heterogeneous masses.

Malignant vaginal masses
Carcinoma *in situ*.
Invasive epidermoid carcinoma.
Melanoma.
Fibrosarcoma.
Leiomyosarcoma.
Sarcoma botyroides (girls under 5 years).
Endodermal sinus tumour.
Metastatic carcinoma – choriocarcinoma, cervix, endometrium, bladder, rectum.

6.2.10 INDICATIONS FOR TRANSLABIAL SONOGRAPHY

This technique can be used in small girls, virgins and in women with a narrow vagina, for the assessment of incontinence and other voiding dysfunctions. It is an excellent alternative for disorders of the lower urogenital tract, that can allow a dynamic examination. A 5 to 7 MHz transducer covered with a condom is placed on the labia minora with a small amount of gel. When a urodynamic study is required scans are also performed in a standing position before, during and after voiding. The technique has been found useful in the following conditions.

Malformations – ureterocoeles, urethral or paraurethral cysts and diverticula, Bartholin gland cyst (this may imitate irreducible hernia).
Tumours – bladder neck, recurrent metastatic ovarian tumour (peritoneal metastases), endometrioma.

Voiding disorders – partial or total bladder obstruction, stress incontinence, vesico-vaginal fistula, urethral duplication.

6.2.11 THE PREGNANT UTERUS

The possibility of pregnancy should be remembered when scanning the abdomen of any woman of child-bearing age. Demonstrating an unexpected pregnancy may prevent further investigation and avoid irradiating the foetus. Pregnancy may be demonstrated as early as 6 weeks after the first day of the last menstrual period (4 weeks after fertilisation). As the foetus develops the following structures become visible.

5.5 weeks the gestational sac is visible.

6-7 weeks the foetal node is visible.

7-8 weeks foetal heart movement becomes visible.

8-10 weeks the placenta is seen as a thickened part of the gestational ring, it is easily seen by 12 weeks.

14 weeks the kidneys are visible.

16 weeks the bladder and stomach are visible (the bladder should be visible by 18 weeks).

In early pregnancy measuring the crown–rump length dates the foetus. As the foetus flexes the accuracy of crown–rump dating decreases and the cranial biparietal diameter is used (the crown–rump length measurement is most accurate for foetal dating in the 6 to 8 week period. After 12 weeks the biparietal diameter is used.) Dating a pregnancy sonographically is important, as 15 to 30 per cent of women cannot accurately remember their last menstrual period and a further 15 per cent have irregular periods.

With a normal pregnancy the human chorionic gonadotrophin (HCG) level correlates with the gestational sac size up to a diameter of 2.5 cm. A foetal node or developing foetus should be visible in all normal sacs of 2.5 cm or greater. Lack of visualisation of a sac or embryo, or the distortion of the sac strongly suggests an abnormal pregnancy. A visible sac with a relatively low HCG level for the sac size occurs in threatened abortions.

Predictors of early failure of pregnancy

Absence of cardiac activity

Absence of cardiac activity in an embryo is a sign of pregnancy failure, however, cardiac activity is often not visualised in embryos less than 4 mm in size. If in doubt a repeat examination should be undertaken.

Yolk sac abnormalities

The absence of a yolk sac on transvaginal ultrasound, when the gestational sac diameter is 8 mm or more, is a sign of failed pregnancy. A calcified gestational sac indicates a poor prognosis. An abnormal-shaped yolk sac or lack of growth over serial scans are further indicators of pregnancy failure.

Gestational sac abnormalities

On transvaginal ultrasound the following characteristics are indicators of pregnancy failure

- mean sac diameter of greater than 8 mm without a yolk sac
- a yolk sac greater than 20 mm (mean sac diameter) without an embryo
- a distorted gestational sac
- a decidual reaction of less than 2 mm
- absence of a double decidual sign
- a weakly echogenic decidual reaction and low position of gestational sac within the uterine cavity.

Abnormalities of the amnion

A collapsed amnion or an amnion with irregular borders with no visible embryo is an indicator of pregnancy failure.

Low foetal heart rate

The normal foetal heart rate at 5 to 6 weeks is 100 beats/min rising to 140 beats/min at 8 to 9 weeks. A heart rate of 85 beats/min at 5 to 8 weeks is a poor prognostic sign.

Oligohydramnios

Oligohydramnios in the embryonic period is regarded as a poor indicator of a successful pregnancy.

Sonographic signs of pregnancy

These begin to occur 5 weeks after the first day of the last menstrual period (i.e. 3 weeks postfertilization).

A decidual reaction is seen in the endometrium with a small hypoechoic area.

A gestational scan becomes visible.

Within the next week the foetal node becomes visible within the sac.

Mimics of a gestational sac

Endometrial bleeding.

Retained products of conception.

Endometriosis.
Incomplete abortion.
Pseudogestational sac of ectopic pregnancy.
Endometrial carcinoma.
Cervical stenosis or obstruction due to carcinoma or previous surgery.

Blighted ovum or anembryonic gestation

The following are features of an anembryonic gestation

A gestational sac may be found without evidence of foetal parts at any time when they should normally be visible.
Any gestational sac greater than 2.5 cm in diameter without a foetal node is suggestive of a blighted ovum.
No embryo is seen in an identified yolk sac.
The HCG level is positive but does not show a rise with time.
A distorted gestational sac with internal echoes due to haemorrhage.
An empty sac at more than 6 to 8 weeks menstrual age.
Gestational sacs small or large for appropriate dates.
Lack of demonstrable growth of the gestational sac on serial scans.
A blighted ovum may occur in a twin pregnancy – one blighted, one normal pregnancy.

Placenta

The placenta is normally easily seen by 12 weeks of gestation. Its echogenicity is similar to that of the myometrium. By 16 weeks the placenta is the same size as the foetus. The appearance of the placenta may be graded as it matures.

Grading of placental maturity

Grade 0 – homogeneous pattern bounded by a straight line of the chorionic plate, usually less than 30 weeks gestation.
Grade 1 – echopattern becomes uneven associated with bright echoes and an undulating chorionic plate. This grading is seen at term in 40 per cent of pregnancies but can occur at any time during gestation.
Grade 2 – 'comma-shaped' bright echoes within the placenta with or without an undulating chorionic plate. This grade of placenta is rarely seen before 32 weeks gestation.
Grade 3 – there is increasing placental calcification in the intercotyledonary septa, which appear to surround echopoor areas. This grading is rarely seen before 34 weeks gestation.

Fifty per cent of placentas show calcification by 33 weeks. The mature placenta is usually up to 4 cm thick. Placentas 5 cm or greater in thickness are pathological and may be oedematous. Premature calcification is associated with smoking, hypertension and intrauterine growth retardation (IUGR). Placental grading does not appear to be clinically very useful, as grading is not precise for foetal dating or to assess foetal lung maturity. A grade 3 placenta before 34 weeks gestation is regarded as premature placental senescence and associated with hypertension and IUGR in almost 50 per cent of cases.

Placenta praevia

The blastocyst can implant in the lower uterine segment causing the siting of the placenta to cover the internal os. Stretching and thinning of the lower uterine segment during the third trimester of pregnancy may sheer off part of the placenta.

As the placenta may migrate cranially during uterine enlargement the diagnosis should only be made late in pregnancy. A posterior placenta praevia is unlikely if the distance from the foetal head to the sacrum is 2 cm or less.

Classification of types of placenta praevia

Type I – the placenta encroaches upon the lower segment but does not reach the internal os.

Type II – the placenta reaches the internal os but does not cover it.

Type III – the placenta covers the internal os before dilatation but not when the os is dilated.

Type IV – the placenta completely covers the internal os even when dilated.

Types I and II are termed as marginal and lateral in contemporary classification respectively, and minor in ultrasound classification.

Types III and IV are termed 'central' in contemporary classification and 'major' in ultrasound classification.

Patients with placenta praevia usually present with painless bleeding, women with bright-red painless vaginal bleeding are considered to have a placenta praevia until proved otherwise. Transvaginal ultrasound is the best technique available for investigating women with possible placenta praevia but, although it has a high sensitivity and specificity for central placenta praevia in the third trimester, it is less sensitive in the late second trimester or for marginal placenta praevia.

Placental infarction

Placental infarcts occur in 25 per cent of pregnancies and are secondary to disorders of maternal vessels and retroplacental haemorrhage. Placental infarction is associated with hypertension and pre-eclampsia. It is difficult to visualise unless haemorrhagic. It results in a variable-sized sonolucent collection within the placenta.

Intervillous thrombosis

Intervillous thrombosis occurs in 36 per cent of pregnancies, usually as a result of intraplacental haemorrhage. It is clinically significant, as it can be the cause of rhesus sensitisation and is a recognised cause of a raised alpha fetoprotein level. The sonographic appearances are those of sonolucent spaces within the placenta.

Abruption of the placenta

A premature separation of the placenta in the second half of pregnancy is a death threat to the foetus and a hazard to the mother. The placenta separates from its bed most probably as the result of a rupture of an ectatic vessel with resultant haematoma, causing a barrier between the placental bed and villi. Placental separation also results in the release of prostaglandins causing a major degree of uterine spasm. Besides the lack of perfusion of the placenta, a major degree of placental separation causes shock in the woman well beyond the amount of blood loss.

Sonographic appearances depend upon the degree of placental separation and the size of the haematoma. The haematoma is seen as a sonolucent or complex collection beneath the placenta. The haematoma may be mistaken for placental thickening.

Chorioangioma

These vascular malformations or placental haemangiomas occur in 1 per cent of pregnancies. They cause placental enlargement and are often an incidental finding. There is an intraplacental mass of variable size, which has a complex echopattern.

Complications of chorioangioma

Maternal – polyhydramnios, premature labour or premature rupture of membranes, placental abruption, elevated alpha fetoprotein, toxaemia of pregnancy, postpartum haemorrhage, retained placenta, dystocia.

Foetal – several foetal complications have been described including intrauterine growth retardation (IUGR), hydrops, prematurity, heart failure and haematological abnormalities.

Pelvic masses during pregnancy

Physiological masses – corpus luteum cyst, bowel loop, pelvic kidney.

Pathological masses – endometrioma, ovarian neoplastic cysts, myomas, solid ovarian tumours, non-neoplastic adnexal tumours, pelvic abscesses (tubo-ovarian, appendiceal or Crohn's).

Miscellaneous cystic masses – mesenteric cysts, enteric cysts, echinococcal cysts, peritoneal inclusion cysts, lymphocoele, hydrosalpinx.

Neurogenic masses – schwannomas.

6.2.12 GYNAECOLOGIC AND OBSTETRIC EMERGENCIES

Pelvic inflammatory disease

The severity of pelvic inflammatory disease ranges from isolated endometritis to tubo-ovarian abscesses and diffuse peritonitis. The clinical presentation can be variable and sometimes non-specific, depending upon the degree of pelvic organ involvement and the type of infective organism. Sonographic findings are again related to the severity of organ involvement. In early pelvic inflammatory disease the sonographic appearances may be entirely normal. Endometritis may be suspected with fluid in the uterine cavity, uterine enlargement and ill-defined central echo complex. The presence of air within the uterine cavity is a further clue to the presence of endometritis although this may be present normally in the post-partum uterus in up to 21 per cent of patients in the first 3 weeks. Tubo-ovarian abscesses appear as tubular folded pelvic structures. Pelvic fluid collections in the cul-de-sac may be septate. With extension of the inflammatory exudate to the ovaries a tubo-ovarian complex mass may be formed and the ovary becomes ill defined and can no longer be identified as a separate structure. Although the ultrasound features are non-specific a fairly confident diagnosis can be made when the clinical presentation is taken into account. In the absence of an appropriate history differentiation from endometrioses, pelvic neoplasm, ectopic pregnancy, adnexal torsion and haemorrhagic ovarian cyst may be difficult on ultrasound alone.

Adnexal torsion

The ultrasound findings of ovarian torsion vary with age. In neonates and young children ovarian masses appear extrapelvic (abdominal), whereas in pubertal girls the ovarian mass is adnexal. One of the most consistent findings in ovarian torsion is the increase in volume of the involved ovary to 26–441 cc (normal volume is 2.5–21.9 cc). In this unilaterally enlarged ovary peripheral cysts are found, which may be up to 2.5 cm in diameter. Other findings include a complex adnexal mass and fluid in the cul-de-sac. Doppler signals can be documented in many twisted ovaries but Doppler ultrasound features are not specific and overlap with a number of other gynaecological and non-gynaecological disorders such as pelvic inflammatory disease, ectopic pregnancy, ruptured ovarian cysts and appendicitis.

Haemorrhagic ovarian cysts

Haemorrhage within luteal and follicular cysts is not uncommon. The majority present in patients under the age of 40 years, with a sudden onset of lower abdominal pain. Haemorrhage may also occur in malignant ovarian cysts, most being serous adenomas usually in postmenopausal women. The ultrasound features depend upon the stage at which an ultrasound examination is performed after the onset of haemorrhage. Increased through transmission is present in 90 per cent of haemorrhagic cysts confirming their background cystic nature. When evaluated in the first few hours most haemorrhagic cysts are hypoechoic although most are heterogeneous. The cysts become increasingly hypoechoic with the passage of time. A fluid–debris level or a septate mass may be seen. A solid hyperechoic mass may occur because of the presence of blood clot. In the event of a cyst rupture the cyst may no longer be visible or it may be seen as a thick-walled irregular ovarian mass. Free peritoneal fluid and fluid in the cul-de-sac may be detected in the event of cyst rupture.

Massive oedema of the ovary

See p. 462.

Ovarian vein thrombosis

Ovarian vein thrombosis is an unusual post-partum complication, and is also associated with endometriosis, abortion, pelvic inflammatory disease and pelvic surgery. It is a potentially life-threatening situation with a risk of pulmonary embolism. Ultrasonically the thrombosed ovarian vein is seen as a tubular retroperitoneal hypoechoic or hyperechoic structure running from the pelvis to the inferior vena cava, parallel to the psoas muscle. The ovary may be enlarged and hypoechoic and associated hydronephrosis may be seen on the ipsilateral side caused by ureteral compression, although the degree of pelvic dilatation may be difficult to assess in the postpartum patient. Ascites may be present. The thrombus may extend into the inferior vena cava, which can be assessed by duplex and colour Doppler.

Intrapelvic haemorrhage

Haematomas should be considered in the differential diagnosis in patients with pelvic pain and fever in the postpartum period. Bladder-flap haematomas following low transverse incisions for caesarian section are seen as solid or complex masses between the uterus and posterior bladder wall. Haematomas anterior to the bladder wall may occur as a result of disruption of the inferior epigastric artery during caesarian section or traumatic vaginal delivery. These haematomas may be seen as complex or echogenic masses anterior to the bladder or posterior to the rectus sheath.

Retained products of conception

The causes of postpartum haemorrhage include uterine atony, focal genital canal laceration and retained products of conception. The value of ultrasound in the diagnosis of retained products of conception has not been defined. An endometrial thickening greater than 5 mm associated with a focal fluid collection has been associated with retained products of conception. A hyperechoic endometrial mass has been shown to have a predictive value of 90 per cent for retained products of conception. Doppler ultrasound has been shown to demonstrate low-impedence flow in the 3 days following a delivery irrespective of the uterine appearance. Low-impedence flow beyond this period may be associated with endometrial debris and endometrial thickening.

Uterine rupture

This is a rare complication of previous uterine surgery or prolonged labour. Patients with a history of previous lower uterine segment incision are more susceptible to uterine rupture during labour, whereas patients with previous high transverse uterine incision are more likely to rupture prior to delivery. The presentation may mimic placental abruption but occasionally symptoms may be minimal. The actual site of rupture may not be identified but the presence of peritoneal or extraperitoneal fluid should suggest the possibility. Occasionally the intra-abdominal contents may be sucked into the uterine cavity producing a bizarre mass. An intrauterine subchorionic haematoma adjacent to the site of a previous caesarian section scar is also said to be suggestive of a uterine rupture.

Inversion of the uterus

This is a rare complication of misplaced pressure on the uterine fundus or traction on the cord of a non-separated placenta, usually occurring in a multiparous women in whom the uterus dimples and inverts. In severe cases the fundus turns inside out and may go through the vagina. This is usually a clinical diagnosis but ultrasound may show the infolding of the uterus with a rather bizarre layered appearance of the uterus. Hydrostatic reduction can be attempted and monitored by sequential sonograms.

Ectopic pregnancy

Ectopic pregnancy accounts for 1 per cent of pregnancies. The classic triad of vaginal bleeding, abdominal pain and an adnexal mass is rarely seen. The majority of patients present with abdominal pain. Transvaginal ultrasound appears to be more sensitive at evaluating an ectopic pregnancy than trans-abdominal ultrasound. A negative ultrasound does not exclude an ectopic pregnancy.

Exclusion of an ectopic pregnancy by demonstration of an intrauterine pregnancy ultrasound demonstration of an intrauterine pregnancy makes the occurrence of an ectopic pregnancy rare (recent estimates are 1 in 4000). The incidence is higher in patients undergoing ovulation induction, and is quoted as 1 in 100 in patients undergoing *in vitro* fertilisation.

Direct demonstration of an ectopic pregnancy on transvaginal ultrasound 15 to 30 per cent of ectopic pregnancies have been shown to demonstrate an embryo in an extrauterine mass. An adnexal 'ring-like' structure in the absence of an embryo has been reported in 14 to 69 per cent of cases and is said to be specific for ectopic pregnancy.

Foetal cardiac activity foetal cardiac activity, when seen in an extra-uterine mass on transvaginal ultrasound and supported by Doppler ultrasound, is a specific sign of an ectopic pregnancy.

Haematosalpinx or complex adnexal mass a complex adnexal mass, when associated with a positive pregnancy test (β-hCG), makes up a high probability of an ectopic pregnancy.

Fluid in the cul-de-sac when associated with an adnexal mass the incidence of ectopic pregnancy rises to 70 per cent. When the quantity of fluid is moderate to large in association with an adnexal mass the incidence is even higher and a figure of 100 per cent is quoted.

Pseudogestational sac a pseudogestational sac that contains *no* embryo, may occur in 20 per cent of ectopic pregnancies. The double decidual sign is a reliable discriminator between a true and a pseudogestational sac.

Quantitative β-hCG a β-hCG level greater than 1800 IU/L in association with an empty uterus in at-risk women is highly suggestive of the presence of an ectopic pregnancy.

Endometrial thickness 0.5–1.7 cm approximately 50 per cent of patients with an ectopic pregnancy may form a decidual cast indistinguishable from normal pregnancy.

Normal sonographic findings with transabdominal ultrasound 20 per cent of patients with an ectopic pregnancy had a normal ultrasound appearance. However the accuracy has improved considerably with transvaginal ultrasound.

Doppler ultrasound in an ectopic pregnancy high-velocity low-impedence flow is the norm both in normal as well as ectopic pregnancies. Luteal flow may be confused with an ectopic pregnancy on spectral Doppler. When colour flow Doppler is used in conjunction with transvaginal ultrasound, it may be possible to separate placental flow in an adnexal mass from ovarian or uterine flow.

Spontaneous resolution of an ectopic pregnancy there is little doubt that this phenomenon occurs although its exact incidence is not known.

Risk groups for ectopic pregnancy

The incidence of ectopic pregnancy has risen from 4.5 per 1000 in 1970 to 16.8 per 1000 in 1987. All females of reproductive age are at risk.

Delayed transit of zygote – tenfold increase past tubal pregnancy, past tubal surgery, previous salpingitis (in particular *Chlamydia* spp.), infertility (shared tubal abnormality).

Infertility – ovulation induction, *in vitro* fertilisation (multiple pregnancy is a contributory factor), gamete intrafollicular transfer (hydrostatic force during transfer).

Intrauterine devices.

History of pelvic inflammatory disease.

Increasing maternal age and parity.

Differential diagnosis of ectopic pregnancy

Any adnexal mass.

All causes of fluid in the cul-de-sac.

Corpus luteum cysts with or without septa.

Ovarian torsion cyst or neoplasm.

Endometriosis.

Tubo-ovarian abscess.

Torsion of a fibroid.

Ovarian neoplasm.

Uterine leiomyoma.

Haemorrhagic subserosal fibroid.

Appendix abscess.

Diverticular abscess.

6.2.13 GESTATIONAL TROPHOBLASTIC DISEASE

Gestational trophoblastic disease is a neoplastic proliferative disorder of the trophoblast that may present in either a relatively benign form (the hydatidiform mole) or more malignant forms (an invasive mole or choriocarcinoma). The moles may also be classified into complete moles, which consist of only trophoblastic tissue, and incomplete moles containing both trophoblastic tissue and foetal parts. The trophoblastic tissue shows an abnormal chromosomal karyotype and is associated with a positive pregnancy test and a markedly raised β-hCG level. They represent less than 1 per cent of all gynaecological malignancies. The at-risk population includes women over 35 or under 20 years of age, and women who have had a previous molar pregnancy or previous spontaneous abortions.

Classification of gestational trophoblastic disease

Hydatidiform mole, molar pregnancy and complete or classic mole

Clinical presentation may be with a uterus that is too large for the dates, severe pre-eclampsia before 24 weeks gestation, first trimester vaginal bleeding, and the passage of grape-like vesicles per vagina. Rarely hyperthyroidism can occur owing to the production of thyroid-stimulating hormone-like activity by the trophoblast. Echogenic material fills the uterus, there is no foetal tissue and the mass is echogenic but does not cause a great deal of ultrasound beam attenuation. Vesicles are usually less than 1.5 cm in the first trimester but may be over 2 cm in diameter in the second trimester. Later confluent hypoechoic areas occur because of haemorrhage. Ovarian cysts are evident in 30 to 50 per cent of patients.

Complete mole with co-existent foetus

This is a rare occurrence and is usually due to molar degeneration of a dizygotic twin. The β-hCG level is markedly elevated and is not explainable on a normal pregnancy. Patients present with vaginal bleeding in the second trimester and a uterus that is large for the dates. Amniocentesis shows a normal karyotype thus eliminating a partial mole. Ultrasound shows a normal foetus and placenta associated by echogenic material, which represents a hydatidiform mole. Ovarian cysts may be apparent.

Invasive mole

Locally invasive hydatiform moles account for up to 15 per cent of cases sonographically. There is often (75 per cent) a history of a previous molar pregnancy or missed abortion. This is seen as an enlarged uterus containing a molar mass with foci of increased echogenicity extending into the myometrium. Anechoic areas may be present caused by areas of haemorrhage and necrosis, and appearances may be indistinguishable from other uterine tumours. Large ovarian cysts may be apparent.

Partial mole

This refers to a co-existent mole and foetal parts. The foetus is severely abnormal with karyotype abnormalities and often associated with IUGR. Clinically there may be early onset of pre-eclampsia. Sonographic demonstration of molar vesicles together with a well-formed foetus and a normal placenta suggest co-existent mole and foetus.

Hydropic degeneration of placenta

Hydropic degeneration is not a variant of a hydatiform mole because it involves the placenta without histologic evidence of trophoblastic proliferation. The overall appearances depend upon the extent of vesicular change, haemorrhage, necrosis and breakdown products of conception. It may be very difficult to differentiate sonographically from a partial mole.

Choriocarcinoma

Choriocarcinoma is the most malignant form of trophoblastic disease. Nearly half the cases of choriocarcinoma are preceded by molar pregnancy, whilst only 3 to 5 per cent of molar pregnancies are complicated by a choriocarcinoma. Choriocarcinoma is also associated with spontaneous abortion (25 per cent), normal pregnancy (22 per cent) and ectopic pregnancy (2.5 per cent). Clinically they present with continued vaginal bleeding and a continued elevation of the β-hCG level after expulsion of a molar pregnancy or normal delivery. Choriocarcinoma metastasises to the liver, lung, brain, bone and the gastrointestinal tract. Ultrasound reveals an echogenic mass enlarging the uterus surrounded by irregular sonolucent areas due to haemorrhage and necrosis. Liver metastases may be detected sonographically. Theca lutein cysts are seen frequently.

Placental site trophoblastic tumour

This is a rare neoplasm considered by some to be a variant of choriocarcinoma. The tumour arises from intermediate trophoblast cells within the placental bed. In the majority of patients the tumour runs a benign course, however disseminated disease may be fatal. The levels of β-hCG are low compared to those found in gestational trophoblastic disease. The tumour can be distinguished from a hydatidiform mole by the absence of chorionic villi and from a choriocarcinoma by the absence of necrosis and haemorrhage. The ultrasound appearances may mimic an invasive mole.

6.2.14 THE FOETUS

Almost any foetal anomaly which causes major structural changes can be detected by ultrasonography. It should be remembered that abnormalities might not be evident until the organ systems are fully developed. A normal ultrasound at 16 weeks cannot therefore exclude major foetal abnormalities. Also, foetal anatomy and physiology changes as the foetus develops and an apparent abnormality seen *in utero* may resolve before birth and may not be evident in the neonate.

The diagnosis of foetal abnormalities is a complex and exacting task requiring experience and expertise. Misdiagnosis of anomalies can have disastrous consequences both for the foetus and its family and thus obstetric sonography should only be undertaken by those fully trained in the field.

6.3 FURTHER READING

Arger PH: Transvaginal ultrasonography in post-menopausal patients. Radiol Clin North Am *30*:759–767, 1992.

Barloon TJ, Brown BP, Abu-Yousef MM *et al.*: Paraovarian and paratubal cysts: preoperative diagnosis using transabdominal and transvaginal sonography. J Clin Ultrasound *24*:117–122, 1996.

Bisset RAL, Khan AN, Thomas NB: Differential Diagnosis in Obstetric and Gynecologic Ultrasound, ed. JM McHugo. London, WB Saunders, 1997.

Brandt KR, Thurmond AS, McCarthy JL: Focal calcification in otherwise ultrasonographically normal ovaries. Radiology *198*:415–417, 1996.

Callen PW (ed.): Ultrasonography in Obstetrics and Gynecology, 3rd edn. Philadelphia, WB Saunders, 82–83, 1994.

Chamberlain G, Steer P: ABC of labour care: obstetric emergencies. Br Med J *318*:1342–1345, 1999.

Crade M: Ovarian cancer: detection by transvaginal ultrasound. A practical approach for clinical practice and review of literature. Ultrasound Quarterly *12*:117–126, 1994.

Dodd GD, Budzik RF: Lipomatous tumors of the pelvis in women: spectrum of imaging findings. Am J Roentgenol *155*:317–322, 1990.

Haber HP, Mayer EI: Ultrasound evaluation of uterine and ovarian size from birth to puberty. Pediatr Radiol *24*(1):11–13, 1994.

Hertzberg BS, Kliewer MA: Sonography of benign cystic teratoma of the ovary: pitfalls in diagnosis. Am J Roentgenol *167*:1127–1133, 1996.

Hricak H, Yu KK: Radiology of invasive cervical carcinoma. Am J Roentgenol *167*:1101–1108, 1996.

Hulka CA, Hall DA: Endometrial abnormalities associated with Tamoxifen therapy for breast carcinoma. Am J Roentgenol *160*:809–812, 1993.

Kurtz AB, Tsimikas JV, Tempany CMC *et al.*: Diagnosis and staging of ovarian cancer: comparative values of Doppler and conventional ultrasound, CT and MR imaging correlated with surgery and histopathologic analysis – report of the radiology diagnostic oncology group. Radiology *212*:19–27, 1999.

Lee AR, Kim KH, Lee BH *et al.*: Massive oedema of the ovary: imaging findings. Am J Roentgenol *161*:343–344, 1993.

Lin MC, Gosink BB, Wolf SI *et al.*: Endometrial thickness after menopause: effect of hormonal replacement. Radiology *180*:427–432, 1991.

Lorion JL, Paula CC, Wacquez M, Connay M: Leiomyoma of the urethra: appearances on transvaginal sonography. Am J Roentgenol *158*:694, 1992.

Martensson O, Duchek M: Translabial sonography in evaluating the lower female urogenital tract. Am J Roentgenol *166*:1327–1331, 1996.

Meilstrup JW, Kasales CJ, Van Hook DM *et al.*: Woman's health case of the day. Am J Roentgenol *162*:1457–1459, 1994.

Oram DH, Jacobs IJ, Prys-Davis MR: Early diagnosis of ovarian cancer. Br J Hosp Med *44*:320–324, 1990.

Parvey HR, Markland N: Pitfalls in transvaginal sonographic diagnosis of ectopic pregnancy. J Ultrasound Med *3*:139–144, 1993.

Quillin SP, Siegel MJ: Transabdominal color Doppler ultrasonography of the painful adolescent ovary. J Ultrasound Med *13*(7):549–555, 1994.

Rasines GL, Gutierrez MR, Abascal FA, de Diego AC: Female urethral diverticula: value of transrectal sonography. J Clin Ultrasound *24*:90–92, 1996.

Reuter KL: Critical uses of intra-operative gynecological sonography. Am J Roentgenol *169*:541–546, 1997.

Roberts CE, Athey PA: Sonographic demonstration of air in the myometrium. A complication of culdocentesis. J Ultrasound Med *11*:7–9, 1992.

Russell SA, Filly RA, Damato N: Sonographic diagnosis of ectopic pregnancy with endovaginal probes: what really has changed? J Ultrasound Med *3*:145–151, 1993.

Sanders R, Genadry R, Yarg A, Mostwin J: Imaging of the female urethra with ultrasound. Ultrasound Quarterly *12*:167–183, 1994.

Schellpfeffer MA: Sonographic detection of free pelvic fluid. J Ultrasound Med *14*:205–209, 1995.

Schiller VL, Raft E, Linde R: Uterine arteriovenous malformation. Am J Roentgenol *170*:219–220, 1998.

Schmahmann S, Haller JO: Neonatal ovarian cysts: pathogenesis, diagnosis and management. Pediatr Radiol *27*:101–105, 1997.

Sivit CJ, Nussbaum-Blask AR, Bulas DI: Pediatric pelvic sonography. Ultrasound Q *11*(1):59–93, 1993.

Sohaey R, Gardner TL, Woodward PJ, Paterson M: Sonographic diagnosis of peritoneal inclusion cysts. J Ultrasound Med *14*: 913–917, 1995.

Stadtmauer L, Grunfield L: The significance of endometrial filling defects detected on routine transvaginal sonography. J Ultrasound Med *14*:169–172, 1995.

Stark JE, Siegel MJ: Ovarian torsion in pre-pubertal and post-pubertal girls: sonographic findings. Am J Roentgenol *163*:1479–1482, 1994.

Stud H, Murala K, Kwabela M *et al.*: Preoperative assessment of myometrial invasion of endometrial cancer by MR imaging and intra-uterine ultrasonography with a high frequency probe: preliminary study. J Ultrasound Med *16*:545–548, 1997.

Tepper R, Lerner-Geva L, Altaras MM *et al.*: Transvaginal color flow imaging in the diagnosis of ovarian tumours. J Ultrasound Med *14*:731–734, 1995.

Thurmond AS: Ultrasound of infertility and uterine anomalies. Ultrasound Quarterly *13*:87–102, 1995.

Triano RN, Quedeni-Case C, Taylor KJW: Correlation of findings on transvaginal sonography with serum CA 125 levels. Am J Roentgenol *168*:1587–1590, 1997.

Varner RE, Sparks JM, Cameron CD *et al.*: Transvaginal sonography of the endometrium in post-menopausal women. Obstet Gynecol *78*:195–199, 1991.

Volpi E, De Grandis T, Zuccaro G *et al.*: Role of transvaginal sonography in the detection of endometriomata. J Clin Ultrasound *23*:163–167, 1995.

Ward HR: O'Sullivan's hydrostatic reduction of an inverted uterus: sonar sequence recorded. Ultrasound Obstet Gynecol *12*(4):283–286, 1998.

Wolman I, Sagi J, Ginat S *et al.*: The sensitivity and specificity of vaginal sonography in detecting endometrial abnormalities in women with postmenopausal bleeding. J Clin Ultrasound *24*:79–82, 1996.

Yacoe ME, Brooke J: Degenerated uterine leiomyoma mimicking acute appendicitis: sonographic diagnosis. J Clin Ultrasound *23*:473–475, 1995.

Yamashita Y, Torashima M, Hatanaka Y *et al.*: Adnexal masses: accuracy of characterization with transvaginal ultrasound and precontrast and postcontrast MR. Radiology *194*(2):557–565, 1995.

7

Abdominal wall, peritoneum, retroperitoneum and miscellaneous gamuts

7.1.1 THE SKIN

High-frequency sonography of the skin provides a simple and non-invasive method for confirming certain dermatological diseases and its relationship to underlying subcutaneous fat and muscle.

Normal appearances of the skin include the following.

1. The epidermis is a strongly echogenic layer 1–3 mm thick. Using 25 MHz and 40 MHz ultrasonic sector probes the malpighian layer of the epidermis can be demonstrated as an echolucent zone under the strongly echogenic, linear corneomalpighian junction. With this technique longitudinal sections of hair follicles and hypertrophic sebaceous glands can also be demonstrated as echolucent structures.
2. The dermis is a homogeneous zone less echogenic than the epidermis and approximately 3.3 mm thick.
3. Subcutaneous fat, connective tissue and subcutaneous fat lie deep to the dermis. Though fat attenuates the ultrasound beam, the degree of attenuation can differ quite remarkably between different patients. Also despite this marked attenuation the fat may appear hypoechoic relative to the skin.

Determination of skin thickness

Ultrasonic skin thickness measurement accuracy compares fairly well with more established methods. Skin thickness measurements can be made using high-resolution real time probes or a pulsed ultrasound technique. Skin thickness may be increased in acromegaly and scleroderma amongst other conditions. A mean dermal thickness of 7.7 mm has been found in patients with scleroderma compared to 3.3 mm in a normal control group, ultrasonic evaluation of skin thickness may be of value in following the natural history of scleroderma or response to treatment. Skin thickness is reduced in osteoporosis, Cushing's syndrome and with ageing, though there is a wide range of appearances.

Necrotising fasciitis

Necrotising fasciitis is one of the most serious infections known to humans. A highly aggressive inoculum of bacteria causes rapid destruction of skin and fascia. It has a high mortality and morbidity because diagnosis is often delayed. The emergence of toxic shock strains of *Streptococcus* spp. leading to fasciitis with organ dysfunction make a rapid diagnosis necessary for the early institution of antibiotic therapy and surgical intervention. Necrotising fasciitis may follow trauma, surgery and abdominal perforations or it may appear *de novo*. Most infections have been reported in and around the neck and limbs, but any part of the body including the abdominal wall and retroperitoneum may be involved. Because the skin is initially spared, early recognition prior to extensive tissue destruction is difficult. Early diagnosis has been achieved using ultrasonography.

Sonographic signs of necrotising fasciitis
Irregularity of fascia.
Abnormal fluid collections along the fascia plane.
Diffuse, distorted thickening of the fascia when compared with the normal opposite side.
Well-defined loculated abscesses may be found.
Ultrasonography can be used to guide aspiration of pus for culture and sensitivity.
In severe infective cellulitis the above findings are not found.

Subcutaneous masses

Ultrasonography provides immediate characterisation of mass size, consistency and anatomical location. It may be the only diagnostic modality required for diagnosing lesions such as cysts and foreign bodies and for characterising fatty, fibrous, cartilaginous, vascular and lymphatic tissue.

AIDS-related subcutaneous masses
Subcutaneous and soft tissue involvement such as pyomyositis, Kaposi's sarcoma and lymphoma is frequent in AIDS patients. Lymph nodes may be

seen in the inguinal regions that are usually hypoechoic and homogeneous with no necrotic centre. These appearances are similar to the lymphoma pattern in non-AIDS patients. Ultrasound-guided aspiration and subsequent histology (lymphoma) and bacteriological examination (pyomyositis) can establish the diagnosis.

Colour flow Doppler in cutaneous and subcutaneous masses

Colour flow Doppler may differentiate between malignant and benign lesions in some instances. Over 90 per cent of malignant lesions show either a hypervascular lesion with multiple peripheral poles or a hypervascular lesion with internal vessels. Benign lesions show an avascular lesion in over 86 per cent of cases. However a peripheral type of blood flow is recorded with abscesses or lymphadenitis. Subcutaneous metastasis may occur from primary sites from a melanoma, colon and lung amongst other sites. Most of these lesions are solid homogeneous and hypoechoic masses; diagnosis is usually achieved by a fine needle aspiration biopsy.

Abdominal wall endometrioma

Endometriosis can occasionally involve the abdominal wall. Usually the symptoms of focal pain associated with menses may be a give away. Sonography may show a cystic or polycystic abdominal wall lesion with septae or minimal debris. Complex solid or cystic lesions may occur, or the endometrioma may be solid with scattered internal echoes. A fine needle aspiration may be sufficient to diagnose the lesion when taken in conjunction with the history.

Abdominal wall haemangioma

Haemangiomas of the abdominal wall present as heterogeneous echoic masses with anechoic spaces, some may, however, appear solid. Hyperechoic foci of calcifications or phleboliths may be detected. Colour flow Doppler may demonstrate flow within the haemangioma.

Adhesion-related abdominal wall varices

Adhesion-related abdominal wall varices may occur in patients with portal hypertension who have undergone laparotomy. These are seen as serpiginous anechoic tubes in or under the abdominal wall. Colour flow Doppler demonstrates flow within the tubes.

Differential diagnosis of solid abdominal wall masses

Abscess.
Haematoma.
Hernia.
Sebaceous cyst.

Lipoma.
Haemangioma.
Endometrioma.
Malignancy – lymphoma, sarcoma, metastases.

Differential diagnosis of cystic abdominal wall masses
Abscess.
Haematoma.
Pyomyositis – abscesses.
Necrotising fasciitis – abscesses.
Abdominal wall varices.
Hernia with ascitic fluid.
Meningocoeles.
CSF leak – lumbar puncture, surgery.

Abdominal wall calcification
Skin – papilloma, neurofibroma, melanoma, naevi, scar, stoma, tattoo.
Soft tissues – idiopathic calcinosis, hypercalcaemic states.
Muscles – cysticercosis, Guinea worm, myositis ossificans.
Injection sites – quinine, bismuth, procaine benzylpenicillin (procaine penicillin), calcium gluconate.
Nodal calcification.
Vein calcification.
Arterial calcification.

7.1.2 THE RECTUS SHEATH

The rectus muscles are easily identified in the anterior abdominal wall. They are enclosed in a fibrotic sheath, which may trap blood if the abdominal wall is injured thus forming a haematoma. Rectus sheath haematoma is uncommon and frequently misdiagnosed as clinically it may mimic any acute abdominal emergency. A varied pathology may be seen as haematomas present in both the upper and lower abdomen. The single most important factor in the diagnosis of rectus sheath haematoma is to be aware of its existence. All age groups may be affected. Haematomas are frequently associated with an underlying abnormality that predisposes to haemorrhage, for example anticoagulation. Spontaneous haemorrhage may occur in pregnancy, in muscular men and in elderly ladies. Most cases present with acute abdominal pain. The cause is most often due to rupture of the inferior epigastric vessels. The haematoma is usually seen as a spindle-shaped or round hypoechoic mass localised to the rectus sheath, although initially the haematoma may be echofree. It is one of the few causes of a cystic mass anterior to the bladder, although as the blood clots the haematoma may rapidly become echogenic or complex.

Differential diagnosis of rectus sheath haematoma

Abscess.
Urachal cyst.
Bladder diverticulum.
Lymphocoele.
Lymphangiomatous cyst.
Necrotic tumour.
Mesenteric or omental cyst.
Enteric duplication.
Exophytic hepatic cyst.
Pancreatic pseudocyst.
Ovarian cyst.

7.1.3 ABDOMINAL WALL HERNIAS

These include inguinal, femoral, umbilical, incisional and spigelian hernias. They usually are diagnosed from the history and clinical examination and normally do not need imaging. One exception is the spigelian hernia where there is an inherent defect in the linea semilunaris, that may pose problems with diagnosis. The hernial sac invaginates between the external oblique and internal oblique or transversus muscles. Because of the intact overlying muscle the herniation may be masked clinically. With high-resolution sonography each muscle of the anterior abdominal wall can be distinguished and the hernia may be identified. With other hernias discontinuity of the fascia with protruding hernial contents may be demonstrated.

7.1.4 THE DIAPHRAGM

The diaphragm is seen as a curved echogenic sheet. The inferior vena cava, oesophagus and aorta at the levels of the 8th, 10th and 12th thoracic vertebral bodies traverse it respectively. The diaphragmatic crura may be seen as slightly sonolucent curvilinear structures anterior to and on either side of the abdominal aorta.

Diaphragmatic movement

To assess diaphragmatic movements the patient is scanned in the supine position. A fixed intercostal position is chosen symmetrically in the midaxillary line to achieve an acceptable view of the diaphragm in full expiration and inspiration. This scanning position should include the maximal renal length. The part of the diaphragm adjacent to the midpoint of the upper kidney is marked both in expiration and inspiration. The excursion of the diaphragmatic movement is measured between these two points and expressed in centimetres. An average of three movements in quiet respiration and maximal excursion should be taken. The right to left ratio of maximum excursion is noted and compared to the normal range of 0.5–1.6. Measurements outside this range are regarded as abnormal.

Impaired diaphragmatic movement

Paralysis.
Pulmonary over-inflation.
Pleural effusion.
Empyema.
Pulmonary inflammation – embolus or infection.
Diaphragmatic hernia or eventration.
Subphrenic abscess.
Abdominal pain.
Peritonism.
Hepatosplenomegaly.
Ascites.

Abnormalities of diaphragmatic position and contour

Polyarcuation
Polyarcuation or scalloped diaphragm is due to hypertrophic muscle bundles, usually seen during deep inspiration or emphysema.

Focal eventration
Localised eventration of the diaphragm because of incomplete musculature seen as focal diaphragmatic bulges is common. These bulges may mimic diaphragmatic hernias or masses above or below the diaphragm. The diaphragm is usually clearly visualised by ultrasound with the liver tissue extending into the bulges on the right-hand side. Localised paradoxical movement may be confirmed on sonography.

Subpulmonic effusion
A basal or subpulmonic pleural effusion with no meniscus sign may mimic an elevated diaphragm on a chest radiograph. Sonography readily confirms the cause as a basal effusion which may appear free or loculated.

Diaphragmatic hernia

Herniation through the diaphragm may be congenital or acquired. Sonography may reveal herniation of abdominal viscera into the thorax through a diaphragmatic defect. Depending upon the type of hernia (i.e. Bochdalek's, Morgagni or traumatic) the herniated organs may include liver, kidney, omentum or bowel. All these structures may be recognisable on sonography. Hiatus hernias may be difficult to see unless outlined by fluid. In case of doubt examining the abdomen while the patient is drinking may demonstrate the anatomy of the distal oesophagus. In traumatic hernias when the diaphragm has ruptured, bowel loops may be identified passing upwards into the thorax although gas within the bowel loops may obscure the diaphragm. If pleural effusion is also present then bowel loops may be identified on both sides of the diaphragm. Peristalsis within the thorax may confirm herniation of bowel loops.

Masses above the diaphragm

These include pulmonary and pleural neoplasms and cysts (hydatid) in close proximity or in contact with the diaphragm that may usually be characterised by ultrasound.

Masses within the diaphragm

These include diaphragmatic tumours such as mesothelioma, fibroma, lipoma, lymphoma and metastases. Sonography cannot usually differentiate between various diaphragmatic tumours although it is possible to characterise a lipoma that is echogenic and may shadow.

Rotation of the diaphragmatic echo

Hepatic cysts may cause displacement of diaphragmatic echo behind the cyst. This is an artefact caused by the differences in acoustic velocity between the cyst fluid and normal solid hepatic tissue. Such artefacts have been described in 58 per cent of all liver tumours, the most common is a counter-clockwise rotation that occurs in 58 per cent of hepatic haemangiomas and a clockwise rotation described in 43 per cent of liver metastases. Recognition of the artefact may be a clue to the underlying liver pathology.

Masses below the diaphragm

These masses may cause the elevation of the whole leaf of the diaphragm or they may cause a localised hump

- liver neoplasms – primary or metastatic
- liver abscess
- hydatid cysts
- benign liver cystic disease.

Fluid collections below the diaphragm

These collections usually cause elevation of the whole leaf of the diaphragm

- ascites
- subphrenic abscess
- pyonephrosis.

Differential diagnosis of disruption of diaphragmatic echoes

Invading bronchial neoplasm.
Invading fibrosarcoma.
Ovarian metastases to the diaphragm.
Aspiration of amoebic debris via thoracentesis.
Diaphragmatic laceration.
Diaphragmatic rupture.
Rupture of liver or splenic abscess through the diaphragm.
Invasion or organisation by adjacent abscess or empyema.

Differential diagnosis of juxta-diaphragmatic masses

Diaphragmatic tumours are rare but juxta-diaphragmatic masses are more common. A chest radiograph is usually sufficient for diagnosis of these masses but ultrasound is the next investigation of choice. There are a variety of juxta-diaphragmatic masses including the following.

Pleuropericardial cyst.
Pericardial pad of fat.
Foregut duplication.
Aortic aneurysm.
Hiatus hernia.
Pulmonary cyst, fluid-filled bulla, abscess, hydatid cyst, sequestration.
Subphrenic abscess.
Hepatic abscess, neoplasm, cyst, hydatid cyst.
Fluid collections – loculated ascites
Hydronephrosis.
Herniated kidney, liver.

7.1.5 SUBPHRENIC ABSCESS

Appendicitis, perforated peptic ulcer or diverticulum, pelvic inflammatory disease and surgery are the commonest causes of intraperitoneal abscesses. The abscess usually forms in a dependent part of the peritoneal cavity such as subphrenic and subhepatic spaces and the pelvis. In the upper abdomen abscesses occur more frequently in the right subphrenic space than in the left. They are seen as fluid collections or complex masses above the liver or spleen closely following the superior contour of these organs. Abscesses may contain debris or even gas giving an echogenic appearance. At times it may be impossible to reliably differentiate a subphrenic abscess from a hepatic abscess. Right-sided subphrenic collections may be divided into anterior and posterior collections by the right triangular ligament but these spaces are continuous laterally.

7.1.6 ABDOMINAL MASSES IN CHILDREN

Differential diagnosis of intra-abdominal cysts in childhood

Omental cyst – greater omentum.
Mesenteric cyst.
Hepatic cyst.
Choledochal cyst.
Renal cyst.
Adrenal cyst.
Meckel's diverticulum.
Enteric duplication cyst.
Intramural bowel tumour.
Pancreatic cyst.
Ovarian cyst.
Pancreatic pseudocyst.
Cystic renal tumour.
Abscess.
Mesenteric lymphoma.
Lymphangioma.

Giant cystic abdominal masses in children

Right upper quadrant – hydronephrosis, gallbladder hydrops, cystic hepatic neoplasm, enteric duplication, polycystic liver.
Left upper quadrant – epidermoid cyst of the spleen, hydronephrosis, enteric duplication.
Mid-abdomen and epigastrium – mesenteric cyst, pancreatic pseudocyst.
Lower abdomen and pelvis – urachal cyst, mesenteric cyst, enteric duplication cyst, serous or mucinous cystadenoma of the ovary.

Upper abdominal masses in children

Echogenic – Wilms' tumour, infantile polycystic renal disease, neuroblastoma, hepatoblastoma, hepatocellular carcinoma.

Echogenic with hypoechoic areas – Wilms' tumour, mesoblastic nephroma, hepatoblastoma, neuroblastoma.

Hypoechoic with echogenic areas – hepatic hamartoma, hepatic adenoma, lymphoma, cystic neuroblastoma, cavernous haemangioblastoma, teratoma, metastases (for example testicular embryonal cell carcinoma), haematoma.

Anechoic – abscess, choledochal cyst, benign cystic hepatoblastoma, lymphoma, urinoma, haematoma.

Neonatal abdominal masses

Renal (55 per cent) – hydronephrosis 25 per cent (for example urethral valves, pelviureteric junction obstruction, ureterocoele), multicystic kidney 15 per cent, infantile polycystic disease, renal vein thrombosis, renal ectopia, Wilm's tumour, mesoblastic nephroma.

Genital (15 per cent) – ovarian cyst, hydro- and haemometrocolpos.

Gastrointestinal – bowel duplication, mesenteric cyst.

Retroperitoneal (non-renal) – adrenal haemorrhage, neuroblastoma, teratoma.

Hepatic, splenic and biliary – hepatoblastoma, hepatic cyst, splenic haematoma, choledochal cyst.

Sonographic appearances of pelvic masses in female children

Cystic adnexal masses – ovarian cyst, teratoma, cystadenoma, cystadenofibroma, hydrosalpinx.

Complex adnexal masses – ovarian cyst, teratoma, tubo-ovarian abscess, haemorrhagic cyst, dysgerminoma.

Solid adnexal masses – haemorrhagic cyst, ovarian torsion, teratoma, dysgerminoma.

Uterine and vaginal masses – pregnancy, hydrometrocolpos, hydatidiform mole, rhabdomyosarcoma.

Non-gynaecological masses – abscess, bowel duplication, ureteral stump, sacrococcygeal teratoma, haematoma, neuroblastoma, distended bowel (for example Hirschsprung's disease), distended bladder, extramedullary haemopoiesis, sacrococcygeal chordoma, ectopic kidney, meconium pseudocyst, cloacal dysgenesis.

7.1.7 COMPLEX CYSTIC MASSES IN THE LOWER ABDOMEN IN ADULTS

A complex cystic mass may have either a cystic appearance with internal septae or debris, or both solid and cystic elements.

Ovarian masses – simple cyst, cystadenoma and cystadenocarcinoma, haemorrhagic cyst, polycystic ovary.

Infection – pyogenic abscess, tuberculous psoas abscess, hydatid cyst.

Haematoma – bowel (intramural), mesentery, rectus sheath, retroperitoneal (trauma, anticoagulants).

Renal masses – ectopic and ptotic kidney, hydronephrosis, polycystic kidney, necrotic tumour, dilated tortuous ureter, ureterocoele.

Bowel masses – adjacent loops of fluid-filled small bowel, inflammatory bowel mass, duplication cyst.

Mesentery – benign mesenteric cyst, cystic mesenteric tumour, cystic lymphangioma of mesentery.

Peritoneum – loculated ascites, inclusion cyst, cystic mesothelioma, pseudomyxoma peritonei, chylous cyst, ventriculoperitoneal pseudocyst.

Retroperitoneum – benign peritoneal cyst, lymphangioma, necrotic retroperitoneal tumour (sarcoma), post-traumatic uriniferous pseudocyst, lymphocoele.

Uterine masses – necrotic endometrial carcinoma, uterine leiomyosarcoma, hydro- and pyosalpinx, haemato- and pyometra.

Adnexal masses – ectopic pregnancy, cystic teratoma or dermoid, endometrioma.

Bladder dome masses – urachal cyst, urachal tumour, bladder diverticulum with tumour, bladder rupture.

Incarcerated Spigelian hernia.

Any large upper abdominal mass extending to the pelvis, for example gastric leiomyosarcoma.

7.2 PERITONEUM

The peritoneum is a thin serous membrane lining the abdominal cavity. It has parietal and visceral layers, the latter being reflected over the abdominal viscera. A thin layer of serous fluid, which acts as a lubricant, separates the two layers. Several intra-abdominal organs are invaginated by visceral peritoneum to such an extent that they are almost completely covered by peritoneum and carry double layers of peritoneum with them as mesenteries and ligaments.

7.2.1 FALCIFORM LIGAMENT

This is a double layer of peritoneum that forms anteriorly near the midline between the umbilicus and oesophagus. It passes backwards and splits to enclose the liver. Superiorly peritoneal layers form the triangular and coronary ligaments, which enclose the bare area of the liver. The layers of peritoneum investing the liver unite on its visceral surface to form the lesser omentum, which passes from the liver to the oesophagus, stomach and the first part of the duodenum. The free edge of the lesser omentum between the porta hepatis and duodenum contains the portal vein with the hepatic artery and common bile duct lying anteromedial and anterolateral respectively. The layers of the lesser omentum split to enclose the stomach and then reunite to form the greater omentum and gastrosplenic and lienorenal ligaments.

7.2.2 ABNORMAL INTRA-ABDOMINAL GAS

Abnormal abdominal gas collections are subdivided by anatomical location which is often the key to the differential diagnosis.

Extraluminal gas: pneumoperitoneum

This results from a perforated abdominal viscus, through the female genital tract or an extension of mediastinal gas from a hyperbaric injury, and is gas within an abscess or fistulous tract. In the appropriate clinical setting gas bubbles within a complex fluid collection suggest an abscess. Gas within a pelvic abscess usually means the abscess is of gastrointestinal origin. Gas within an abscess of pelvic inflammatory disease is unusual. Gas within the paracolic gutter is usually associated with gastrointestinal perforation. Diverticulitis may produce extraluminal gas trapped within the adjacent mesentery.

Intraluminal gas

This may be normal or abnormal. Abnormal intraluminal gas includes intra-tumoural (within a neoplasm with infection or bowel communication), intramural, gas within a paralysed loop of bowel, gas within an obstructed Meckel's diverticulum (secondary infection) or gas within the biliary tree. Normal intraluminal gas can be differentiated by the presence of gas within the bowel lumen associated with visible peristalsis.

Intraparenchymal gas

Intraparenchymal gas may sometimes be seen within the portal vein as gas microbubbles moving through the liver on real time sonography. Gas may be seen in a liver abscess. Differential diagnosis between liver micro-abscesses and microcalcification may be difficult on sonography. In most other organs intraparenchymal gas usually indicates an abscess.

Intratumoural gas

This typically occurs in a gastric leiomyoma or leiomyosarcoma where gas may be seen extending from the lumen of the stomach into the tumour. Intratumoural gas may also be seen in hepatic tumours following chemo-embolisation where differentiation from an abscess may be difficult on imaging alone.

Intramural gas

This may be related to ischaemia or infection. The distinct ultrasound features include high amplitude echoes that do not change with patient position or with peristalsis, there is often adjacent bowel wall thickening. Crohn's disease and cytomegalovirus are less common causes of intramural bowel gas. Pneumatosis coli is often better shown with CT. Acute emphysematous cholecystitis which often occurs in diabetic and elderly patients shows ultrasound evidence of intramural gas. Confusion may occur with mural calcification which is often curvilinear but which does not have the characteristic ring-down artefact associated with air bubbles. Adenomyosis of the gallbladder may also cause a comet-tail artefact.

Ultrasonic detection of intra-abdominal gas

Total sound reflection at interface of soft tissue and air.

Reverberation of ultrasound between gas and the transducer.

High-amplitude linear echoes with distal artefactual reverberation echoes which may be periodic.

The reverberation echoes are 'dirty' as compared to clear shadowing from calculi.

Small reverberation artefacts have a characteristic comet-tail appearance.

Small gas collections may show little or no distal reverberation artefacts with standard abdominal transducers (3.5–5.0 MHz).

At times the small gas bubbles are difficult to differentiate from microabscesses or microcalcification.

Location of the gas collection is often the key to the differential diagnosis.

Pneumoperitoneum is best seen on ultrasound around the perihepatic space in the supine or lateral decubitus position.

Gas collection in the paracolic gutter is usually due to gastrointestinal perforation.

Gas in a fistulous tract is usually due to Crohn's disease.

Gas within a pelvic abscess is usually of gastrointestinal origin; gas is unusual in pelvic inflammatory disease.

Diverticulitis may produce extraluminal gas trapped within the adjacent mesentery.

Portal venous gas may be seen as discrete gas bubbles moving with the blood stream towards the periphery of the liver.

Apart from the liver gas within other organs is usually secondary to an abscess.

Normal intra-abdominal gas is intraluminal, with surrounding bowel usually seen and associated with bowel peristaltic movements.

Mimics of pneumoperitoneum

Shadowing from a rib.

Ring-down artefacts from adjacent air-filled lung.

Colonic gas anterior to the liver–colonic interposition.

Mimics of acute emphysematous cholecystitis

Mural calcification.

Porcelain gallbladder.

Adenomyosis.

7.2.3 ASCITES

Ascitic fluid is seen as echofree fluid between the bowel loops. With small volumes the location of the fluid is very dependent upon the patient's position. In these cases the fluid tends to gravitate into the pelvis or paracolic gutters. Traces of fluid may frequently be seen in the flanks, around the liver and between the liver and right kidney. With larger volumes of fluid the bowel loops float rising to the centre of the abdomen which is obscured by bowel gas. Pseudomyxoma peritoneii may give a similar appearance but may encase the bowel or lie anterior to the bowel, which does not float in the fluid to the same extent as with ascites. The presence of debris within ascites is suggestive of tuberculosis or haemoperitoneum. Septations may occur in chronic pyogenic peritonitis, pseudomyxoma peritoneii or peritoneal–atrial shunt whilst mottled or thick-walled bowel loops suggest malignancy or bowel inflammation.

Aetiology of intra-abdominal fluid collections

Transudate   cardiac failure, hypoalbuminaemia, hypoproteinaemia, inferior vena cava obstruction, portal hypertension and cirrhosis.

Exudate   peritoneal inflammation (tuberculous peritonitis), peritoneal malignancy, polyserositis, pancreatitis and Meigs' syndrome.

Urine   due to intraperitoneal rupture of the urinary tract. In the neonate urinary ascites may be related to upper urinary tract rupture because of pelviureteric junction obstruction or obstruction of the lower urinary tract, i.e. urethral valves.

Chylous ascites secondary to congenital or acquired lymphatic obstruction though slight chylous ascites is not uncommon in neonates. Acquired chylous ascites may be secondary to lymphatic obstruction that may complicate malignancy, trauma, radiotherapy and filariasis.

Blood due to trauma, penetrating injury, hepatic and splenic laceration or spontaneous rupture of an intra-abdominal structure such as an ovarian cyst, hydrometrocolpos.

Cerebrospinal fluid location of cerebrospinal fluid around a shunt usually occurs in the presence of peritoneal adhesions which reduce the peritoneal surface available for resorption. The ventriculoperitoneal shunt tubing may be identified within the collection.

Meconium peritonitis this is a chemical peritonitis caused by a foetal meconium leak from the bowel into the peritoneum. Inflammation may block the bowel leak thus evidence of previous meconium peritonitis may be the only sign of an earlier bowel abnormality. Other causes of meconium peritonitis such as bowel atresia or stenosis may also be evident. The peritoneal meconium calcifies giving rise to a curvilinear and irregular appearance. Detection *in utero* may be associated with polyhydramnios, ascites and bowel abnormalities. A 'snow-storm' appearance has been recorded because of the presence of multiple fine calcified particles floating in the ascitic fluid. These abnormalities may persist after birth giving rise to abdominal cysts and calcifications.

Causes of neonatal ascites

Haemolytic disease – hydrops foetalis.
Bowel perforation – meconium ileus.
Obstructive uropathy – urinary tract rupture.
Cardiovascular disease.
Chylous ascites – inflammatory, traumatic, neoplastic or idiopathic.
Intrauterine infection – congenital syphilis.
Ruptured intra-abdominal or pelvic cyst.
Bile peritonitis.
Portal venous obstruction, cirrhosis or biliary atresia.

Causes of echogenic ascites

Pseudomyxoma peritonei.
Meconium peritonitis.
Tuberculous peritonitis.
Peritoneal haemorrhage.

Pyogenic peritonitis.
Peritoneal carcinomatosis.

7.2.4 PERITONEAL CARCINOMATOSIS

Peritoneal metastases may arise from any primary site but they occur more commonly as a result of gastrointestinal tract, kidney, pancreas, breast and pelvic organ malignancy. When visible the peritoneum is seen as the peritoneal line, which comprises both the peritoneum and the deep abdominal fascia. This is most clearly demonstrated by scanning with a high-frequency probe. When extraperitoneal fat is abundant the peritoneum and fascia are seen as two separate lines. Peritoneal metastases may present as follows.

1. Ascites, with or without debris, with peritoneal metastases projecting as polypoid masses into the ascitic fluid. The masses may be nodular, sheet-like or irregular (Figure 7.1)
2. Omental involvement, this is frequent and is easily seen because of its superficial location when not obscured by bowel gas or rib cage. The omentum is often fixed to the bowel posteriorly and to the peritoneum anteriorly. Three patterns of involvement have been described:
   - nodular   single or multiple nodules with varying echogenicity
   - pancake   these have an irregular, lobular contour and are often hyperechoic
   - interstitial   these present as firm omental bands seen as nodular structures with subtle irregularity in the presence of ascites, they may indent the anterior peritoneum when compressed.
3. Mesenteric involvement, the fat between mesenteric vessels or bowel loops becomes heterogeneous, firm, fixed and nodular.
4. Interruption of the anterior hyperechoic peritoneal line, irrespective of the presence or absence of ascites.
5. Masses between bowel loops.
6. Bowel fixation, firm pressure with a transducer fails to displace bowel loops.
7. Extensive adhesions may obliterate part of the peritoneal cavity.
8. Gallbladder wall thickening greater than 3 mm.
9. Liver metastases are often associated with peritoneal metastases.
10. The primary site may be detectable on ultrasound.

Differential diagnosis of peritoneal metastases

Peritoneal mesothelioma.
Sclerosing peritonitis.

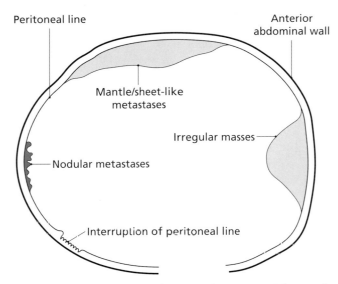

Figure 7.1 Sonographic appearances of peritoneal metastases. When small, peritoneal metastases are difficult to identify and are easily missed. The presence of ascites makes it easier to visualise small metastatic deposits which may show the pattern in this figure.

All causes of echogenic ascites.
Pseudomyxoma peritoneii.

7.2.5 PERITONEAL MASSES

Solid – mesothelioma, metastases, sclerosing peritonitis.
Infiltrative – mesothelioma.
Cystic – cystic mesothelioma (benign), pseudomyxoma peritoneii, pyogenic and tuberculous peritonitis, peritoneal inclusion cyst.

Sclerosing peritonitis

This is one of the most serious complications of ambulatory peritoneal dialysis that carries a high mortality. The peritoneum often encapsulates the small bowel. Sclerosing peritonitis should be suspected in patients being treated with ambulatory peritoneal dialysis, who present with increasing abdominal pain and progressive loss of ultrafiltration. Sonography shows increased peristalsis associated with fixation or tethering of the bowel to the posterior abdominal wall, intraperitoneal echogenic strands and, in the late stages, membrane formation. The bowel loops may be dilated; this may be seen on ultrasound when fluid filled.

Peritoneal mesothelioma

This is a rare primary neoplasm of the peritoneum originating in the mesothelial cells. There is a known association with asbestos exposure. The prognosis is poor as cases present late with few surviving over a year. There is thickening of the peritoneum, mesentery, omentum and bowel wall. Nodular or cake-like masses may be seen arising from the anterior peritoneum usually associated with a streak of ascites. Occasionally areas of calcification may be detected.

Cystic peritoneal mesothelioma

This is a rare primary benign peritoneal neoplasm, which has a tendency to recur in 27–50 per cent of cases. The tumour has no known association with asbestos exposure. The tumour most often affects the omentum or pelvic peritoneum where, because of its cystic nature, it may be difficult to differentiate from a lymphangioma or ovarian cystic neoplasm. The tumour may present as a thin-walled multiloculated cystic mass arising from the omentum or pelvic peritoneum.

Peritoneal inclusion cysts

These cysts develop because of impaired peritoneal fluid drainage as a result of extensive pelvic adhesions that are usually secondary to previous pelvic surgery. The most common presentation is with pelvic pain. An ovary surrounded by septations and fluid is the most common ultrasound appearance with low resistive flow in the septations on Doppler ultrasound. The diagnosis is important because it should encourage the use of more conservative therapy.

7.2.6 THE OMENTAL BURSA (LESSER SAC)

The lesser sac is a peritoneal recess lying behind the stomach. It communicates with the peritoneal cavity via the foramen of Winslow and is bound anteriorly by the liver, lesser omentum, stomach and greater omentum from above downwards. The posterior abdominal wall, duodenum, inferior vena cava and pancreas lie posteriorly. The lesser sac may be visualised when distended by pathological fluid collections such as loculated ascites or a pancreatic pseudocyst.

Omental masses

Solid masses

Benign – leiomyoma, lipoma, neurofibroma, dermoid (teratoma), endometriosis of omentum, myofibromatosis, torsion of the omentum.

Malignant – metastases, primary carcinoma, leiomyosarcoma, liposarcoma, haemangiopericytoma, fibrosarcoma, lymphoma, mesothelioma, leiomyoblastoma.

Cystic masses

Haematoma.
Cystic teratoma.
Lymphangioma.
Cystic mesothelioma.
Hydatid cyst.

Torsion of the omentum

This is a spontaneous occurrence of unknown aetiology although torsion has been reported with omental tumours. Presentation is with acute abdominal pain and leucocytosis. Differentiation from other causes of an acute abdomen may be difficult on clinical grounds and diagnosis is usually made at laparotomy. Ultrasound findings have been described in a few cases. The appearances are those of a solid complex omental mass, a streak of ascites may be present, Doppler ultrasound findings have not been described.

7.2.7 THE MESENTERY

Normal mesentery is an elongated structure with an echogenic surface with small blood vessels at its centre; it is usually 0.5 to 1 cm thick. Lymph nodes may be seen as solid masses. The mesentery may be the seat of ischaemia, trauma, inflammation, solid tumours and cysts of various aetiologies.

Causes of mesenteric calcification

Calcified infarcts – trauma, ischaemia, polyarteritis nodosa, pancreatitis.
Mesenteric haematoma.
Dystrophic fat calcification.
Tuberculous peritonitis.
Tumour calcification – carcinoid, lipoma, metastases, teratoma, following irradiation.
Cyst – lymphangioma.
Hydatid cyst.

Meconium peritonitis.
Pseudomyxoma peritonei.

Mesenteric tumours

Mesenteric tumours are common, the majority being metastases seen in middle-aged and elderly patients. In adults peritoneal and mesenteric metastases may arise from peritoneal seeding of an abdominal malignancy such as bowel or ovarian carcinoma, or they may have spread from distant tumours such as bronchial carcinoma. Primary mesenteric tumours are rare but they include mesothelioma, neurofibroma, lipoma, benign fibromatosis, fibrous histiocytoma, benign mesenchymoma, lymphomas, leiomyoma and leiomyosarcoma, desmoid tumours, haemangioma, etc. In children mesenteric metastases usually arise from neuroblastoma or lymphosarcoma.

Mesenteric masses are not visible sonographically when small or when visible it may not be possible to differentiate them from bowel, lymph nodes, retroperitoneal masses or exophytic bowel lymph nodes, retroperitoneal masses or exophytic bowel tumours. Mesenteric tumours are frequently associated with ascites which may aid the visualisation of bowel loops. When visualised mesenteric tumours may have a well-defined or ill-defined nodular appearance.

Diffuse mesenteric disease

The mesentery can be affected with inflammatory processes such as sclerosing mesenteritis, retractile mesenteritis, mesenteric panniculitis and mesenteric lipodystrophy. There is no gender predilection, patients in the age range of 23 to 87 years usually present with abdominal pain or a palpable abdominal mass. The most common presentation (70 per cent) on imaging is with a single mass over 10 centimetres in size involving the small bowel mesentery. The remaining cases may present with multiple masses or with diffuse mesenteric thickening. Some authorities believe that all these conditions represent histologic variants of one clinical entity. Imaging can detect a mass or diffuse thickening but definitive preoperative diagnosis is not usually possible. Mesenteric amyloidosis has been shown to present as diffuse infiltration. The CT, ultrasound and operative findings mimicked abdominal carcinomatosis. Infections causing peritonitis will also affect the mesentery but actinomycosis has been reported to present a solitary solid abdominal mass mimicking a mesenteric tumour with desmoplastic reaction. Castleman's disease, which is a relatively rare lymphoproliferative disorder, has been reported as presenting as a solid mass with peripheral vascularity on colour flow Doppler affecting the mesentery and mimicking a malignant mass.

Mesenteric infarction

The incidence of ischaemic bowel disease is rising in proportion to the ageing population. Acute mesenteric ischaemia may present as an acute abdomen that may pose a difficult diagnostic problem. Plain abdominal radiographs may reveal dilated loops of bowel, thickening of bowel loops, intramural gas, gastric distension and a gasless abdomen. Sonographic features are again those of dilated thickened loops of bowel, intraperitoneal fluid and intramural or portal venous gas. Doppler interrogation in acute mesenteric ischaemia is fraught with difficulty because of gaseous distension of the bowel, but it may show superior mesenteric vein occlusion in a minority of patients.

Mesenteric trauma

Bowel and mesenteric injuries make up 20 per cent of injuries in blunt abdominal trauma. As abdominal ultrasonography is now routinely used as an initial examination for most abdominal trauma it is becoming more important to be able to recognise signs of mesenteric injuries on sonography. Free peritoneal fluid is identified in 58 per cent of mesenteric and bowel injuries. Bowel haematomas may be directly visualised and associated renal, splenic and hepatic injuries may be identified. Mesenteric haematomas may result from blunt abdominal trauma such as handle-bar injuries. Sonography reveals an echogenic mass with echogenic walls in the centre of the abdomen. Colour flow Doppler may reveal vascularity at the periphery originating from the superior mesenteric artery. Colour Doppler may help to differentiate mesenteric haematoma from intramural intestinal haematoma, since no Doppler signals are found at the periphery of an intramural haematoma, but mesenteric haematoma can be associated with mesenteric vessels coursing the periphery of the lesion.

Differential diagnosis of mesenteric cysts

The first step in diagnosing a cystic lesion is to determine the organ from which the mass originates. Giant mesenteric cysts may mimic ascites.

Lymphangioma.
Non-pancreatic pseudocyst.
Hydatid cyst.
Müllerian cyst.
Mesothelial cyst.
NB *The above fine cysts are often multiloculate.*

Chylous cyst.
Haematoma.
Enteric duplication cysts – relatively thick-walled merging with bowel.
Enteric cyst.
Cystic mesothelioma.
Cystic teratoma.
Cystic spindle cell tumour.

Mesenteric lymphangioma

Lymphangiomas are thought to represent localised malformations of the lymphatics. Three types have been described characterised by the size of the lymphatic channels and their wall composition, they include capillary, cavernous and cystic types. Over 80 per cent present in the first 5 years of life, the majority are in the neck, axilla, mouth, mediastinum and thoracic wall. Only 5 per cent of lymphangiomas involve the retroperitoneum, omentum or mesentery. Patients with abdominal lymphangioma may be asymptomatic or present with an acute abdomen as a result of bowel obstruction, infarction, and volvulus. Larger cysts may mimic ascites both clinically as well as on ultrasonography. Ultrasonography shows a characteristic multilocular cystic appearance. The lesion may occasionally be solid as a result of multiple tissue interfaces provided by tiny cysts (analogous to autosomal recessive polycystic renal disease).

Solid mesenteric masses

Metastatic tumours.
Primary tumours.
Haematoma.
Infarct.
Infection – actinomycosis.
Endometrioma.
Amyloid.
Diffuse mesenteric disease – lipodystrophy, sclerosing mesenteritis, panniculitis, etc.
Castleman's disease.

7.3 RETROPERITONEUM

The retroperitoneum comprises the organs and fascial spaces lying posterior to the peritoneal cavity and anterior to the muscles of the posterior abdominal wall. Retroperitoneal structures include the major vessels and adjacent lymphatics, kidneys, adrenal glands, pancreas and psoas muscles. Disease of any of these organs may affect the retroperitoneum and disease from other areas may affect the retroperitoneum either by direct spread or indirectly via the blood vessels or lymphatics.

7.3.1 ANECHOIC RETROPERITONEAL MASSES

Retroperitoneal varices – serpiginous anechoic structures, colour Doppler is diagnostic.

Sarcoma – most appear as anechoic or hypoechoic masses.

Lymphadenopathy – lymphoma, metastatic or inflammatory.

Haematoma – anechoic or hypoechoic, septate or complex depending upon the size and age of the haematoma.

Abscess – this may indistinguishable from a haematoma.

Aortic aneurysm – lymphadenopathy wrapped around the aorta may mimic an aneurysm.

Renal artery aneurysm – colour Doppler may be diagnostic.

Renal vein aneurysm – varix-colour Doppler may be diagnostic.

Renal vein leiomyosarcoma and fibrous histiocytoma.

Retroperitoneal fibrosis – this may give rise to a retroperitoneal mantle of tissue of low or moderate echogenicity around the major vessels, that has a well-defined anterior margin. It is not easily separated from adjacent structures and tends to envelop the inferior vena cava and aorta without causing displacement. Hydronephrosis is invariably associated with retroperitoneal fibrosis.

Retroperitoneal lymphangiomatosis and lymphangiomyomatosis – present as multi-loculate cystic structures around the aorta and inferior vena cava.

Urinoma – this may follow ureteric colic or trauma.

Lymphocoele – this is often related to previous surgery, particularly for Crohn's disease, it may be multiseptate.

Psoas or iliacus abscess – corresponds to the anatomical boundaries of these muscles.

Psoas haematoma – the echogenicity depends upon the age of the haematoma.

Double inferior vena cava – colour Doppler may be diagnostic.

Inferior vena cava leiomyosarcoma – intravascular, intramural.

Pancreatic pseudocysts – they may appear at a distance to the pancreas and may be septate.

Hydatid cysts can affect any organ – retroperitoneal hydatid cysts are rare.

Adrenal tumours – particularly metastases may be hypoechoic or echopoor.

Adrenal gland cysts.

Adrenal gland haemorrhage – echogenicity depends upon the age of the haematoma.

Renal tumours, cysts and inflammatory masses.

Inflammatory pseudo-tumours – these are inflammatory masses of uncertain aetiology that mimic true neoplasms often resulting in a diagnostic dilemma.

Castleman's disease – this is a disorder of abnormal lymph node proliferation, the aetiology is uncertain.

7.3.2 EXTRAMEDULLARY HAEMOPOIESIS

Retroperitoneal extramedullary haemopoiesis appears as fatty masses, hyperechoic on ultrasound but CT demonstrates a combination of soft tissue and fatty elements. The masses are usually located in the retroperitoneal space posterior to the kidney.

7.3.3 AORTA

The aorta can easily be identified throughout most of its abdominal course by an anterior approach in slim patients, but in obese patients a left posterior oblique approach may be required scanning through the left kidney. Ultrasonography is now the initial investigation of choice in patients with pulsatile abdominal masses, it allows the clinician to

- measure accurately the diameter of the aneurysm
- identify the configuration of the aneurysm, fusiform or saccular
- see the involvement of the iliac arteries
- identify clot within the aneurysm, this may make the aneurysm artificially small on angiography
- measure the aneurysm wall thickness, the wall is thicker in inflammatory and infective aneurysms than in atheromatous aneurysms
- identify dissection
- identify haematoma around a leaking aneurysm
- differentiate a normal aorta with an overlying mass from an aneurysm, echopoor lymph nodes in lymphoma may mimic an aneurysm
- perceive aortic aneurysms more easily by colour flow mapping, to differentiate them from other anechoic retroperitoneal masses
- use ultrasonic contrast agents to observe percutaneous aortic stent placements for aortic aneurysm.

Normal maximum aortic diameters

The normal maximum aortic diameter varies with site

- at the diaphragm   2.5 cm
- mid-abdomen   2.0 cm
- at the bifurcation   1.8 cm
- iliac arteries   1.0 cm.

The aorta should always be examined in both transverse and longitudinal sections as oblique sections exaggerate the aortic dimensions. Imaging in multiple planes is particularly important if the aorta is tortuous.

Aortic aneurysms

An aortic aneurysm is seen as a dilatation of the aorta. The aneurysm may contain a variable amount of clot which is relatively hypoechoic but is more echogenic than the remaining aortic lumen, which is anechoic. The majority of aortic aneurysms are fusiform although they may be saccular or eccentric. They frequently extend into the iliac arteries although proximally they usually arise below the level of the renal arteries. Turbulent flow may be seen within an aneurysm and blood or clot may be seen outside the aortic lumen in cases of leaking or false aneurysms. An anechoic crescent in an abdominal aortic aneurysm peripheral to echogenic intraluminal thrombus is not a sign of dissection. This pattern of layered thrombus, which may mimic dissection, is usually caused by liquefaction of clot adjacent to intima.

Aortic aneurysms with a diameter less than 6 cm have a

- 1 year survival rate of 75 per cent
- 5 year survival rate of 47.8 per cent.

Aortic aneurysms with a diameter greater than 6 cm have a

- 1 year survival rate of 50 per cent
- 2 year survival rate of 25 per cent
- 5 year survival rate of 6 per cent.

NB overall the risk of rupture is 43 per cent, other deaths occur from related cardiovascular episodes.

Differential diagnosis of aortic aneurysms
Anechoic para-aortic lymph nodes.
Para-aortic or paravertebral haematoma.
Psoas abscess or haematoma.
Oblique sections through a tortuous aorta.
Fluid-filled small bowel loops over the anterior aortic wall.
Loculated ascites in the mid-abdomen.

Pseudoaneurysms of the abdominal aorta
Pseudoaneuryms of the abdominal aorta are rare and account for only 1 per cent of all abdominal aortic aneurysms. They represent an organised para-aortic haematoma that has a lumen in continuity with the aortic lumen. They are caused by surgery, catheterisation or abdominal trauma. They are best seen on colour duplex Doppler, which may show continuous bidirec-

tional flow in the neck of the aneurysm. On grey scale ultrasound they appear as anechoic spaces adjacent to the aorta. Pulsed Doppler shows turbulent or arterial-like flow within the pseudoaneurysm and the classic 'to-and-fro' spectral wave pattern in the communicating channel.

Mycotic aneurysms

Mycotic aortic aneurysms, 20 to 35 per cent of which are caused by infection with *Salmonella* spp., may not be palpable despite their size and there may be no fever. The signs of mycotic aneurysms include

- an aneurysm in the presence of limited atheroma
- an encasing or contiguous inflammatory mass
- an adjacent inflammation such as a psoas abscess.

A CT scan is complimentary and may show additional features such as spinal pathology in association with a psoas abscess.

Sonographic screening for aortic aneurysm

Rupture of an abdominal aortic aneurysm is a major cause of death in men over the age of 60 years. The annual rupture rate of the abdominal aorta in men older than 60 years has been estimated at 7 per 100 000, and the incidence is rising. The mortality from an abdominal aortic rupture is approximately 85 per cent. Abdominal aortic aneurysm is often without symptoms, but those diagnosed opportunistically and given the option of elective surgery have a 5-year survival rate similar to the population with high cardiovascular risk. Therefore a strong case can be made for mass screening of men aged 65 to 75 years. When screening is introduced it is important to choose an aortic diameter beyond which regular surveillance may be instituted. Recent work has shown that changes in diameter of the abdominal aorta occur with age. Beyond the age of 60 years the normal mid-abdominal aortic diameter of 2 centimetres does not usually apply. The threshold aortic diameter, beyond which it is thought to be abnormal, varies with age. These threshold diameters have been estimated at 25 mm at the age of 60 years, 28 mm at 65 years, 32 mm at 70 years and 35.5 mm at 75 years. Although further work is required in this field, at present, in order to reduce unnecessary follow-up scans, only patients with aortic diameters over 25 mm at the age of 60 years and over 31 mm in those aged over 70 years will be offered follow-up scans. These scans are usually performed every 3 months in the first year and thereafter twice yearly.

Neonatal aortic thrombosis

Acute thrombosis is a rare phenomenon in adults and may occur as a complication of trauma or myeloproliferative disorders. Neonates develop aortic thrombosis as a complication of catheterisation of the umbilical artery. The thrombus within the aorta may be directly visualised by ultrasonography, the echogenicity of the thrombus depends upon the age of the thrombus. Colour flow mapping may be useful in demonstrating lack of flow in the aorta and in showing collateral pathways. Sonography is the investigation of choice for follow up of fibrinolytic therapy for aortic thrombosis.

7.3.4 INFERIOR VENA CAVA

The inferior vena cava forms by the union of the common iliac veins at the level of the 5th lumbar vertebral body. It ascends on the right side of the aorta to the level of the 2nd lumber vertebral body at which point it is directed slightly forwards through the liver. The right renal artery can usually be seen passing behind the inferior vena cava just before it enters the liver and the inferior vena cava usually shows posterior indentation at this point. The wall of the inferior vena cava is not usually visible. Calibre changes are frequent during examination. Inferior vena cava distension varies with respiration, position and cardiac cycle. Distension occurs in cases of right heart failure, fluid overload and other causes of raised central venous pressure. As the inferior vena cava distends calibre changes normally seen with respiration become less marked and eventually cease.

Transposition of the inferior vena cava

A left-sided inferior vena cava is the commonest congenital anomaly of the inferior vena cava with an incidence of 0.2 to 0.5 per cent. The inferior vena cava usually ends at the left renal vein then crosses anterior to the aorta to join the normally placed prehepatic segment of the inferior vena cava. Alternatively the inferior vena cava may cross the spine posterior to the aorta to join an enlarged lumbar plexus of veins, the hemiazygos vein, and the coronary sinus, or it may drain into the left atrium. There is a higher incidence of congenital heart disease in association with a transposed inferior vena cava. Diagnosis is important to avoid confusion with pathological retroperitoneal masses and when planning inferior vena cava ligation, shunt placement for portal hypertension filter placement and aneurysm repair. Sonography readily confirms a left-sided inferior vena cava crossing to the right behind or in front of aorta. Doppler ultrasound will demonstrate a venous pattern of flow within the aberrant inferior vena cava.

Inferior vena cava interruption – azygos continuation

The incidence of azygos continuation is 0.6 per cent. In the majority of cases it represent an isolated anomaly but it can be associated with visceral and cardiac defects. The inferior vena cava is normal to the level of the kidneys but the intrahepatic part of the inferior vena cava is absent. Two large veins, the azygos and/or hemiazygos are seen on both sides of the aorta as they ascend in the retrocrural space.

Inferior vena cava duplication

Duplication of the inferior vena cava occurs in 0.2 to 0.3 per cent of the population. The two inferior vena cavas appear smaller than normal and are placed on each side of the aorta, they ascend to the level of the renal veins where they join either anterior or posterior to the aorta. The differential diagnosis includes a dilated gonadal vein which continues into the inguinal canal. Large lymph nodes are non-continuous and are unlikely to cause confusion.

Inferior vena cava obstruction

Differential diagnosis of inferior vena cava obstruction

Intrinsic neoplastic causes
Renal cell carcinoma.
Wilms' tumour.
Adrenal carcinoma.
Renal angiomyolipoma.
Phaeochromocytoma.
Pancreatic carcinoma.
Caval leiomyoma.
Caval leiomyosarcoma.
Caval endothelioma.

Thrombosis
Extension of thrombus – from ileofemoral veins, from hepatic veins (Budd–Chiari syndrome).
Haematologic and metabolic causes of thrombosis – coagulopathy, dehydration, severe exertion.
Inflammatory causes of thrombosis – pelvic inflammatory disease, sepsis, postoperative causes, traumatic phlebitis, cardiac failure.

Extrinsic compression
Hepatomegaly.
Aortic aneurysm.
Retroperitoneal haematoma.
Massive ascites.
Retroperitoneal fibrosis.

Hepatic, adrenal and renal tumours.

Retroperitoneal sarcoma.

Retroperitoneal lymphadenopathy.

Tumour-induced desmoplastic reaction.

Castleman's disease.

Miscellaneous causes

Congenital – congenital webs or membranes.

Idiopathic.

Functional obstruction – valsalva manoeuvre, pregnant uterus, straining or crying (in children), supine position in association with a large abdominal mass.

Iatrogenic – inferior vena cava filters (echogenic foci within the inferior vena cava, that shadow), inferior vena cava plication, inferior vena cava ligation, inferior vena cava clips.

Sonographic diagnosis of inferior vena cava obstruction

The inferior vena cava shows a loss of kinetics – the loss of calibre changes with respiration.

Solid pattern in the lumen.

Decreased or absent Doppler signal.

Abnormal Doppler signal or turbulent flow.

Collateral channels.

Extrinsic compression, for example nodes or retroperitoneal masses.

Hepatic, renal or adrenal tumour extending into the inferior vena cava.

Retroperitoneal fibrosis.

Caval leiomyosarcoma – an echopoor endoluminal mass dilating the inferior vena cava with arterial vascularity and high diastolic flow.

Calcified thrombus in the inferior vena cava – uncommon but may be found in asymptomatic children. Appears as an echogenic mass vertically orientated to the right of the midline with shadowing. Colour Doppler ultrasound may show flow around or peripheral to the echogenic focus.

Masses that elevate the inferior vena cava

The cranial section of the inferior vena cava is nearly always visible although the caudal part is frequently obscured by bowel loops. It may be elevated by the following retroperitoneal masses.

Right adrenal tumour.

Neurogenic tumour.

Hepatic mass in the posterior aspect of the caudate and right lobes.

Right renal artery aneurysm.

Renal mass.

Dilated retrocaval ureter – non-dilated retrocaval ureter does not usually elevate the inferior vena cava.

Retroperitoneal tumour.
Lumbar spine disease.
Tortuous aorta.
Haematoma.
Abscess.
Retroperitoneal fibrosis.

7.3.5 RETROPERITONEAL TUMOURS

Malignant retroperitoneal tumours

Common tumours – liposarcoma, leiomyosarcoma, malignant fibrous histiocytoma.
Rare tumours – haemangiopericytoma, spindle cell sarcoma, neurofibrosarcoma, teratocarcinoma, fibrocytoma, malignant paraganglioma, extra-adrenal neuroblastoma, mesenchymomas.

Liposarcoma

This represents the most common primary tumour of the retroperitoneum. It is sub-classified according to the degree of cellular differentiation

1. the myxoid form, this is the most common form and it has a mixture of varying amounts of mucinous, fibrous and rather sparse fatty tissue (intermediate differentiation)
2. the lipogenic form has relatively large malignant lipoblasts and a scanty myxoid matrix (highly differentiated)
3. the pleomorphic form is poorly differentiated with marked cellular/pleomorphism and relatively little fat and mucin.

Computed tomography is a better imaging modality than ultrasound for the detection of liposarcomas. However ultrasound may reveal a retroperitoneal mass of varying echogenicity depending upon the cell type. Calcification, which occurs in 12 per cent of cases, may be difficult to differentiate from focal fat. The secondary effects of the tumour may be much more readily seen on ultrasound, these are hydronephrosis, renal displacement, aortic displacement, inferior vena cava invasion, displacement and thrombosis. Doppler ultrasound may be invaluable in the appropriate setting when vascular occlusion is suspected.

Leiomyosarcoma

This is the second commonest primary tumour of the retroperitoneum, it may be extravascular (62 per cent), a combination of intravascular and extravascular (33 per cent), intravascular (6 per cent) and rarely intramural. Ultrasound may show a solid mass that may be hypoechoic, hyperechoic or complex with irregular cystic spaces. Vascular invasion may be demonstrated using duplex Doppler.

Malignant fibrous histiocytoma

These are very aggressive retroperitoneal tumours which tend to be hypervascular and frequently recur after resection. These tumours occasionally calcify. Ultrasonography shows a solid hypoechoic or complex mass which may cause vascular invasion or displace retroperitoneal organs.

Benign retroperitoneal tumours

Retroperitoneal teratoma

Most retroperitoneal teratomas are benign and usually found in children. These tumours have multiple tissue elements and therefore have ultrasound appearances that may vary from hypoechoic to hyperechoic to complex or cystic. Fat–fluid levels and debris have been described in complex cystic teratomas.

Neurogenic tumours

These mostly represent benign nerve sheath tumours such as schwannomas and neurofibromas. They may be solitary or multiple as part of von Recklinghausen neurofibromatosis. Ultrasonically they are solid dumbbell-shaped hypoechoic masses.

7.3.6 ABDOMINAL LYMPHATICS

The lymphatics of the anterior and lateral abdominal walls drain to the axillary, anterior mediastinal and superficial inguinal lymph nodes. The lymphatics of the abdominal viscera drain to the lymph nodes around the aorta. The lymph nodes around the aorta lie around the origins of the coeliac axis, superior and inferior mesenteric arteries anteriorly and around the paired lateral aortic branches. Tumour infiltration or inflammatory diseases may enlarge any or all the pre-aortic and para-aortic lymph nodes. Early lymphadenopathy is most easily identified when the pre-aortic nodes are involved, since masses around the origins of the anterior aortic branches distort and elevate these vessels. Enlarged lymph nodes are usually hypoechoic in relation to adjacent retroperitoneal tissue but they may be echogenic. Lymphoma in particular gives rise to large anechoic nodes. When enlarged pre- and para-aortic nodes are identified the bowel mesentery should be reviewed for evidence of lymphadenopathy and the abdominal organs should be examined for evidence of an occult malignancy.

If an occult primary tumour is suspected then examination of the thyroid and testes should also be undertaken.

The common causes of retroperitoneal lymphadenopathy are lymphoma and renal cell, testicular, cervical and prostatic carcinomas.

7.3.7 PSOAS MUSCLE

For the purpose of the sonographic appearance the psoas muscle can be divided into three sections. The psoas, like other muscles, demonstrates hyperechoic striations on a hypoechoic background. The upper section of the psoas from its origin to the lower pole of the kidney also contains echogenic planes in 10 per cent of adults. The middle third of the psoas extending from the lower pole of the kidney to the iliac crest, demonstrates prominent echogenic planes and focal areas of increased and decreased echogenicity in 46 per cent of individuals. The lower third of the psoas muscle, extending from the iliac crest to the fusion with the iliacus muscle, demonstrates a single echogenic plane in 70.05 per cent of individuals running obliquely in the transverse plane, and in 29.5 per cent of cases there are more complex echogenic planes or focal areas of increased or decreased echogenicity. The psoas minor is not identified as a separate structure on routine ultrasonography.

Psoas abscess

A psoas abscess may complicate discitis, Crohn's disease, stage horn renal calculi (with urinary infection), aortic surgery, aortic graft infection and pelvic inflammatory disease. Psoas abscesses are rare in children, although they may be secondary to the causes given above, they are usually a primary occurrence resulting from pyogenic infection. A psoas abscess is exceptionally rare in the neonate. Clinically these patients may present with pyrexia, leucocytosis and a flexion deformity at the hip on the affected side. There is usually a hypoechoic, complex or cystic mass in the distribution of the psoas muscle that may extend from behind the kidney into the groin. The abscess may also be seen posterolateral to the bladder. Particulate fluid movement may be seen within the abscess on real time scanning particularly in tuberculosis psoas abscess.

Necrotising fasciitis of the psoas muscle

Necrotising fasciitis of the psoas from group A streptococci has been reported as a complication in patients with colonic cancer perforation and peritonitis.

Lymphoma of the psoas muscle

The psoas muscle is an infrequent site of extranodal lymphoma. Sonography may reveal a hypoechoic enlargement of the psoas and paravertebral muscles or an anechoic featureless paravertebral mass indistinguishable from an abscess or haematoma on sonographic features alone. Metastatic lymphadenopathy, vertebral metastases with soft-tissue extension and primary retroperitoneal sarcomas may give rise to similar imaging features.

Psoas sheath haematoma

A psoas sheath haematoma may result from coagulopathy, anticoagulant therapy, and abdominal aortic and other surgery on the retroperitoneum. Although the sonographic features may be indistinguishable from an abscess the appropriate history should lead to the correct diagnosis.

Psoas muscle hypertrophy

Psoas muscle hypertrophy is frequently found in marathon runners and is usually of no clinical significance. The psoas muscle being examined may appear hypertrophied because of an atrophic opposite psoas muscle (as a result of neuromuscular disease). These conditions usually should not mimic pathology. Pelvic venous thrombosis may cause diffuse swelling of all abdominal muscles because of oedema and should not be confused with a psoas abscess or other retroperitoneal pathology.

7.3.8 ABDOMINAL WALL RELAXATION

Most abdominal wall lumps and bumps can easily be evaluated clinically. However abdominal wall relaxation can often be confused with an incisional hernia. Abdominal wall relaxation occurs subsequent to renal, aortic or iliac vessel surgery when a lateral retroperitoneal approach is used resulting in an abdominal wall bulge. This bulge can easily be confused with an incisional hernia. Diagnosis is important as treatment is non-surgical.

The three flat flank abdominal muscles, i.e. the external oblique, the transverse and the internal oblique, can be identified by ultrasound. These muscles can be distinguished as three layers separated by thin highly echogenic aponeuroses. The abdominal wall muscles are separated from the abdominal viscera by the thin echogenic peritoneum. In abdominal wall relaxation all the three abdominal wall layers appear intact but when compared to the opposite normal side the overall thickness of the three muscles is reduced. This decrease in muscle thickness is at least 33 per cent of the normal thickness.

7.4 FURTHER READING

Allen HA 3rd, Vick CW, Messmer JM, Parker GA: Diffuse mesenteric amyloidosis: CT, sonographic, and pathologic findings. J Comput Assist Tomogr 9(1):196-198, 1985.

Anderson JF, Cunah BA: Group A streptococcal necrotising fasciitis of the psoas muscle. Heart Lung 28(3):219-221, 1999.

Baird D, Radvany MG, Shanley DJ, Fitzharris GA: Mesenteric cyst with milk of calcium. Abdom Imaging 19(4):347-348, 1994.

Buckingham R, Dwerryhouse S, Roe A: Rectus sheath haematoma clinically mimicking splenic enlargement. J R Soc Med 88(6):334-335, 1995.

Chadha D, Kedar RP, Malde HM: Sonographic detection of pneumoperitoneum an experimental and clinical study. Australas Radiol 37:182-185, 1993.

Chan YL, Cheng CS, Ng PW: Mesenteric actinomycosis. Abdom Imaging 18(3):286-287, 1993.

Chao HC, Kong MS: Sonographic diagnosis of mesenteric hematoma. J Clin Ultrasound 27:284-286, 1999.

Chao HC, Kong MS, Lin TY: Diagnosis of necrotising fasciitis in children. J Ultrasound Med 18(14):277-281, 1999.

Chou YH, Tiu CM, Lui WY, Chang T: Mesenteric and omental cysts: an ultrasonographic and clinical study of 15 patients. Gastrointest Radiol 16(4):311-314, 1991.

Emory TS, Monihan JM, Carr NJ, Sobin LH: Sclerosing mesenteritis, mesenteric panniculitis and mesenteric lipodystrophy: a single entity? Am J Surg Pathol 21(4):392-398, 1997.

Erturk H, Erden A, Yurdakul M et al.: Pseudoaneurysm of the abdominal aorta: diagnosed by color Duplex Doppler sonography. J Clin Ultrasound 27:202-205, 1998.

Fujita N, Noda Y, Kobayashi G et al.: Chylous cyst of the mesentery: ultrasound and CT diagnosis. Abdom Imaging 20(3):259-261, 1995.

Giovagnorio F, Andreoli C, De Cicco ML: Color Doppler sonography of focal lesions of the skin and subcutaneous tissue. J Ultrasound Med 18(2):89-93, 1999.

Goerg C, Schwerk WR: Ultrasound of extra-nodal abdominal lymphoma: a review. Clin Radiol 44:92-97, 1991.

Gollub MJ, Friedweld JP, Sceusa D: Sonographic diagnosis of transposition of the inferior vena cava. J Clin Ultrasound 18:502-506, 1990.

Gordon MJ, Sumner TE: Abdominal ultrasonography in a mesenteric cyst presenting as ascites. Gastroenterology 69(3):761-764, 1975.

Grimshaw GM, Thompson JM: Changes in diameter of the abdominal aorta with age: an epidemiological study. J Clin Ultrasound 25:7-13, 1997.

Guivarc'h M: Tumors of the mesentery: apropos of 102 cases. Ann Chir 48(1):7-16, 1994.

Hardisson D, Limeres MA, Jimenez-Heffernan JA et al.: Solitary fibrous tumour of the mesentery: Am J Gastroenterol 91(4):810-811, 1996.

Hollman AS, McMillan MA, Briggs JD et al.: Ultrasound changes in sclerosing peritonitis following continuous ambulatory peritoneal dialysis. Clin Radiol 43:176-179, 1991.

Houston JG, Morris AD, Howie CA et al.: Technical report: quantitative assessment of hemidiaphragmatic movement. A reproducible method using ultrasound. Clin Radiol 46:405-407, 1992.

Houston JG, Fleet M, Cowan MD, McMillan NC: Comparison of ultrasound and fluoroscopy in assessment of suspected hemidiaphragmatic movement abnormality. Clin Radiol 50:95-98, 1995.

Houston JG, Fleet M, McMillan NC, Cowan MD: Ultrasonic assessment of hemidiaphragmatic movement: an indirect method of evaluating mediastinal invasion in non-small cell lung cancer. Br J Radiol 68:695–699, 1995.

Ishida H, Yagisawa H, Naganuma H et al.: Rotation of the diaphragmatic echo behind the liver tumour: clinical significance and computer analysis: Eur J Ultrasound 3:267–275, 1996.

Jimenez JM, Poustchi-Amin M, Leonides JC, Pena A: Extraperitoneal abdominopelvic inflammatory pseudotumor: report of four cases. Pediatr Radiol 27:170–174, 1997.

King AD, Hine L, McDonald C, Abraham P: The ultrasound appearance of the normal psoas muscle. Clin Radiol 48:316–318, 1993.

Konno K, Ishida H, Hamashima Y et al.: Color Doppler findings in Castleman's disease of the mesentery. J Clin Ultrasound 26(9):474–478, 1998.

Lagalla R, Iovane A, Caruso G et al.: Color Doppler ultrasonography of soft-tissue masses. Acta Radiol 39(4):421–426, 1998.

Latifi HR, Siegel MJ: Color Doppler flow imaging of pediatric soft tissue masses. J Ultrasound Med 13(3):165–169, 1994.

Lee J, Song SY, Park CS, Kim B: Mullerian cysts of the mesentery and retroperitoneum: a case report and literature review. Pathol Int 48(11):902–906, 1998.

Li Yuk-Pui, Guico R, Parikh S, Chiu S: Cystic mesothelioma of the retroperitoneum. J Clin Ultrasound 20:65–68, 1992.

Loble PN, Puylaert JB, Coerkamp EG, Herman ET: Non-palpable rectus sheath haematoma clinically masquerading as appendicitis, ultrasound and CT findings. Abdom Imaging 20(2):152–154, 1995.

Mentzel H-J, Schramm D, Vogt S et al.: Intra-abdominal lymphangioma in a newborn. J Clin Ultrasound 26:320–322, 1998.

Mesurolle B, Sayag E, Meingan P et al.: Retroperitoneal extramedullary hematopoiesis: sonographic CT and MR imaging appearance. Am J Roentgenol 167:1139–1140, 1996.

Moon W, Kim Y, Rhim H et al.: Coexistent cystic teratoma of the omentum and ovary: report of two cases. Abdom Imaging 22(5):516–518, 1997.

Muller M, Truong SN, Schumpelick V: Sonographic diagnosis of abdominal wall relaxation. J Clin Ultrasound 27:183–186, 1999.

Neumann DP, Henken M: Lymphangioma of the jejunal mesentery. J Ultrasound Med 16:563–564, 1997.

Pattison P, Jeffrey RB, Mindelzum RE, Sammer FG: Sonography of intra-abdominal gas collections. Am J Roentgenol 169:1559–1564, 1997.

Paya K, Hayek BF, Rebhandl W et al.: Retroperitoneal necrotizing fascitis in a 4-year-old girl. J Pediatr Surg 33(5):778–780, 1998.

Richards JR, McGahan JP, Simpson JL, Tabar P: Bowel and mesenteric injury: evaluation with emergency abdominal ultrasound. Radiology 211(2):399–403, 1999.

Rioux N, Michaud C: Sonographic detection of peritoneal carcinomatosis: a prospective study of 37 cases. Abdom Imaging 20:47–51, 1995.

Ros PR, Olmsted WW, Moser RP et al.: Mesenteric and omental cysts: histologic classification with imaging correlation: Radiology 164(2):327–332, 1987.

Rudas G, Bors S: Aortic thrombosis diagnosed by ultrasound. Pediatr Radiol 18:77–78, 1988.

Santeusanio G, Ventura L, Partenzi A et al.: Omental endosalpingiosis with endometrial-type stroma in a woman with extensive hemorrhagic pelvic endometriosis. Am J Clin Pathol 111(2):248–251, 1999.

Schut JM, Meradji M, Oranje AP et al.: Double sided psoas abscess in a young infant: sonographic and radiographic findings. Pediatr Radiol 18:176–177, 1988.

Shibuya T, Ishida H, Konno K et al.: Sonographic findings of malignant histiocytoma of the mesentery: report of two cases. Eur J Ultrasound 8(3):207–212, 1998.

Singh-Panheal S, Karenik TJ, Wachberg RH, Baker SR: Inferior vena caval leiomyosarcoma: diagnosis and biopsy with color Doppler sonography. J Clin Ultrasound 25:275–278, 1997.

Sistrom CL, Abbitt PL, Feldman PS: Ultrasound guidance for biopsy of omental abnormalities. J Clin Ultrasound 20:27–36, 1992.

Sohaey R, Gardner TL, Woodward PJ, Peterson CM: Sonographic diagnosis of peritoneal inclusion cysts. J Ultrasound Med 14(12):913–917, 1995.

Stoupis C, Ros PR, Abbitt PL et al.: Bubbles in the belly: imaging of cystic mesenteric or omental masses. Radiographics 14(4):729–737, 1994.

Suchet IB: Colour-flow Doppler artifacts in anechoic soft-tissue masses of infants. Can Assoc Radiol J 45(3):201–203, 1994.

Tsutsumi H, Ohwada S, Takeyoshi I et al.: Primary omental liposarcoma presenting with torsion: a case report. Hepatogastroenterology 46(27):2110–2112, 1999.

Turig PS, Cooperberg PL, Madigar SM: The anechoic crescent in abdominal aortic aneurysm: not a sign of dissection. Am J Roentgenol 146:345–348, 1986.

Verhagen HJ, Tolenaar PL, Sybrandy R: Haematoma of the rectus abdominis muscle. Eur J Surg 159(6–7):335–338, 1993.

Wolf C, Obrist P, Ensinger C: Sonographic features of abdominal wall endometriosis. Am J Roentgenol 169:916, 1997.

Index